Clinical Manual for Treatment of Schizophrenia

Clinical Manual for Treatment of Schizophrenia

Edited by

John Lauriello, M.D.
Stefano Pallanti, M.D.

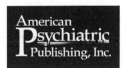

Washington, DC
London, England

Copyright © 2012 American Psychiatric Association
ALL RIGHTS RESERVED
Manufactured in the United States of America on acid-free paper
16   15   14   13   12   5   4   3   2   1
First Edition
Typeset in Adobe AGaramond and Formata

American Psychiatric Publishing, a Division of American Psychiatric Association
1000 Wilson Boulevard
Arlington, VA 22209-3901
www.appi.org

Library of Congress Cataloging-in-Publication Data
Clinical manual for treatment of schizophrenia / edited by John Lauriello, Stefano Pallanti. — 1st ed.
    p. ; cm.
Includes bibliographical references and index.
ISBN 978-1-58562-394-5 (pbk. : alk. paper)
I. Lauriello, John. II. Pallanti, Stefano. III. American Psychiatric Association.
[DNLM: 1. Schizophrenia—therapy. 2. Schizophrenic Psychology. WM 203]
LC classification   not assigned
616.89′8—dc23

2011032532

British Library Cataloguing in Publication Data
A CIP record is available from the British Library.

Contents

12 Remission in Schizophrenia 433

Laine M. Young-Walker, M.D.
Alan J. Mendelowitz, M.D.
John Lauriello, M.D.

List of Tables and Figures

Contributors

Gaurava Agarwal, M.D.
Instructor, Department of Psychiatry and Behavioral Sciences, Northwestern University Feinberg School of Medicine, Chicago, Illinois

Mario Álvarez-Jiménez, Ph.D.
Research Fellow, Orygen Research Centre, The University of Melbourne, Victoria, Australia, and University Hospital "Marqués de Valdecilla," Department of Psychiatry, University of Cantabria School of Medicine, Santander, Spain

Pamela B. Arenella, M.D.
Assistant Professor, Department of Psychiatry, University of New Mexico, Albuquerque

Stephanie D. Bagby-Stone, M.D.
Assistant Professor of Clinical Psychiatry, Department of Psychiatry, University of Missouri School of Medicine, Columbia, Missouri

Tara K. Biehl, M.S.
Senior Program Manager, Department of Psychiatry, University of New Mexico, Albuquerque, New Mexico

Michael P. Bogenschutz, M.D.
Professor, Department of Psychiatry, University of New Mexico, Albuquerque

Andrea Cantisani, M.D.
Psychiatry Resident, Department of Psychiatry, University of Florence, Italy

Will J. Cronenwett, M.D.
Instructor, Department of Psychiatry and Behavioral Sciences, Northwestern University Feinberg School of Medicine, Chicago, Illinois

John G. Csernansky, M.D.
Lizzie Gilman Professor and Chair, Department of Psychiatry and Behavioral Sciences, Northwestern University Feinberg School of Medicine, Chicago, Illinois

Lisa B. Dixon, M.D., M.P.H.
Professor and Director, Division of Services Research, Department of Psychiatry, University of Maryland School of Medicine, College Park, Maryland; Acting Director, VA Capitol Health Care Network (VISN 5), Mental Illness Research, Education, and Clinical Center (MIRECC), Baltimore, Maryland

Amy L. Drapalski, Ph.D.
Administrative Core Manager, VA Capitol Health Care Network (VISN 5), Mental Illness Research, Education, and Clinical Center (MIRECC), Baltimore, Maryland; and Clinical Assistant Professor, Department of Psychiatry, University of Maryland School of Medicine, Baltimore, Maryland

W. Wolfgang Fleischhacker, M.D.
Professor of Psychiatry, Department of Psychiatry and Psychotherapy, Medical University Innsbruck, Innsbruck, Austria

Eóin Killackey, D.Psych.
Associate Professor, Department of Psychiatry; Senior Research Fellow and Clinical Psychologist, Orygen Youth Health Research Centre and Centre for Youth Mental Health, The University of Melbourne, Victoria, Australia

John Lauriello, M.D.
Professor and Chancellor's Chair of Excellence in Psychiatry, Department of Psychiatry, University of Missouri School of Medicine; and Medical Director, University of Missouri Psychiatric Center, Columbia, Missouri

Patrick D. McGorry, M.D., Ph.D.
Professor, Department of Psychiatry; Executive Director, Orygen Youth Health Research Centre; and Clinical Director, Centre for Youth Mental Health, The University of Melbourne, Victoria, Australia

Alan J. Mendelowitz, M.D.
Associate Professor of Psychiatry, Albert Einstein College of Medicine, Bronx, New York; Associate Professor of Psychiatry, Hofstra North Shore–LIJ [Long Island Jewish Health System] School of Medicine at Hofstra University, Hempstead, New York

Seiya Miyamoto, M.D., Ph.D.
Associate Professor, Department of Neuropsychiatry, St. Marianna University School of Medicine, Kawasaki, Kanagawa, Japan

Tamiko Mogami, Ph.D.
Professor, Department of Clinical Psychology, Graduate School of Medical Sciences, Tottori University, Tottori, Japan

Kazuyuki Nakagome, M.D., Ph.D.
Senior Expert, National Center of Neurology and Psychiatry, Tokyo, Japan

Barnaby Nelson, Ph.D.
Ronald Phillip Griffith Senior Research Fellow, Orygen Youth Health Research Centre and Centre for Youth Mental Health, The University of Melbourne, Victoria, Australia

Stefano Pallanti, M.D.
Professor of Psychiatry, Department of Psychiatry, University of Florence, Florence, Italy; Visiting Associate Professor, Department of Psychiatry, Mount Sinai School of Medicine, New York, New York

Leonardo Quercioli, M.D.
Psychiatrist, Istituto di Neuroscienze, Florence, Italy

Ilaria Riccardi, Ph.D.
Clinical Psychologist, Department of Experimental Medicine, Section of Psychiatry and Clinical Psychology, University of L'Aquila, Coppito, L'Aquila, Italy

Volker Roder, Ph.D.
Assistant Professor of Clinical Psychiatry, University Hospital of Psychiatry, Bern, Switzerland

Alessandro Rossi, M.D.
Professor of Psychiatry, Department of Experimental Medicine, Section of Psychiatry and Clinical Psychology, University of L'Aquila, Coppito, L'Aquila, Italy

Stephanie Schmidt, M.Sc.
Research Associate, Department of Psychiatry, University Hospital of Psychiatry, Bern, Switzerland

Paolo Stratta, M.D.
Doctor of Psychiatry, Department of Mental Health, National Health Service, L'Aquila, Italy

Werner Strik, M.D.
Full Professor and Chairman, University Hospital of Psychiatry, Bern, Switzerland

Laine M. Young-Walker, M.D.
Clinical Assistant Professor of Psychiatry, Department of Psychiatry, and Division Chief, Child and Adolescent Psychiatry, University of Missouri School of Medicine, Columbia, Missouri

Alison R. Yung, M.D.
Professor, Department of Psychiatry; Consultant Psychiatrist, Orygen Youth Health Research Centre and Centre for Youth Mental Health, The University of Melbourne, Victoria, Australia

Disclosure of Competing Interests

The following contributors to this book have indicated a financial interest in or other affiliation with a commercial supporter, a manufacturer of a commercial product, a provider of a commercial service, a nongovernmental organization, and/or a government agency, as listed below:

Will J. Cronenwett, M.D.   *Research Support:* Novartis.

W. Wolfgang Fleischhacker, M.D.   *Research Grants:* Alkermes, Eli Lilly, Janssen, Otsuka, Pfizer. *Consulting Honoraria:* Bristol-Myers Squibb, Janssen, Lundbeck, MedAvante, Merck, Otsuka, Pfizer, Roche, Sunovion, United BioSource. *Speaker Honoraria:* AstraZencca, Eli Lilly, Janssen, Lundbeck, Otsuka, Sunovion. *Stocks:* MedAvante.

John Lauriello, M.D.   *Consultant:* Eli Lilly.

Patrick D. McGorry, M.D., Ph.D.   *Research Support:* AstraZeneca, Eli Lilly, Janssen-Cilag, Pfizer.

Alan J. Mendelowitz, M.D.   *Speakers Bureau:* Janssen (Jan.–April 2011); AstraZeneca (ended Jan. 2011).

Kazuyuki Nakagome, M.D., Ph.D.   *Grant Funding/Honoraria:* Eli Lilly, Glaxo SmithKline, Otsuka, Pfizer.

The following contributors to this book have no competing interests to report:

Mario Álvarez-Jiménez, Ph.D.
Pamela B. Arenella, M.D.
Stephanie D. Bagby-Stone, M.D.
Tara K. Biehl, M.S.
Michael P. Bogenschutz, M.D.
Andrea Cantisani, M.D.
John G. Csernansky, M.D.
Lisa B. Dixon, M.D., M.P.H.
Amy L. Drapalski, Ph.D.
Tamiko Mogami, Ph.D.

Barnaby Nelson, Ph.D.
Stefano Pallanti, M.D.
Leonardo Quercioli, M.D.
Volker Roder, Ph.D.
Alessandro Rossi, M.D.
Stephanie Schmidt, M.Sc.
Werner Strik, M.D.
Laine M. Young-Walker, M.D.
Alison R. Yung, M.D.

Preface

Several years ago, the editors of this textbook were asked by our mutual friend and respected colleague Dr. Robert Freedman to create a clinical manual for the treatment of schizophrenia. We had never worked on any project together, nor had we even met. We did have in common our Italian heritage, a shared network of valued colleagues, and a career-long passion for improving the lives of individuals with this devastating illness. Dr. Freedman's directive could have been approached from a variety of perspectives. One could imagine a "cookbook" of treatments or a handy pocket guide to treatment algorithms. Somewhat surprisingly, we immediately agreed on a guiding principle—a desire to provide the reader with a comprehensive view of schizophrenia, grounded in a thorough understanding of the illness: diagnosis, comorbidity, and treatment options.

This book is divided into 12 chapters. Chapter 1, a general introduction to the illness, focuses on the history, etiology, and current diagnostic schema. Chapter 2 describes the basic science underlying the illness, expanding the usual focus on the dopamine hypothesis to encompass other neurotransmitters, as well as the evolving study of the biological markers of schizophrenia. Chapter 3 surveys one of the cutting-edge challenges in schizophrenia, acquiring an understanding of the prodromal or prediagnostic features of the illness as well as the unique demands of treating schizophrenia in the early years postdiagnosis. Chapter 4 considers clinical assessment, not just in terms of differential diagnosis but also the role of early trauma and stress; according to an European phenomenology of the subjective schizophrenic experience, the need for empathy and understanding and the gathering of information are emphasized. Dysfunction in cognitive processes and its clinical assessment are the subject of Chapter 5; the cognitive domain in schizophrenia appears to be most tightly correlated to overall functioning and is currently the subject of intense treatment research. An often-overlooked area in many textbooks on schizophrenia, that of comorbidity, is dealt with in Chapter 6. The authors here do not limit their discussion to substance abuse, but also address a number of other conditions that can co-occur with schizophrenia. Clinicians rarely encounter a patient with symptoms solely of schizophrenia; instead, mood, anxiety, and other disorders are also present. This reminds us that schizophrenia does not confer immunity to other mental and physical difficulties affecting the rest of society. Also, these comorbid symptoms have the potential to impact the course of the disease and therefore represent a specific treatment target. Chapter 7 focuses on the substance use disorders that co-occur with schizophrenia in many patients and offers approaches to diagnosing and treating this uniquely challenging population. Chapters 8, 9, and 10 comprehensively cover the major aspects of schizophrenia treatment: the use of pharmacological and psychosocial interventions for the various domains of the illness, as well as approaches to intervening in the significant minority of treatment-resistant cases. Chapter 11 looks at the role of families and the use of family treatments to improve outcome not only for patients but also for their families. The book concludes with Chapter 12, a review of our current understanding of remission in schizophrenia. This final chapter emphasizes that far from contenting ourselves with merely managing the worst ravages of this disorder, we should expect and strive for a robust reduction in symptoms and a return of functionality in our patients. This concept of remission is slowly becoming reality for many people with schizophrenia.

We wanted this manual to have international contributors, a global outlook, and hopefully an international readership. Toward this end, we approached colleagues we admired in the United States, Europe, Australia, and Asia to write chapters. We endeavored to assemble chapters that could stand alone as independent works but also fit together to form a coherent and comprehensive picture of schizophrenia and its treatment. We believe that we have met these goals, and that the resulting volume is timely and thought-provoking. We hope that you, the reader, agree.

John Lauriello, M.D.
Stefano Pallanti, M.D.

Acknowledgments

We would like to express our gratitude to several people whose contributions were vital to the development and writing of this book:

Ms. Tara Biehl, who not only a coauthored Chapter 1 but also helped review and format the entire text.

Ronald Rieder, who generously shared his thoughtful conversation on the book's topics.

Nancy Andreasen, for the understanding of remission she offered to the field.

1

Introduction to Schizophrenia

John Lauriello, M.D.
Tara K. Biehl, M.S.
Stephanie D. Bagby-Stone, M.D.

Charles had been an exemplary student. As the youngest child of a middle-class family, his parents felt he was a happy but somewhat shy child. He received a prestigious scholarship to a national university with the hopes of studying engineering. The first semester at the university, Charles worked hard but found it increasingly difficult to study. He often stayed up late at night reading the same text again and again, trying to comprehend and retain information. Always uncomfortable with new acquaintances, he began to suspect that his roommate was somehow poisoning him, and he became increasingly agitated. One day, the dormitory supervisor was notified that Charles had locked himself in his room and refused to come out. The school intervened, and he was brought to the school infirmary. There, Charles reported that he was hearing Gabriel the Archangel warning him of the impending end of the world. Charles was admitted to the university psychiatric hospital and was eventually diagnosed with schizophrenia. His symptoms improved with treatment, but he decided to return home to try to complete his studies at a local college.

Brief History of the Diagnosis of Schizophrenia

Schizophrenia is an illness that for many is difficult to grasp. The average person often describes schizophrenia as "split personality" or uses the word *schizophrenic* to describe an inconsistent opinion on a topic. The 2001 movie *A Beautiful Mind,* based on the biography by Sylvia Nasar, chronicled the life of John Nash, the Nobel Prize–winning mathematician. Nash experienced debilitating hallucinations and delusions, which had a profound effect on his life. The movie was a first in portraying a more widely accessible depiction of the illness.

Illnesses resembling schizophrenia have been described throughout the ages, with their causations usually given mystical and religious explanations. In 1911, Eugen Bleuler, the Swiss psychiatrist and director of the renowned Burghölzli Psychiatric Hospital at the University of Zurich, Switzerland, first introduced the term *schizophrenia* to describe adult patients who have profound disturbances of thinking, behavior, and mood. Bleuler did intend schizophrenia to denote a split, but the schism is "a split in the meaning and emotion of one's thoughts and behaviors" rather than a split personality (Kuhn 2004).

In his definition of schizophrenia, Bleuler emphasized observed symptoms of the illness rather than its course. Bleuler's "four A's" (autism, ambivalence, affect inappropriateness, and association defect) remain critical to our modern definition of the illness. Bleuler also divided symptoms of schizophrenia into positive and negative symptom clusters, which has had significant implications in modern schizophrenia treatment and research.

We owe much of our current notion of schizophrenia to the work of Bleuler and another groundbreaking psychiatrist, Emil Kraepelin, in the early twentieth century. Kraepelin was a German psychiatrist working at the Munich University Psychiatric Hospital, alongside Alois Alzheimer. Both physicians began to differentiate those patients with profound mental illness and dementia characteristics with an earlier onset from those whose onset occurred later in life. Alzheimer's patients had a late-onset dementia, a dementia that would eventually bear his name. On the other hand, Kraepelin (1919) described the early-onset patients as having either "dementia praecox," or precocious dementia, or a "manic depression." Kraepelin's conception of an early dementia had a profound influence on the next century's view of patients with schizophrenia. In general, however, he was incorrect. Little clinical or pathological evidence supports dementia because patients with schizophrenia do not have a dementing process or a linear cognitive decline. However, Kraepelin was correct that the illness is biological in nature and that most patients have some progressive worsening of their symptoms, although this worsening is not necessarily continuous. Kraepelin was also correct in implicating cognitive function as an integral part of schizophrenia as an illness. Cognitive dysfunction has become the domain most closely linked to overall functioning for those with schizophrenia (Green 2009) and is discussed in greater detail by Strik and colleagues in Chapter 5, "Cognition and Schizophrenia."

In the late 1950s, Kraepelin's successor in Munich, Kurt Schneider (1959), attempted to refine the definition of schizophrenia. His "first-rank symptoms" of schizophrenia emphasized symptoms that he considered indicative of the illness. The first-rank symptoms include hearing one's thoughts out loud, hearing voices arguing or commenting on one's actions, feeling one's body is being influenced, thought withdrawal, thought insertion, thought broadcasting, and delusions of being controlled by an external force. Schneider believed that these symptoms were specific for schizophrenia, a belief later proven incorrect.

Kraepelin's, Bleuler's, and Schneider's work has had a pronounced influence on our modern definition of schizophrenia. Their ideas are still evident in today's diagnostic psychiatric criteria, both in DSM-IV-TR (American Psychiatric Association 2000) and in the *International Statistical Classification of Diseases and Related Health Problems,* 10th Revision (ICD-10; World Health Organization 1992), described later in this chapter.

Schizophrenia Lexicon

To better understand schizophrenia, understanding the terminology describing it can be very helpful. In this section, we define some of the key terms that underpin the diagnostic criteria for schizophrenia. The first important term is *psychosis.* The word *psychosis* is derived from the Greek words *psykhe* ("mind") and *osis* ("diseased"). Specifically, it denotes a disease state in which there are distortions of reality. These can include false beliefs, or *delusions,* and misperceptions of the senses, or *hallucinations.*

Delusions are culturally bound. If a belief system is shared by a large number in a society, it is often termed an *ideology* or a religious belief. However, if the belief system is idiosyncratic to one person, then it can be construed as delusional. For example, some religious groups believe they can speak in "tongues" to God. This is in contrast to an individual who believes he alone speaks to God or is in fact God himself. Likewise, someone could believe she is being followed by the police, and this may or may not be true. However, a person who believes that aliens from another planet are stalking him would not be believed and would be deemed delusional. Keeping in mind the degree to which delusions affect functioning can help discern those that may be more difficult to identify.

Hallucinations also must be differentiated from the range of normal experiences. An individual may report hearing a voice in her head. It can sometimes be difficult to differentiate the patient's own train of thought from a voice independent of his or her own normal thoughts. *Ruminations* can often be described as foreign to the patient's own thoughts but are actually the patient's train of thought stuck in a repetitive loop. Contrast this to a patient who describes a voice or several voices, distinct and sometimes with identifiable names. Often these "auditory hallucinations" involve a gender or an age that differs from the patient's own thoughts. Visual hallucinations are usually less well defined than auditory hallucinations. In addition, patients may describe seeing shadows or vague images but seldom report visions as clear as what they normally see. Olfactory and tactile hallucinations are often elicited by asking if the patient smells odors that others cannot or, in the case of tactile hallucinations, if he or she experiences electrical jolts or other unusual physical sensations.

Charles returned from the university to live at home. He began to see a local psychiatrist and for the first time related his experiences in greater detail. He described hearing his roommate's voice in his head and would often turn to see if the roommate was hiding somewhere. He became increasingly panicked by this, but he was reassured by Gabriel the Archangel, who told him not to be afraid. He also began to experience a physical sensation of "electrical tingling in his body," which he believed was coming from God and creating a "protective force field." Throughout his recollections of these events, Charles consistently reported that these experiences were as real as any he had had in his life.

It is important to keep in mind that psychotic symptoms are hallmark experiences of schizophrenia but are not exclusive to it. Psychotic symptoms are seen in other psychiatric illnesses and can be mental aberrations of a multitude of neurological and medical illnesses, as well as side effects of medications and illicit substances.

Earlier in this chapter, we referred to Eugen Bleuler's "four A's" (autism, ambivalence, affect inappropriateness, and association defect). Let us now define them in detail. *Autism* is a familiar term and now a diagnostic category of childhood developmental disorders. However, Bleuler was describing *autism* within the context of schizophrenia as the tendency for patients to retreat into their own world, often preoccupied by their hallucinations and delusions. This inhibits the individual from the social interactions necessary to function successfully in society. A classic notion of schizophrenic *ambivalence* is that of having grossly contradictory, simultaneous thoughts that can immobilize the patient. *Affect* refers to the range of emotion shown by individuals. In schizophrenia, affect can be reduced (blunted or even flat) or grossly inappropriate to the topic being discussed. *Associations* refer to the connection of thoughts. In schizophrenia, patients may have disconnected thought processes making tracking what they say difficult. This is often referred as a *looseness of associations* and in the extreme can be so disjointed as to be an incomprehensible "word salad." Patients with schizophrenia can often create "neologisms"— made-up words or a unique combination, truncation, or distortion of real words that conveys a special meaning to its creator.

> As part of his recovery, Charles was referred to a local day treatment program. Charles found it difficult to attend. He preferred staying in his room for many hours at a time. He told his psychiatrist that he knew he needed to go to the program, but he felt that he was better off at home. On days when he was having a particularly difficult time, his family noted that he was hard to understand because his speech jumped from one topic to another. He described having "panxiety," a sudden wave of nervousness when he entered the day treatment building.

Another useful construct in classifying patients is developing an understanding of the positive and negative symptoms of schizophrenia. Table 1–1 shows a list of these symptom clusters.

Table 1–1.   Positive and negative symptoms of schizophrenia

Positive symptoms	Negative symptoms
Delusions	Blunted or flat affect
Hallucinations	Avolition
Disorganization	Alogia
Agitated or bizarre behavior	Attentional problems
Suspiciousness or paranoia	Anhedonia

In essence, positive symptoms are those that would not be experienced by a well person. These include hallucinations, delusions, and inappropriate or bizarre behavior. The positive symptoms can be seen as the extroverted manifestations of schizophrenia. These will capture society's attention in the community and are often the primary reason for hospitalization. In contrast, negative symptoms are the "lack" of experiences that well individuals routinely use in their daily life. These include lack of motivation, sociality, and even production of words in conversation. These are the introverted manifestations of the illness. If these symptoms predominate or precede the positive symptoms, society often will not notice these individuals until they reach a point that they cannot care for themselves. Families especially are keenly aware of this symptom cluster, but parents will often misconstrue that their child is depressed or even lazy and may be slow to recognize that schizophrenia could be a factor.

Finally, schizophrenia has its own unique glossary for describing the course of the illness. These terms are often confused and misapplied to patients. The terms include *premorbid functioning, prodromal schizophrenia, first onset of psychosis, first episode of schizophrenia,* and *early-* and *late-onset schizophrenia.* Table 1–2 defines each term. In Chapter 3, "Prodromal Phase and First-Episode Schizophrenia," Nelson et al. describe the prodrome and first-episode schizophrenia in greater detail. Here we simply define the terms.

Premorbid functioning describes the level of functioning prior to the onset of symptoms and the eventual diagnosis of schizophrenia. Premorbid functioning varies widely. Some individuals have an unremarkable or even stellar level of functioning but are later diagnosed with schizophrenia. However, other individuals have had a very difficult time leading up to a diagnosis and

Table 1–2. Terms used to describe the course of schizophrenia

Premorbid functioning	Level of functioning before onset of symptoms
Prodromal schizophrenia	Initial unusual experiences prior to developing frank psychosis
First onset of psychosis	Manifestation of first psychotic symptom
First episode of schizophrenia	First time the patient receives the diagnosis of schizophrenia
Early-onset schizophrenia	A diagnosis of schizophrenia early in life (i.e., before age 16)
Late-onset schizophrenia	A diagnosis of schizophrenia later in life (i.e., after age 45)

may receive other diagnoses such as attention-deficit disorder or oppositional defiance or merely have a character style that is noteworthy.

> Charles had always been a shy child. As the youngest of the family, his parents described him as sensitive and "their baby." Despite his shyness, Charles was able to go to school and make close friends. However, he was never eager to join athletic teams or attend large gatherings. When asked to consider his level of adjustment, his parents felt he was a happy child but less gregarious than his siblings. They admired his ability to "entertain himself" and found him easy to manage.

Prodromal schizophrenia or *prodromal signs* are those unusual experiences that patients will have prior to developing frank psychosis. These may include magical thinking, unusual perceptions but not overt hallucinations, anxiety, and concentration difficulties. The "prodrome" often occurs in adolescence and lasts 1–2 years before either resolving, being diagnosed as another illness, or progressing to psychosis and a diagnosis of schizophrenia.

First onset of psychosis is the time that the individual first experiences clearly describable psychotic symptoms. This first onset may be sudden, or symptoms may appear gradually and evolve for some time before they come to the attention of family or caregivers. Many patients have described hiding their symptoms during this phase or simply not voicing their concerns out of fear, denial, or paranoia. The *first episode of schizophrenia* is usually defined as the time that the patient first receives the diagnosis. Sometimes there is enough background information to make the diagnosis retrospectively, but first diagnosis most often occurs when the patient reaches the attention of a psychiatric professional. If the symptoms have been present for less than 6 months, the patient should be given the diagnosis of schizophreniform disorder, which can be—and often is—later modified to the diagnosis of schizophrenia when the illness exceeds the 6-month duration.

Early-onset schizophrenia is a term used to describe children who meet the diagnosis of schizophrenia earlier than expected. This will include latency and very early teenagers, typically younger than 16. Some evidence indicates that these patients have a more severe form of the illness and a poorer prognosis. It is certain that they have an earlier disruption of their development because of the illness. *Late-onset schizophrenia* was an "official" subdiagnosis of schizophrenia in earlier versions of the DSM, but age differentiation is not included in DSM-IV-TR. However, this category of patients, who by all accounts are well until age 45 or older, remains an active descriptor. Studies have supported a better prognosis for late-onset patients and their propensity to be a more paranoid type (Harris and Jeste 1988).

Diagnosing Schizophrenia

Now that we have discussed variations regarding the course of schizophrenia, it is important to understand the diagnostic process and possibilities of the illness. Considering the average person's understanding of schizophrenia, it is imperative that clinicians feel comfortable when making such a diagnosis and in relaying the information to the patient and family in a realistic yet delicate manner. Clinicians should have a thorough understanding of the diagnostic criteria and exclusions.

As mentioned earlier in this chapter, essentially two tools are used by clinicians and researchers to aid in the diagnostic evaluation of schizophrenia and schizophrenia spectrum illnesses. DSM-IV-TR is most widely used in the United States. ICD-10 is used most often in Europe and in other parts of the world. In both, it can be seen that the underlying descriptions first provided by Kraepelin and Bleuler are still applicable.

DSM-I, originally published in 1952 by the American Psychiatric Association, is currently in its fourth revision, with a fifth revision pending. The ICD-10 is published by the World Health Organization and is in its tenth revision, having added mental disorders for the first time in 1949 (Houts 2000). Both tools were originally designed to accumulate statistical information to help classify a wide va-

Table 1–3. DSM-IV-TR multiaxial assessment

Axis I   Clinical disorders and other conditions that may be a focus of clinical attention

Axis II   Personality disorders and mental retardation

Axis III General medical conditions

Axis IV Psychosocial and environmental problems

Axis V   Global assessment of functioning

riety of disease states, symptoms, and circumstances. However, their use has extended far beyond simple classification purposes to more practical diagnostic applications used to help identify specific illnesses and their course and severity for individuals. The coding systems used to classify various mental disorders for both DSM and the ICD-10 are intended to correspond with each other, but differences do exist. Unlike the ICD-10, DSM provides a framework for a multiaxial assessment, one that is often required by insurance providers and health care administration. This five-axis approach is detailed in Table 1–3.

For the purpose of this chapter, we focus on the DSM-IV-TR diagnosis of schizophrenia, which is the framework used in the United States and in most scientific publications on the illness. In DSM-IV-TR, one must satisfy Criteria A through E. These criteria are included in Table 1–4.

The diagnosis of schizophrenia begins with the collection of its hallmark symptoms. In Criterion A, all of the characteristic symptoms are detailed for the clinician to review. At least two or more of these symptoms must be present for 1 month or longer. As described previously, the symptoms may include delusions (false beliefs), hallucinations (misperceptions), disorganization (speech and behavior are each coded separately), and negative symptoms (affective flattening, alogia, or avolition). One can imagine a large number of combinations that can be made from these symptoms. This accounts for the varied diagnostic presentation of patients with schizophrenia. A patient with severe positive symptoms and no negative symptoms may require a different set of treatment interventions from a patient with disorganization and negative symptoms alone. An important caveat is that any given patient may express a different set of these symptoms over time. In a bow to Schneiderian first-rank symptoms, an individual may meet Criterion A with only one symptom if that symptom is a bizarre delusion or a "complex" auditory hallucination.

Table 1–4   DSM-IV-TR diagnostic criteria for schizophrenia

A. *Characteristic symptoms:*   Two (or more) of the following, each present for a significant portion of time during a 1-month period (or less if successfully treated):

(1) delusions

(2) hallucinations

(3) disorganized speech (e.g., frequent derailment or incoherence)

(4) grossly disorganized or catatonic behavior

(5) negative symptoms, i.e., affective flattening, alogia, or avolition

Note: Only one Criterion A symptom is required if delusions are bizarre or hallucinations consist of a voice keeping up a running commentary on the person's behavior or thoughts, or two or more voices conversing with each other.

B. *Social/occupational dysfunction:*   For a significant portion of the time since the onset of the disturbance, one or more major areas of functioning such as work, interpersonal relations, or self-care are markedly below the level achieved prior to the onset (or when the onset is in childhood or adolescence, failure to achieve expected level of interpersonal, academic, or occupational achievement).

C. *Duration:*   Continuous signs of the disturbance persist for at least 6 months. This 6-month period must include at least 1 month of symptoms (or less if successfully treated) that meet Criterion A (i.e., active-phase symptoms) and may include periods of prodromal or residual symptoms. During these prodromal or residual periods, the signs of the disturbance may be manifested by only negative symptoms or two or more symptoms listed in Criterion A present in an attenuated form (e.g., odd beliefs, unusual perceptual experiences).

D. *Schizoaffective and mood disorder exclusion:*   Schizoaffective disorder and mood disorder with psychotic features have been ruled out because either (1) no major depressive, manic, or mixed episodes have occurred concurrently with the active-phase symptoms; or (2) if mood episodes have occurred during active-phase symptoms, their total duration has been brief relative to the duration of the active and residual periods.

E. *Substance/general medical condition exclusion:*   The disturbance is not due to the direct physiological effects of a substance (e.g., a drug of abuse, a medication) or a general medical condition.

F. *Relationship to a pervasive developmental disorder:*   If there is a history of autistic disorder or another pervasive developmental disorder, the additional diagnosis of schizophrenia is made only if prominent delusions or hallucinations are also present for at least a month (or less if successfully treated).

Table 1–4. DSM-IV-TR diagnostic criteria for schizophrenia *(continued)*

Classification of longitudinal course (can be applied only after at least 1 year has elapsed since the initial onset of active-phase symptoms):

Episodic With Interepisode Residual Symptoms (episodes are defined by the reemergence of prominent psychotic symptoms); *also specify if:* **With Prominent Negative Symptoms**

Episodic With No Interepisode Residual Symptoms

Continuous (prominent psychotic symptoms are present throughout the period of observation); *also specify if:* **With Prominent Negative Symptoms**

Single Episode In Partial Remission; *also specify if:* **With Prominent Negative Symptoms**

Single Episode In Full Remission

Other or Unspecified Pattern

Source. Reprinted from the *Diagnostic and Statistical Manual of Mental Disorders, 4th Edition, Text Revision.* Washington, DC, American Psychiatric Association, 2000, pp. 312–313. Copyright © 2000 American Psychiatric Association. Used with permission.

The remaining criteria for diagnosing schizophrenia include the presence of impairments in social and/or work functioning. Most often, the impairments are obvious to all, such as the person being unable to continue school, maintain friendships, or find or keep employment. Rarely, the patient can function at a relatively high level. It is critical to determine whether this functioning is consistent with the patient's highest attained level. For example, having a job is a positive, but if the job is inferior to previous work, the individual has had a decline in functioning. A good reference point is to ask the patient what his or her parents and siblings do for a living. If the patient's work is consistent with that of his or her family, then there may not be impairment. However, if the family has been able to maintain higher levels of occupational functioning than the patient has, this is a possible indication of impairment. Patients also may report adequate social functioning, but this should be further explored. For example, a middle-aged patient once cheerfully described his best friend as being an important part of his life. However, when asked when he had last seen or talked to his friend, he replied, "in high school"!

The symprom presentation and disturbance must be present for a minimum of 6 months, and other possible mental Illnesses, such as schizoaffective disorder and mood or possible substance-induced disorders, along with medical explanations, must be ruled out. Individuals with autism diagnoses can be dually diagnosed with schizophrenia, but only if prominent delusions or hallucinations develop. This criterion avoids counting preexisting autistic symptoms as the only criteria for schizophrenia.

In DSM-IV-TR, once the diagnosis of schizophrenia is made, a subtyping of the diagnosis is determined based on the predominant symptoms elicited. These subtypes are listed in Table 1–5.

In addition to the selection of the appropriate subtype, DSM-IV-TR also classifies the course of the illness. This classification can be made only after the patient has met criteria for the illness for 1 year. This classification includes differentiating an episodic and a continuous manifestation of symptoms, with or without prominent negative symptoms. It also allows for a single episode with partial or full remission. In our experience, these course specifiers are not used by most clinicians. The proposed DSM-5 criteria for schizophrenia are very similar to the DSM-IV-TR criteria, with one notable exception: the removal of the schizophrenia subtypes. This is because of their lack of use and questionable validity.

Table 1–5.   DSM-IV-TR schizophrenia subtypes

Paranoid type	Delusions or frequent hallucinations predominate.
Disorganized type	Disorganized speech and disorganized behavior and flat or inappropriate behavior predominate.
Catatonic type	At least two catatonic symptoms predominate, including motoric immobility, purposeless excessive motor activity, extreme negativism or mutism, posturing and stereotyped movements, and echolalia (repeating what is just heard) or echopraxia (repetition of others' movements).
Undifferentiated type	No one type predominates.
Residual type	Absence of prominent symptoms but continued evidence of impairments

The above information outlines criteria for making the diagnosis of schizophrenia via DSM-IV-TR. More specific information related to evaluating a patient's first episode of schizophrenia is discussed further in Chapter 3.

Epidemiology of Schizophrenia

Schizophrenia is a relatively common illness. Conventional wisdom states that it affects all classes, sexes, and nationalities equally at an approximately 1% worldwide prevalence. Recently, new information and systematic reviews on the epidemiology of schizophrenia paint a much more complex and varied picture. Schizophrenia can no longer be viewed as an "equalitarian" or "exceptional" disorder. It varies across locations, cultures, and genders in much the same way as most other diseases (McGrath 2005; Messias et al. 2007).

Incidence

The incidence of a disease refers to the disease frequency or rate. It is the number of newly diagnosed cases during a specific time period in a population. In 1992, the WHO 10 Nation study found "strong support for the notion that schizophrenic illnesses occur with comparable frequency in different populations" (Sartorius et al. 1986, p. 909). More recent reviews have found substantial variation in the incidence of schizophrenia across multiple studies and locations worldwide (McGrath et al. 2004). The median incidence rate has been found to be 15.2 per 100,000, with a range of 7.7–43 and with the 10%–90% quartiles covering more than a fivefold range of rates (McGrath et al. 2004; Messias et al. 2007). The incidence of schizophrenia is showing variation among locations and in a positively skewed distribution—not the equalitarian incidence across countries and cultures as was once believed.

Although the male-to-female ratio in schizophrenia was long believed to be identical, recent data from several reviews report incidence differences between the sexes. Current analyses show that the male-to-female ratio is 1.4:1, which indicates that for about every three men given the diagnosis of schizophrenia, two women will be given the diagnosis (McGrath et al. 2008). Narrative reviews also depict the variation in the illness course as being more severe in men than in women (McGrath et al. 2008). Additionally, males with schizophrenia tend to have a slightly younger age at onset than females (Saha et al. 2005). In general, the earlier the onset of schizophrenia, the more virulent the disease presents. Children who receive the diagnosis at age 5 or 6 years, although uncommon, face a long struggle with fulfilling developmental milestones necessary for adequate adult functioning. The later the illness presents, the more experience and strengths the person can use to deal with the illness.

Prevalence

The prevalence of an illness is the proportion of the population having a disease; it is the number of individuals alive with a disease at a certain time. Data from a recent systematic review found the median lifetime prevalence of schizophrenia to be 4.0 per 1,000. The lifetime morbid risk median was 7.2 per 1,000, so it can be thought that "about 7 individuals per 1000 will be affected" (McGrath et al. 2008). The mean lifetime morbid risk was found to be 11.9 per 1,000, which is consistent with the teaching that "schizophrenia affects one in one-hundred" (McGrath and Susser 2009).

The most recent prevalence data on schizophrenia do not show variance between men and women, which is consistent with the differences in course of illness observed between sexes; nor do the data show a difference in urban and nonurban inhabitants. However, the prevalence is higher in immigrants than in nonimmigrants (Saha et al. 2005). Interestingly, the prevalence of schizophrenia is also significantly higher in developed countries as compared with developing countries. Furthermore, no evidence indicates that the incidence of schizophrenia varies by economic status (Saha et al. 2006). This leads to the question: Does schizophrenia have a more favorable outcome in developing countries? And if so, what are the reasons?

Mortality

Comparing the overall incidence and prevalence figures, it is clear that contemporary treatments for schizophrenia are not curing the disease. Also, individuals with schizophrenia have a two- to threefold increase in mortality risk compared with the general population (Auquier et al. 2006). It is troubling that this risk has shown a worsening gap in recent decades (Saha et al. 2007). Suicide is one cause of this mortality risk, as are the multiple medical comorbidities that affect schizophrenic patients, including conditions such as cardiovascular disease, smoking, diabetes, obesity, and substance abuse. There is also concern with regard to the effect of atypical antipsychotics precipitating metabolic syndrome and perhaps exacerbating this trend in mortality risk (McEvoy et al. 2005; McGrath et al. 2008; Meyer et al. 2008).

Risk Factors for Schizophrenia

The exact cause of schizophrenia is not fully understood, but it is generally accepted that patients have an abnormality involving neurotransmitters in the brain, especially dopamine and probably glutamate. These hypotheses are discussed at length by Cronenwett and colleagues in Chapter 2, "Basic Science Underlying Schizophrenia." Complicating etiology and potential risk factors is the possibility that schizophrenia comprises multiple individual illnesses under the collective banner. For example, one might imagine that one patient has an inheritable disorder and another patient a substance-induced disorder, each meeting the criteria for schizophrenia. Given that caveat, there appear to be some general proposed risk factors for developing schizophrenia. These risk factors are presented in Table 1–6.

Genetics

Genetic factors are involved in the vulnerability to the development of schizophrenia, yet clearly schizophrenia is not an entirely genetic disease. Family, twin, and adoption studies have been consistent in supporting a high degree of heritability in schizophrenia. The incidence of schizophrenia in third-degree relatives is 2%, in second-degree relatives is 2%–6%, and in first-degree relatives is 6%–17% (Lewis and Lieberman 2000). The concordance is 40%–50% in monozygotic twins. Heritability describes the amount of phenotypic variability among individuals that can be attributed to genes; in schizophrenia, the heritability is high at about 80% (Gejman 2010).

Table 1–6. Proposed risk factors for developing schizophrenia

Genetics	Older paternal age
Winter birth	Marijuana use
Infections	Urbanicity
Obstetric complications	Immigration

In gathering more history on Charles, his parents reported that Charles's uncle had experienced a "nervous breakdown" soon after he was drafted into the military. Charles's parents did not know the details, except that he had been institutionalized for some time for hearing voices and paranoia. Charles had no known infectious or perinatal risk factors, but his college roommate told his parents that Charles had been smoking marijuana regularly while at school.

Schizophrenia is a complex genetic disorder. The search for susceptibility genes has not been a simple process. Numerous candidate genes have been identified and researched, including *DISC1, DTNBP1, NRG1, DRD2, HTR2A,* and *COMT,* just to name a few of the nearly 800 genes that have been tried. However, none of these genes are fully established. It is currently believed that several genes contribute to the susceptibility of schizophrenia, each with a small effect and none having full responsibility for the disease (Gejman 2010).

Winter Birth and Latitude Effect

Season of birth and geographic location have been indicated as risk factors given that winter births and higher latitudes seem to convey a greater risk for schizophrenia. According to recent epidemiological data, it appears that there is a 10% increase in schizophrenia diagnosed in persons born in the winter months as compared with summer months (Messias et al. 2007). In the late 1980s, researchers acknowledged the possibility of a north-south gradient, as well as special populations with higher incidences of schizophrenia (Torrey 1987). A trend shows that at higher latitudes, there tends to be a higher incidence of schizophrenia in males. These variations have been hypothesized as perhaps related to genes, environment, weather conditions, and socioeconomic factors (McGrath et al. 2008). The shape of the seasonality in schizophrenia births varies by latitude. Possible explanations of this gradient may be related to seasonal changes in the patterns of viral illnesses and prenatal vitamin D exposure (Davies et al. 2003).

Infectious Agents

Infectious agents that have been implicated in schizophrenia risk include influenza (specifically exposure in the second trimester), rubella, *Toxoplasma gondii,* herpes simplex 2, and meningitis (McGrath et al. 2008; Messias et al.

2007). Exposure to infection during pregnancy is consistent with neurodevelopmental conceptualizations of schizophrenia (Messias et al. 2007).

Pregnancy and Birth Complications

Increased schizophrenogenic risk has been found to be related to pregnancy difficulties, abnormal fetal growth and development, and delivery complications. Risk can begin early in development, as prenatal famine has been shown to increase risk for schizophrenia, leading some to consider the possibility of problems emerging as a result of nutritional deficits in vitamin D or folate (McGrath and Susser 2009). Results from prospective population studies have shown specific exposures with increased risk to include antepartum hemorrhage, diabetes, Rh factor incompatibility, preeclampsia, low birth weight, congenital malformations, reduced head circumference, uterine atony, asphyxia, and emergency cesarean delivery (McGrath and Susser 2009). Proposed possible mechanisms of these obstetric complications may be related to poor nutrition, extreme prematurity, or hypoxia/ischemia (Messias et al. 2007).

Older Paternal Age

Advanced age in the father has been recently more supported in the literature as a risk factor for the development of schizophrenia. Several population-based studies in multiple countries have supported the link between increased paternal age and schizophrenia. One study showed that the relative risk of developing schizophrenia rose consistently in each 5-year group of paternal age. Furthermore, advanced maternal age did not seem to be a risk factor (Malaspina et al. 2001). Current population-based cohort research suggests that this trend was observed only among those individuals with no family history of schizophrenia, which may suggest the possibility of spontaneous sperm mutations (Messias et al. 2007).

Cannabis

The use of cannabis has been indicated as another strong risk factor for schizophrenia. Persons with schizophrenia are more likely to have used or currently use marijuana. Recent research has shown that the risk for developing schizophrenia is 2–25 times higher among cannabis users (Messias et al. 2007). Moreover, several reviews have shown a dose effect, meaning that the greater the exposure to marijuana, the greater the risk of developing schizophrenia

(McGrath and Susser 2009). These findings lead to speculation as to whether these individuals are using marijuana to treat their illness or whether the cannabis use itself is causing or precipitating symptoms (Messias et al. 2007).

Urbanicity

City living increases one's risk of developing schizophrenia. The incidence of schizophrenia is higher in urban than in rural dwellers (McGrath and Susser 2009). The relative risk is about two to four times higher to those born in urban areas. Although the reasons for this risk are not completely understood, some look to a possible biological etiology associated with the physical or cultural environment, birth practices, or overcrowding (Messias et al. 2007).

Immigration

The risk of schizophrenia is increased among individuals immigrating to another country, and country of origin also may be a factor. As was mentioned previously, the prevalence and incidence of schizophrenia in immigrants have been shown to be higher than in native-born individuals (McGrath and Susser 2009; Saha et al. 2005). Both first- and second-generation immigrants have an increased risk of developing schizophrenia. The effect is most pronounced in immigrants from areas where most of the population is black (McGrath and Susser 2009). In a study done in the United Kingdom, those immigrating from Africa or the Caribbean had rates of schizophrenia up to 10 times greater than in the general population (Messias et al. 2007). Possible causes of this increased risk may be related to social stress or defeat, nutrition, infection, or race and ethnicity factors (McGrath et al. 2008).

The currently understood risk factors for schizophrenia weave a complicated web of genetic and environmental interactions. Further research linking risk factors to neurobiology, neurogenetics, and early development as well as elucidating relative risk will help to further untangle the causative mechanisms of this complex disease.

Social Effects of Schizophrenia

Charles made steady progress at home. He continued to see his psychiatrist and continued taking his medication. He was no longer paranoid and gradu-

Table 1–7.   Direct and indirect costs of schizophrenia

Direct costs

Inpatient and outpatient visits

Frequent hospitalizations

Police costs

Medication

Public assistance, including long-term psychosocial and economic support

Indirect costs

Lifetime lost productivity (both talent and employment)

Continued financial support by families

Reduced employment of caregivers

---

ally became more comfortable at his day program. He began to take classes at his local college and did well, and he was able to continue his engineering major, although he could not take on a full course load. His mother reduced her job to part time to better help Charles in his pursuits. As it became apparent that his studies would require some time, and his means for independent support would be reduced, his family and he applied for government disability, which he now receives.

Financial Costs

The financial costs of schizophrenia is heavy whether one looks at it from the individual, family, or community level. These direct and indirect costs are detailed in Table 1–7.

Direct costs are defined as the up-front costs associated with the treatment of the disease, such as those for mental health facilities and operations; inpatient, outpatient, and long-term care; physician costs; as well as general medication, legal, and support costs. In 2002, it was estimated that the total cost of schizophrenia in the United States was $62.7 billion per year (Wu et al. 2005). Similar high costs have been found in other industrialized nations (Fitzgerald et al. 2007).

Indirect costs are often hidden costs that include the loss of potential wages from those with schizophrenia, as well as their families and caregivers.

Indirect costs also include in-kind support from family and general family and community burden expenses (McEvoy 2007).

Vocational Loss

The ability to work and to be self-sufficient is an important element of most people's lives. People with schizophrenia experience a major impairment in developmental skills, often dependent on the age at onset of their illness, and in their ability to work. Competitive employment (i.e., jobs acquired without the support of government programs) is estimated to be held by fewer than 20% of persons with schizophrenia (Lehman et al. 2002). A person's severity of symptoms plays an important role in his or her ability to work, but taking a job also has external disincentives, including a reduction or loss of government stipends and associated insurance programs. Great strides have been made to generate work opportunities for patients that will not jeopardize the financial and supportive safety net they need (Cook and Razzano 2000). Programs with a psychosocial or vocational rehabilitation component, such as Ticket to Work, have been shown to help patients both secure and maintain employment, as well as their benefits.

Note that vocational loss is often experienced by families and caregivers as well as they struggle to maintain consistent hours and to manage the stress that can be associated with caring for someone with schizophrenia.

Family Burden

Families are an essential support system for patients with schizophrenia, but historically, families were also "blamed" for malnurturing and causing schizophrenia in their children. Fromm-Reichmann (1948) coined the term *schizophrenogenic mother* to describe a cold, rigid, and maladaptive parenting style believed to be common in families with schizophrenic children. Bateson et al. (1956) described the double-bind hypothesis of schizophrenia: the notion that families created a no-win environment for their children, which leads to psychosis. Bateson et al. believed that psychosis was an expression of distress and mixed communications experienced early in family life. These past theories laid responsibility for the illness on the families and damned the very people obliged to care for their children. With the acknowledgment of the biological underpinnings of schizophrenia, families today are no longer considered the cause of the disorder.

Today what is commonly referred to as the "burden of care," a rather negative construct, is a very real phenomenon that is difficult to quantify in dollars, but its effect on families and communities is large and widespread. The role of caring for someone with schizophrenia, with its varying presentations and severity of illness, can be complex. The financial burden on families can be enormous, caring for their children far into adulthood, with a myriad of medical and health care expenses. In addition, the day-to-day carrying out of basic tasks can be cumbersome, as well as the perceived burden that many caregivers experience. Families can, however, improve the outcome of their children by reducing stressful interactions in the household. Brown and colleagues (Brown and Rutter 1966; Brown et al. 1966) identified the concept of *expressed emotion* (EE) to describe conscious or unconscious criticism and blaming of the patient by parents. Although evidence indicates that family interventions designed to improve the overall family environment and to reduce relapse are effective, these interventions are often not well integrated into care plans and tend to be underfunded (Awad and Voruganti 2008).

Sometimes even the best supportive efforts of family and the community are not enough. The very nature and variable course, along with complex issues of insight and medication compliance, make schizophrenia a difficult illness to contend with for some families. Some members, either the person who has the illness or the family providing support, may end up alienated, or the family system may become generally fragmented. In Chapter 11, "Family Issues and Treatment in Schizophrenia," Drapalski and Dixon provide more details on the challenges families encounter dealing with a loved one with schizophrenia. Fortunately, there has been a great deal of progress in family education and support that is proven to help both the patient and the family do better.

Conclusion

In this chapter, we have highlighted the history, diagnosis, risk factors, and effect of schizophrenia. Schizophrenia is a hallmark disorder; it sweeps over many individuals just as they are entering adulthood, leaving dramatic changes in its wake. In the following chapters, specific topics on schizophrenia are presented, including the underlying pathology, subtypes of the illness, comorbidity, and treatment.

Suggested Readings

Andreasen NC, Carpenter WT Jr: Diagnosis and classification of schizophrenia. Schizophr Bull 19:199–214, 1993

Bromet EJ, Fennig S: Epidemiology and natural history of schizophrenia. Biol Psychiatry 46:871–881, 1999

Crow TJ: How and why genetic linkage has not solved the problem of psychosis: review and hypothesis. Am J Psychiatry 164:13–21, 2007

Lauriello J: Great(er) expectations. Am J Psychiatry 164:377–379, 2007

Palmer BA, Pankratz VS, Bostwick JM: The lifetime risk of suicide in schizophrenia: a reexamination. Arch Gen Psychiatry 62:247–253, 2005

Selten JP, Cantor-Graae E, Kahn RS: Migration and schizophrenia. Curr Opin Psychiatry 20:111-115, 2007

Tandon R, Nasrallah HA, Keshavan MS: Schizophrenia, "just the facts" 4. Clinical features and conceptualization. Schizophr Res 110(1-3):1–23, 2009

Toda M, Abi-Dargham A: Dopamine hypothesis of schizophrenia: making sense of it all. Curr Psychiatry Rep 9:329–336, 2007

White T, Anjum A, Schulz SC: The schizophrenia prodrome. Am J Psychiatry 163:376–380, 2006

References

American Psychiatric Association: Diagnostic and Statistical Manual: Mental Disorders. Washington, DC, American Psychiatric Association, 1952

American Psychiatric Association: Diagnostic and Statistical Manual of Mental Disorders, 4th Edition, Text Revision. Washington, DC, American Psychiatric Association, 2000

Auquier P, Lançon C, Rouillon F, et al: Mortality in schizophrenia. Pharmacoepidemiol Drug Saf 15:873–879, 2006

Awad AG, Voruganti LN: The burden of schizophrenia on caregivers: a review. Pharmacoeconomics 26:149–162, 2008

Bateson G, Jackson D, Haley J, et al: Toward a theory of schizophrenia. Behav Sci 1:251–264, 1956

Bleuler E: Dementia Praecox or the Group of Schizophrenias (1911). Translated by Zinkin J. New York, International Universities Press, 1950

Brown GW, Rutter M: The measurement of family activities and relationships: a methodological study. Hum Relat 19:241–263, 1966

Brown GW, Bone M, Palison B, et al: Schizophrenia and Social Care. London, Oxford University Press, 1966

Cook JA, Razzano L: Vocational rehabilitation for persons with schizophrenia: recent research and implications for practice. Schizophr Bull 26:87–103, 2000

Davies G, Welham J, Chant D, et al: A systematic review and meta-analysis of northern hemisphere season of birth studies in schizophrenia. Schizophr Bull 29:587–593, 2003

Fitzgerald PB, Montgomery W, de Castella AR, et al: Australian Schizophrenia Care and Assessment Programme: real-world schizophrenia: economics. Aust N Z J Psychiatry 41:819–829, 2007

Fromm-Reichmann F: Notes on the development of treatment of schizophrenics by psychoanalysis and psychotherapy. Psychiatry 11:263–273, 1948

Gejman PV: The role of genetics in the etiology of schizophrenia. Psychiatr Clin North Am 33:35–66, 2010

Green MF: New possibilities in cognition enhancement for schizophrenia. Am J Psychiatry 166:749–752, 2009

Harris MJ, Jeste DV: Late-onset schizophrenia: an overview. Schizophr Bull 14:39–55, 1988

Houts AC: Fifty years of psychiatric nomenclature: reflections on the 1943 War Department Technical Bulletin, Medical 203. J Clin Psychol 56:935–967, 2000

Kraepelin E: Dementia Praecox and Paraphrenia. Translated by Barclay RM. Edited by Robertson GM. Edinburgh, Scotland, E & S Livingstone, 1919

Kuhn R: Eugen Bleuler's concepts of psychopathology. Hist Psychiatry 15:361–366, 2004

Lehman AF, Goldberg R, Dixon LB, et al: Improving employment outcomes for persons with severe mental illnesses. Arch Gen Psychiatry 59:165–172, 2002

Lewis DA, Lieberman JA: Catching up of schizophrenia: natural history and neurobiology. Neuron 28:325–334, 2000

Malaspina D, Harlap S, Fennig S, et al: Advancing paternal age and the risk of schizophrenia. Arch Gen Psychiatry 58:361–367, 2001

McEvoy JP: The costs of schizophrenia. J Clin Psychiatry 68 (suppl 14):4–7, 2007

McEvoy JP, Meyer JM, Goff DC, et al: Prevalence of the metabolic syndrome in patients with schizophrenia: baseline results from the Clinical Antipsychotic Trials of Intervention Effectiveness (CATIE) schizophrenia trial and comparison with national estimates from NHANES III. Schizophr Res 80:19–32, 2005

McGrath JJ: Myths and plain truths about schizophrenia epidemiology—the NAPE lecture 2004. Acta Psychiatr Scand 111:4–11, 2005

McGrath J[J], Susser ES: New directions in the epidemiology of schizophrenia. Med J Aust 190 (suppl 4):S7–S9, 2009

McGrath J[J], Saha S, Welham J, et al: A systematic review of the incidence of schizophrenia: the distribution of rates and the influence of sex, urbanicity, migrant status and methodology. BMC Med 2:13, 2004

McGrath J[J], Saha S, Chant D, et al: Schizophrenia: a concise overview of incidence, prevalence and mortality. Epidemiol Rev 30:67–76, 2008

Messias EL, Chen C, Eaton W: Epidemiology of schizophrenia: review of findings and myths. Psychiatr Clin North Am 30:323–338, 2007

Meyer JM, Davis VG, Goff DC, et al: Change in metabolic syndrome parameters with antipsychotic treatment in the CATIE Schizophrenia Trial: prospective data from phase 1. Schizophr Res 101:273–286, 2008

Saha S, Chant D, Welham J, et al: A systematic review of the prevalence of schizophrenia. PLoS Med 2:413–433, 2005

Saha S, Welham J, Chant D, et al: Incidence of schizophrenia does not vary with economic status of the country: evidence from a systematic review. Soc Psychiatry Psychiatr Epidemiol 41:338–340, 2006

Saha S, Chant D, McGrath J: A systematic review of mortality in schizophrenia: is the differential mortality gap worsening over time? Arch Gen Psychiatry 64:1123–1131, 2007

Sartorius N, Jablensky A, Korten A, et al: Early manifestations and first-contact incidence of schizophrenia in different cultures: a preliminary report on the initial evaluation phase of the WHO Collaborative Study on determinants of outcome of severe mental disorders. Psychol Med 16:909–928, 1986

Schneider K: Clinical Psychopathology. New York, Grune & Stratton, 1959

Torrey EF: Prevalence of schizophrenia. Br J Psychiatry 150:598–608, 1987

World Health Organization: International Statistical Classification of Diseases and Related Health Problems, 10th Revision. Geneva, World Health Organization, 1992

Wu EQ, Birnbaum HG, Shi L, et al: The economic burden of schizophrenia in the United States in 2002. J Clin Psychiatry 66:1122–1129, 2005

2

Basic Science Underlying Schizophrenia

Will J. Cronenwett, M.D.

Gaurava Agarwal, M.D.

John G. Csernansky, M.D.

Introduction: Schizophrenia Has a Biological Basis

Since the earliest days of scientific medicine, people have been searching for explanations for insanity, "madness," and the mental illness that today we call schizophrenia. Many ideas competed in the beginning. Some held that insanity was a derangement of the spirit, a psychological disturbance, or an illness caused by a failure of the human will to maintain itself against the exigencies of the world. Religious explanations for madness persisted into the nineteenth century (Palha and Esteves 1997). But alongside these notions, the idea that insanity could be traced back to dysfunction in the brain was always present. "Insanity, then, I believe to be always caused by irritation of some portion of the brain," wrote physician Beverly R. Morris (1844). Similarly, W.A.F. Browne, contemporary of Morris and notable reformer of asylums in Scotland, declared his confidence that insanity was "a disease of the afferent parts of the tissues of which the mental phenomena are symptoms" (1859, in Jacyna 1982).

Many causes of mental status changes came to be associated with observable changes in the brain and body. Endocrine dysfunction, infection, fever, and tumors were all implicated in psychosis. Although this was encouraging to early physicians, similar evidence was notably absent for some types of insanity, including the illness that came to be called schizophrenia; still, the search for biological causes went on, and in the twentieth century, that evidence finally began to appear. The changes in schizophrenia are subtle. Innovative modalities that used advanced technology were required before they became visible. Still, study after study has determined that structural, functional, molecular, and genetic changes are associated with this illness. Sadly, no single biological finding is yet of great enough magnitude to be used clinically as a test. But one can still make useful generalizations when looking at people with schizophrenia as a population. There is indeed much noise, as it were, but the signal is beginning to come through.

In this chapter, we review the basic science underlying schizophrenia. We begin with a description of the brain changes seen in the illness and then discuss some of the competing and complementary theories that explain how these changes came about. Although treatment is discussed elsewhere in this volume, it will be clear that a tight link exists between theories of the illness and some of the treatments. That particular arrow points both ways: effective treatments have suggested hypotheses about the illness, which have suggested new treatments. The twentieth century marked enormous progress in neuroscience research, and our understanding of schizophrenia has grown immensely. It is our fervent hope that the twenty-first century will see even more progress, to the betterment of the millions of human beings whose lives are disrupted by this frequently catastrophic disease.

Biological Markers of Schizophrenia

Biological Markers Inform About Illness

A biological marker, or "biomarker," is an objective indicator of a particular biological state of an organism. A biological marker of an illness, for example, is a measurable change in the state of an organism that should be present if the illness is present and absent if the illness is absent. Biomarkers are helpful in several ways. First, they can form the basis for clinical tests, allowing us to divide a population into healthy and sick based on the presence or absence of the marker. Two such diagnostic biomarkers in neuropsychiatry are a CAG-repeat mutation in the short arm of chromosome 4, which if present, is diagnostic for Huntington's disease; and periventricular white matter lesions seen with magnetic resonance imaging (MRI), which are associated with plaques in multiple sclerosis. These two examples also serve to illustrate the distinction between state and trait markers. The CAG-repeat mutation in Huntington's disease is typical of a biomarker for an illness *trait:* the mutation is present long before symptoms emerge, and the marker stable over time. In contrast, the white matter lesions seen on MRI in multiple sclerosis correlate with inflammation. The lesions wax as the illness flares and regress as the acute inflammation resolves. This type of imaging marker indicates the *state* of the patient and his or her illness. Biomarkers thus can also inform about illness severity, progression, or response to treatment. We now review some of the most promising biomarkers for schizophrenia, with an eye toward what these objective, measurable markers tell us about the biology of the illness.

Brain Structure Is Different in Schizophrenia

The first investigations into the biology of schizophrenia involved the examination of brains at autopsy (see subsection "Brain Cytology Is Different in Schizophrenia," later in this chapter). This line of inquiry was fraught with obvious disadvantages, most notably, that the subjects were deceased at the time of the examination. This meant that the subjects had generally been alive long enough for the findings to be confounded by the processes of normal aging and by any comorbid illnesses such as dementias or cerebrovascular disease. Longitudinal studies were clearly impossible, thus leaving unexamined the question of whether brain changes were present at the onset of illness or developed progressively over time. Therefore, in vivo brain imaging was eagerly embraced as soon as it became available.

The first brain imaging modality that showed changes in schizophrenic populations was pneumoencephalography (PEG). In this complicated, risky, and painful procedure, the patient's cerebrospinal fluid (CSF) is extracted via a needle inserted into the spine, and air or another gas is introduced into the spinal column in its place. Standard X-ray photographs are then taken of the head. The brain/air interface is visible on the films, which allows for the description of the size and shape of ventricular spaces. Jacobi and Winkler (1927) noted that individuals with schizophrenia tended to have enlarged ventricles. Subsequent PEG studies in the middle of the twentieth century confirmed this finding, and several studies were able to correlate the severity of the clinical symptoms with the degree of ventricular enlargement. The studies, however, were plagued with methodological and technical difficulties, not the least of which was the stated opinion of the American Roentgen Ray Society in 1929 that the use of healthy volunteers in PEG studies was unjustifiable because the procedure exposed them to unacceptable risks (Lawrie et al. 2004).

Today, the PEG procedure itself is only of historical interest; however, the early findings are still notable because PEG illustrated for the first time that schizophrenia is associated with objective and measurable changes in the structure of the brain. Indeed, the original pneumoencephalographic findings of enlarged ventricles have been confirmed by all subsequent imaging modalities and remain among the most durable and widely reproduced findings in schizophrenia research.

The advent of computed tomography (CT) removed the most urgent hazards of PEG and ushered in a new enthusiasm for neuroimaging research. The first CT study of schizophrenia (Johnstone et al. 1976) confirmed the PEG findings of enlarged ventricles. Subsequent studies also benefited from the rigorous consensus definitions of schizophrenia that emerged in that era, including the publication of DSM-III in 1980 (American Psychiatric Association 1980). Some variability remained in methodology and sample characteristics; for example, the size of ventricles was still calculated mostly by hand and thus subject to problems with interrater variation. Still, collecting CT data was easy enough that investigators began to benefit from larger sample sizes in their studies. This allowed them to control for medication history, exposure to electroconvulsive therapy (ECT) or insulin coma, as well as race and gender. The finding of enlarged ventricles withstood correction for the influences of all of these factors (Seidman 1983). Duration of illness appeared not to be a factor because changes were present in subjects scanned in the initial episode of their illness.

Studies in this period profited not just from consensus definitions of schizophrenia but also from standardized clinical assessments. For the first time, research groups began to use standardized instruments for the description and quantification of clinical symptoms. This allowed for more rigorous correlations between brain anatomy and clinical presentations. One important finding was that large ventricles tended to correlate with negative symptoms, such as affective flattening, avolition, and alogia. Smaller ventricles, on the other hand, were associated with positive symptoms such as delusions, hallucinations, and bizarre behavior (Andreasen and Olsen 1982). In general, larger ventricles also correlated with more severe illness and poorer outcome. Note that although enlarged ventricular space is a highly consistent finding in imaging and postmortem research, the absolute amount of increase is still fairly small. People with schizophrenia as a population, in other words, have larger ventricles, especially those with severe illness, but very few indeed have such large spaces that this information could be used for diagnostic purposes. Furthermore, ventricular enlargement is a nonspecific finding that is common to many pathological processes besides schizophrenia. Even the mechanism and significance remain unclear because ventricle size is influenced by both genetic and environmental factors (Peper et al. 2007).

Other neuroimaging findings emerged as well, although not as consistently as ventricular enlargement. These included a relative thinning of some portions of the cerebral cortex, widening of the cerebral sulci, and atrophy of the cerebellum. These measures are particularly variable across studies because of inconsistent methodologies. As one might expect, both negative and positive findings are reported in the CT literature (see Seidman 1983 for a review).

The invention of CT imaging renewed interest in the application of neuroimaging to schizophrenia with a resultant expansion in the number of studies published, but as we have seen, the findings remained inconsistent except for ventricular size. But then the field took a quantum leap forward with the arrival of MRI. Like CT scanning, MRI is noninvasive, but it has the added advantage of sparing the participants from potentially harmful X rays. Early MRI already had higher resolution than CT and could elaborate contrast between cerebral gray and white matter. The first paper to report MRI data in schizophrenia was published in 1984 (Smith et al. 1984). Despite using a 0.3-tesla magnetic field, which is weak by the standards of today, they were able to present higher-resolution images with better contrast than in any previous schizophrenia study published to date. MRI has continued to provide impressive data in the nearly 30 years since that landmark study.

The findings have been of great scientific value. First, MRI experiments were able to confirm the enlargements that were seen in the lateral and third ventricles with previous imaging modalities. This was not surprising. More interesting is that MRI has been able to describe changes in regions such as the prefrontal cortex (PFC). The PFC is the major integrative association area of the brain; it is involved in complicated cognitive tasks such as planning, shifting and maintaining attention, decision making, and behavioral self-control. People with injuries or illnesses affecting the PFC have shown cognitive deficits, avolition, poverty of speech, emotional withdrawal, and inappropriate affect, all of which are commonly seen in schizophrenia (Weinberger 1995).

Initial MRI studies of the frontal regions were equivocal, possibly because they tended to look at the frontal lobes in their entirety (Shenton et al. 2001). More recent studies have parceled the frontal lobe into smaller separate and discrete areas. This makes empirical sense because the PFC contains regions that can be differentiated histologically on the basis of cell type, number, and distribution. Approached this way, the PFC does begin to show regional changes in schizophrenia. Sullivan et al. (1998) reported volume loss in prefrontal regions, and Buchanan et al. (1998) reported volume loss in schizophrenia in the inferior region of the PFC. Some evidence suggests that deficits in this area are associated with more profound negative symptoms and that this pattern of volume loss is specific to schizophrenia (Sullivan et al. 1998). Furthermore, the discovery of changes in the PFC makes sense based on what we know of schizophrenia because people with the illness tend to have problems with cognitive tasks that rely on intact prefrontal neural circuitry.

In contrast to imaging studies of the frontal cortex, which found changes in only selected regions, most studies of the temporal lobes have reported low volumes across the entire structure. In fact, temporal lobe changes are among the most consistently reported findings in MRI studies in schizophrenia (see Shenton et al. 2001 for a review). Regional volume loss also has been localized to the superior temporal gyrus (STG) and its posterior third, the planum temporale, as well as the medial temporal structures. The STG and the planum temporale are intimately involved in auditory processing and language, likely serving as integration areas for language and speech-related processes (Hickok 2009). Deficits here have been clinically correlated with both increased auditory hallucinations and more severe formal thought disorder, which is generally measured by looking at language content and output. Medial temporal structures including the hippocampus, amygdala, and parahippocampal gyrus are similarly affected, with volume reductions reported in most studies. Again, these results are not surprising, given the role that these structures play in encoding and retrieving memories and emotional processing.

Most investigations of cortical changes have focused on the regions described earlier; that is, the parts of frontal and temporolimbic cortex that govern executive function, memory, emotional regulation, communication, and the sorts of complex cognitive activities that both make us human beings and are so grievously disrupted in schizophrenia. However, neuroimaging shows changes in thickness throughout the cortex as well and in complex patterns (Schultz et al. 2010). Studies performed at the onset of psychotic symptoms have shown that cortical thinning might begin in the parietal regions and progress briskly through adolescence toward the front of the brain, culminating in prefrontal and temporal changes. This pattern of progressive cortical loss correlates with worsening symptoms of psychosis and increasing cognitive deficits as time passes (Thompson et al. 2001).

Subcortical structures are similarly affected. The thalamus has attracted much research attention because of its unique role in the coordination of mental activity. All incoming sensory information passes through the thalamus and receives modulation there, as does all information passing from one region of the cortex to another. As many as 95% of the synapses in the thalamus belong to neurons that affect this flow of information (Reichova and Sherman 2004; Sherman and Guillery 1998). Lesions confined to the thalamus, such as from stroke, can result in neuropsychiatric syndromes similar to schizophrenia. Thalamic strokes can cause hallucinations, confusion, impaired insight, attention disturbances, poverty of speech, apathy, and confabulation (Schmahmann 2003). Therefore, it is perhaps not surprising that structural changes are seen in the thalamus in schizophrenia. Imaging studies are not in full agreement, but most show reduced thalamic volume (Konick and Friedman 2001; Sim et al. 2006) with changes perhaps localized to the portions of the thalamus that project to prefrontal cortical areas (Csernansky et al. 2004). Because these cortical areas also show volume loss, the illness may cause structural changes that are not localized to particular regions but are instead distributed across interconnected neural networks.

Although the studies referenced thus far have looked at gray matter structures, changes are seen in white matter as well. White matter consists of myelinated axons of neurons. It forms the infrastructure over which neuronal impulses are carried from one point to another in the brain. The earliest studies of white matter were able to measure only relative volume, and these did not identify differences in schizophrenia. However, the recent introduction of diffusion tensor imaging (DTI) has begun to detect some interesting changes. DTI is a method of measuring the diffusion of water, which is helpful because the characteristics of water diffusion in white matter are thought to be related to the integrity of axonal tracts. The most consistent findings to date implicate the white matter tracts in frontotemporal regions (Kubicki et al. 2007). The assumption is that complex diffusion patterns correlate with reduced integrity of the axonal tracts. The implication for schizophrenia is once again that pathological changes might not be localized to one particular region but instead might be spread across interconnected networks.

Most of these neuroimaging findings have been seen at the onset of illness, implying that they are neither artifacts of treatment nor the result of chronic disease. The regions that are most consistently different are frontal structures such as the dorsolateral PFC (DLPFC), temporal structures such as the hippocampus and STG, and the thalamus; these structures are implicated in executive functioning, working memory, episodic memory, and the smooth coordination of neural and cognitive processes. However, contradictory and negative studies also exist, likely because of differences in methodology and because of the small magnitude of the changes themselves. The correlations between structural findings and clinical symptoms have been inconclusive. However, similar structural findings are usually present to an attenuated degree in the healthy relatives of people with schizophrenia, which is evidence that at least part of the underlying process is genetically determined and heritable.

Brain Function Is Different in Schizophrenia

In the previous section, we reviewed evidence from neuroimaging studies that points toward structural anomalies in the brain. In this section, we look at brain function, beginning with functional neuroimaging, and then review other objective measures of cognitive and neurophysiological processes.

Functional neuroimaging was introduced in the second half of the twentieth century with positron emission tomography (PET), in which metabolically active, radiolabeled tracers were used to locate regions of neuronal activity. This was invasive and cumbersome, however, and so was largely supplanted in the

1990s by functional MRI (fMRI), which is noninvasive and uses changes in cerebral blood oxygenation as a marker for metabolic activity. The most consistent findings from PET and fMRI are that glucose metabolism and cerebral blood flow are not globally altered in schizophrenia. Regional differences do exist, however, with the most compelling evidence being for decreased activity in the DLPFC, so-called hypofrontality. Decreases in fMRI signal here correlate well with other cognitive markers of DLPFC dysfunction, such as measures of working memory and executive function. Hypofrontality also appears to be associated with psychomotor poverty and increased negative symptoms. These results have been well replicated; additionally, the differences are visible at the onset of illness, appear to be stable over time, and are independent of the effects of psychotropic medication (Andreasen et al. 1997; Bunney and Bunney 2000; Taylor 1996).

Findings in other regions are conflicting and not as consistent but still quite interesting. This includes temporal and limbic overactivity, as well as sensory-specific regional activation during periods of hallucinations. Subcortical differences are also seen, as is evidence that prefrontal and temporolimbic changes are actually present in concert with differences in the basal ganglia and thalamus. This provides yet more evidence that the abnormalities in schizophrenia are not localized to one brain region but instead are distributed across interconnected networks (Andreasen 1997; Siegel et al. 1993).

One can also measure brain function by looking at reactions to various sensory stimuli. People with schizophrenia tend to have deficiencies in sensory gating or the way in which the brain receives, prioritizes, and filters sensory input. With impaired sensory gating, it is difficult to assign the correct level of importance to perceptions from the environment, and this makes it difficult to filter out stimuli that are less relevant. One example of a sensory gating phenomenon is prepulse inhibition (PPI), which refers to the attenuation of an involuntary startle response when a test stimulus is preceded by a weaker "prepulse." Typically, this is demonstrated with acoustic stimuli. A sound, the prepulse, is given about 30–300 ms before the test stimulus, and electrodes on the face near the eye measure the subject's startle response by tracking movement of the muscles involved in blinking. Healthy individuals will startle less when a prepulse is given, but in people with schizophrenia, this attenuation is impaired. Although not specific for any one illness, PPI is a useful marker for the functioning of complex prefrontal, limbic, and subcortical neural circuitry. It is also easily demonstrated in animal models, which show that PPI can be manipulated both by drugs and by developmental, anatomical, and genetic interventions (Swerdlow et al. 2008). PPI appears to be a heritable trait in both animals and humans, and healthy relatives of people with schizophrenia have PPI at an intermediate level between that of people with the illness and that of healthy control subjects (Turetsky et al. 2007).

P50 suppression is a sensory gating phenomenon that is conceptually similar to PPI but neurologically distinct. In a typical P50 testing paradigm, two auditory stimuli are presented 500 ms apart, and the amplitude of the P50 wave is measured on an electroencephalogram (EEG) after the second stimulus. The EEG response to the second stimulus is smaller in healthy people. This is because the first stimulus activates a section of the brain, conditioning it, such that subsequent activity in that region is suppressed. Similar to PPI, this suppression is not as strong in people with schizophrenia. The affected circuitry appears to involve the STG and the hippocampus (Freedman et al. 1996), and as is the case with PPI, functional changes appear to be heritable. In the case of P50 gating, the changes are inherited in an autosomal dominant fashion, which further suggests a genetic basis (Adler et al. 1998). Furthermore, reduced P50 suppression appears to be state-independent because it is seen in high-risk individuals before the onset of psychosis or prodromal symptoms (Brockhaus-Dumke et al. 2008).

Investigations of analogous animal models have implicated the nicotinic cholinergic system because it modulates sensory input passing from heteromodal association areas through the entorhinal cortex and into the hippocampus. This would have profound implications for learning and memory, and defects here could plausibly make it difficult for people with schizophrenia to create proper associations around their perceptions. This might lead to fundamental difficulties in making sense of the world.

In another neuropsychological test, participants are shown a series of visual targets on either their left or their right and are asked to look in the direction opposite the displayed target. This requires that they inhibit a natural tendency to look toward the target; that is, they should try to inhibit natural saccadic eye movements in the direction of the target. The test measures the number of times the patients look in the incorrect direction (i.e., antisaccades); it requires intact working memory and the ability to maintain attention. Participants with schizophrenia and people at high risk for psychosis both have higher error rates than do healthy people. People with neurological damage to the frontal lobes also make more errors on antisaccades tests (Nieman et al. 2007).

The previous procedures test involuntary responses to stimuli. The P300 event-related potential (ERP), in contrast, is a marker of deliberate cognitive activity in response to a stimulus. In the P300 test, subjects are presented with a series of similar targets and are told to press a button when they see a target that is different. Thus, they must decide whether each target is an irrelevant distracter or an important "oddball" stimulus. EEG recordings are obtained while the subject evaluates the target and makes the decision, with the result that oddball stimuli (as opposed to the distracters) evoke an EEG wave that occurs about 300 ms after presentation. The amplitude of this P300 wave is decreased in schizophrenia, and in some studies the latency appears to be increased as well. These findings also appear to be heritable and are present regardless of the state of the illness. Decreased P300 amplitude is not specific for schizophrenia, however, but is present in a variety of other illnesses including Alzheimer's disease and bipolar disorder (Turetsky et al. 2007). Thus, although nonspecific, it is nevertheless a robust marker for some of the brain changes that are seen in people with schizophrenia and their relatives.

Another neurophysiological performance indicator is mismatch negativity (MMN). To detect MMN, a subject is presented with a constant train of auditory pulses that are infrequently interrupted by a tone that differs in pitch, duration, or intensity. The individual tones evoke EEG waves rapidly, within about 50 ms. When there is a mismatch between a novel tone and the repetitive background train, the waveform at 50 ms is deflected sharply in the negative direction. This response is impaired in schizophrenia (first reported in Shelley et al. 1991). MMN is particularly interesting because the impairment is much more specific to this illness; for example, MMN deficits are not seen in bipolar disorder, depression, or schizoaffective disorder (Umbricht et al. 2003). MMN also stands out for the briskness of the response: because the evoked potential develops just 50 ms after the mismatched stimulus, there is no time for conscious cognitive processing to take place.

MMN responses thus occur independent of any conscious mental activity. In fact, participants will show MMN when they are actively focusing their attention on some other task. Alho et al. (1990) documented MMN responses in sleeping newborn infants. Animal models exist as well. The MMN phenomenon has been associated with N-methyl-D-aspartate (NMDA) receptor activity because psychotomimetic NMDA receptor antagonists such as keta-mine produce schizophrenia-like MMN changes in humans (Turetsky et al. 2007). Unlike the biological markers discussed earlier, MMN may not be present at illness onset but may instead develop as the illness progresses.

These neuropsychological experiments are informative in that they show differences in schizophrenia beyond the traditional clinical symptom domains. By testing specific subcomponents of cognition, they can also be helpful in characterizing and localizing deficits to specific regions of the brain. Because they are heritable, there is great hope that a genetic basis for the deficits can be discovered. For example, one gene implicated in schizophrenia is neuregulin-1 (*NRG1*), which is important for many types of neural growth, connectivity, and signaling. One recent study reported that mice bred to be missing one copy of *NRG1* show reduced MMN but normal PPI (Ehrlichman et al. 2009). Further work should clarify the linkage between genes associated with schizophrenia and the precise neurological differences attributed to them (see also "Genetic Factors" subsection later in this chapter).

One final neurophysiological abnormality seen in schizophrenia is in smooth pursuit eye movements. This abnormality is easy to elicit and is present with a large effect size (see O'Driscoll and Callahan 2008 for a review). It is so easily apparent that researchers first noticed the differences more than 100 years ago. When tracking a target, people with schizophrenia move their eyes less smoothly than healthy comparison subjects; their eyes show more sudden saccadic jumps. This has been consistently observed in both patients and their first-degree relatives (Levy et al. 1994). Despite many efforts, smooth pursuit anomalies have yet to be correlated with any other neuropsychological performance measures, and the underlying neural mechanism remains unclear (Zanelli et al. 2009); still, it is a consistent and repeatable marker and has been observed since the earliest days of schizophrenia research.

Cognitive markers have been proposed for schizophrenia as well, especially in the domain of executive functioning. One component of executive functioning is goal maintenance, or the ability to hold attention on a particular goal such that automatic responses are overcome and behavior is directed in a consistent direction. Another component is rule selection, which refers to the activity of modifying goal-directed behavior to accommodate changing rules. People with schizophrenia have deficits in these dimensions of executive functioning. The deficits are easily identified with neuropsychological exam-

inations such as the Wisconsin Card Sorting Test and the Stroop Test. Perfor
mance on these tasks depends on healthy functioning in neural circuits extending from the DLPFC to the basal ganglia (Kerns et al. 2008), regions seen
on imaging studies to be sites of pathology in schizophrenia.

Cognitive markers have special clinical relevance because functional outcome in schizophrenia correlates more strongly with the degree of cognitive
impairment than with other types of symptoms (Kurtz et al. 2008; Milev et al.
2005). Thus, improvement on cognitive markers would be an excellent and
useful method for tracking response to therapeutic interventions.

In summary, brains perform differently in schizophrenia. This is seen in
functional imaging studies examining differences in brain metabolism while
cognitive tasks are being performed. It is also seen in circumstances when subjects are providing completely preconscious and involuntary responses to
stimuli. The pattern of deficits is informative. First, metabolic activity appears
to be reduced in the regions subserving working memory and executive function, whereas it is increased in areas associated with contextual knowledge and
emotional processing. Second, people with schizophrenia have marked deficits in sensory gating, or the ability to appropriately filter unimportant stimuli. This suggests an overinclusive cognitive style in which the signal-to-noise
ratio of cognitive events is skewed: too much noise is experienced as signal.

Brain Cytology Is Different in Schizophrenia

The earliest studies of brain changes in schizophrenia began with the examination of brains at autopsy. Alois Alzheimer pioneered the postmortem investigation of schizophrenic brains with two studies published in 1897 and 1913
(discussed in Heckers 1997). He described generalized decreases in the volume
of gray matter with specific volume loss in the layers II and III of the cortex, layers that contain neurons projecting to other cortical regions. This volume loss
was associated with a decrease in the neuropil, the portion of gray matter between neurons that contains synaptic connections. He also noted alterations in
the shape and orientation of excitatory pyramidal cells. These neurons are present throughout the cortex but are much more morphologically complex in the
prefrontal regions and are thought to be critical for executive function and cognition in humans (Elston 2003).

These and indeed most other early studies of the neuroanatomy of schizophrenia were carried out without the methodological rigor that is seen as nec-

essary today. For example, until the second half of the twentieth century, it was uncommon to include matched, healthy brains in the sample for comparison. Furthermore, Alzheimer and other early investigators were not blind to the diagnoses of their subjects. Therefore, it is perhaps all the more remarkable that these early findings have remained durable throughout the years.

In 1987, Bente Pakkenberg carried out a high-quality, rigorous, blinded study of postmortem brains with matched healthy control subjects and confirmed that the schizophrenic population indeed had less gray matter and larger cerebral ventricles (Pakkenberg 1987), by a factor of approximately 10%. Ventricles also were relatively larger in people with schizophrenia whose illness was characterized by more profound negative symptoms. These volume decreases are widespread throughout the cortex, with changes apparent in all four lobes and in the limbic system (Bogerts et al. 1985). In a subsequent study, Pakkenberg (1993) reported that the number of neurons was not different in schizophrenia. This finding was rather remarkable, suggesting that differences in volume were caused by something other than loss of neuronal cells. Further investigation indicated that both neuronal and glial size was reduced in schizophrenia, most significantly in the pyramidal cells in layer III of the cortex (Rajkowska et al. 1998). The finding that cortical thinning can be explained through reduced pyramidal cell volume, rather than decreased number of cells, provides strong evidence against a degenerative process.

Indeed, no study has found evidence of neuronal degeneration in schizophrenia: gliosis, the pathological hallmark of neuronal injury and scarring, has always been absent. This sets schizophrenia apart from other disorders in which neurons degenerate with time, such as Alzheimer's disease, Parkinson's disease, and Huntington's disease.

Here two lines of evidence converge: first, the number of neurons is not reduced in schizophrenia, and second, in the face of decreased cortical volume, there is no evidence for neuronal degeneration or cellular destruction. This implies an increase in neuronal density, and this has indeed been confirmed independently (Selemon et al. 1995). If the number of neurons is the same, then volume loss in the cortical gray matter must be a result of reduced neuropil, as Alzheimer originally observed in 1913. Intriguingly, the neuropil contains components of cells that underlie intercellular connectivity and facilitate communication between regions of the brain.

The major neuron type in the cerebral cortex is the pyramidal cell, named for the triangular shape of its cell body. It receives signals from other cells on synapses that are located on thousands of spines on the neuron's dendrites. These spines increase in number rapidly as synapses are formed in the developing human brain, and then many are lost, or "pruned" away, in adolescence. The number of dendritic spines remains fairly constant through adult life, until the total starts to fall off again as the brain approaches old age. The number of spines changes on a shorter time scale as well and is believed to be affected by learning and experience (Bhatt et al. 2009). Dendritic spines are reduced in number in schizophrenia, specifically in layer III of the cortex, which is where pyramidal cells receive synaptic input from other cortical neurons. This appears to be one mechanism whereby the neuropil is reduced (Garey 2010).

The relative strengthening and weakening of synapses in neural networks is called synaptic plasticity. This process is fundamental to the creation of long-term memories and had been demonstrated experimentally in the hippocampus. More recently, evidence also has emerged that the PFC shows synaptic plasticity throughout life. In some animal models of schizophrenia, markers for plasticity appear to be enhanced (Goto et al. 2010). This suggests a mechanism by which corticocortical synaptic connectivity may be altered, leading to the disrupted cognitive processes that are hallmarks of the disorder.

In contrast to the cortex, which does not seem to have lowered numbers of neurons, careful examinations have suggested that the thalamus has reductions in the number of cells. Specifically, Pakkenberg (1990) found a 40% reduction in the number of neurons in the thalamic mediodorsal nucleus. Differences were not present in comparison regions. This is interesting because the mediodorsal nucleus receives projections from the DLPFC, the higher-order association area involved in working memory and executive function. Studies looking at markers for axon terminals have also reported evidence of reduced connectivity between the thalamus and the cortex (Lewis and Lieberman 2000).

Parvalbumin-staining γ-aminobutyric acid (GABA)ergic interneurons are reduced in the DLPFC in schizophrenia (Lewis 2000). This is fascinating because these interneurons regulate the functioning of the pyramidal cells, applying inhibition and disinhibition in a way that balances neuronal tone. Interneurons are thought to be important for salience detection and sensory gating because their inhibitory properties would allow the brain to filter unwanted responses so that attention can be focused properly. One type of GABAergic interneuron is the aptly named chandelier cell, which has multiple synapses on the bodies of pyramidal cells close to where the action potential is generated. These axon terminals, called cartridges, are rich in the GABA membrane transporter 1 (GAT-1). Immunochemical studies have shown repeatedly that these GAT-1-containing cartridges are significantly less dense in individuals with schizophrenia. The regions most notable for such changes are those regions subserving corticocortical and thalamocortical communication, and the changes here may disrupt executive functioning (Pierri et al. 1999).

Pathological studies of white matter in the brain show decreased number and size of oligodendrocytes (Kubicki et al. 2005). Oligodendrocytes are the cellular component of the central nervous system (CNS) that supports neuronal communication by providing myelin sheaths around axons, in a way that is analogous to the plastic insulation around electrical wires. In addition to changes seen in oligodendrocytes, several laboratories have reported changes in associated cellular proteins, as well as lower levels of the messenger RNA that codes for them. Oligodendrocytes are particularly susceptible to injury, so it is unclear if this is a primary finding or the result of a disease process elsewhere in the brain or even perhaps a result of an environmental insult. Still, taken with the DTI studies showing altered white matter macrostructure (see subsection "Brain Structure Is Different in Schizophrenia," earlier in this chapter), this provides convincing evidence that brain changes in schizophrenia are not limited to cortical and subcortical regions containing neuronal cell bodies. Instead, the changes also extend to the machinery of intercellular connectivity and signal transduction.

Evidence also indicates disturbances in neuronal migration. For example, in schizophrenia, there appear to be more neuronal cell bodies located in lower (deeper) layers of the cortex. Indeed, higher numbers of cell bodies are present in the white matter itself, a region deep to the cortex with traditionally many fewer cell bodies. This suggests a disturbance in the migration of cells from the ventricular zone to their final intended destinations. This has been seen in regions of the cortex already implicated in schizophrenia such as the entorhinal cortex, hippocampus, and PFC (Akbarian et al. 1993; Falkai et al. 2000; Kovalenko et al. 2003). Furthermore, interstitial neurons in the white matter are distributed abnormally (Eastwood and Harrison 2003). These findings argue strongly for a developmental pathology in schizophrenia because neuronal migration is a prenatal event (see subsection "Disconnection or Dysconnection?" later in this chapter).

Taken as a body of evidence, abnormal markers are found throughout the microcircuitry of the brain, including smaller cell bodies, reduced dendritic spines, differences in myelination and oligodendrocytes, changes in marker proteins, fewer interneurons, and evidence for disrupted neuronal migration. Significant cytological differences are present in the cortex, white matter, and subcortical structures. These changes belong in part to some of the earliest findings in schizophrenia research. We turn next to how disrupted neural functioning might produce some of the clinical hallmarks of the illness and how some of these functional and physical changes might come about.

Cells and Signaling: The Dopamine Hypothesis and Beyond

Dopamine Hypothesis of Schizophrenia

Dopamine was first synthesized in 1910 and was noted then to have mild physiological activity that was "adrenaline-like" (Barger and Dale 1910; the authors introduced the word "sympathomimetic" to describe this activity). Arvid Carlsson (1959), in work for which he later shared the 2000 Nobel Prize in physiology or medicine, subsequently established that dopamine is an agent of neurotransmission in the brain. Proposed by van Rossum (1966) and building on Carlsson's previous work, the "dopamine hypothesis" of schizophrenia is one of the oldest and most widely known scientific theories in psychiatry (Baumeister and Francis 2002; Carlsson 1978; Howes and Kapur 2009). It has undergone much revision since its original form, which postulated quite simply that the symptoms of schizophrenia were caused by excess synaptic activity at the dopamine receptor.

The strongest evidence came from the clinical observations that dopamine-blocking medications effectively treated some components of psychosis. Many biological theories of mental illness developed after compounds were serendipitously discovered to be useful against certain symptoms. In the case of the antipsychotics, chemists in the middle of the twentieth century were trying to synthesize molecules with antihistaminic properties when they found to their surprise that they had discovered a medication that could treat psychiatric agitation and hallucinations (Healy 2004). Investigations eventually showed that this compound, chlorpromazine, worked by modifying the dopamine system in the brain. The development of other medications quickly followed, and Seeman and Lee reported in 1975 that the efficacy of this class of agents was directly correlated with the ability to block dopamine receptors. To this day, every available medication with antipsychotic properties exerts its desired effects by modulating dopaminergic activity. Specifically, antipsychotic efficacy correlates with the ability to block the dopamine type 2 (D_2) receptors in the striatum, with between 65% and 80% receptor occupancy needed to achieve clinical efficacy (Farde et al. 1992). Blockade at higher levels correlates with increased undesirable movement-related side effects.

The second main line of support for the dopamine hypothesis came from observation of the psychoactive effects of compounds such as amphetamine and cocaine. These two drugs work by different mechanisms, but ultimately both increase the concentration of synaptic dopamine in the frontal lobes and in the nucleus accumbens (Wise 1996). Both drugs can cause psychotic symptoms such as delusions, paranoia, and hallucinations. When given to patients with schizophrenia, both drugs provoke relapse or worsening of their psychosis (Lieberman et al. 1987).

Thus, drugs that increase dopamine can cause psychosis, and drugs that block D_2 receptors can treat psychosis; this gives the dopamine hypothesis an enormous amount of strength and credibility. D_2 antagonists also can reverse the psychotic symptoms caused by amphetamine and cocaine, once again confirming that their mechanisms of action were tightly bound. The final piece of support for the dopamine hypothesis came from observations that reserpine, a dopamine-depleting agent, reduced the intensity of psychotic symptoms. With these lines of evidence in place, the dopamine hypothesis was born, and schizophrenia has been associated ever since with abnormally increased dopamine-mediated neuronal signal transduction. (See Baumeister and Francis 2002 for an intellectual history of the dopamine hypothesis.)

It was soon clear, however, that schizophrenia was not simply a disease of "too much" dopamine. Investigators looked for dopamine metabolites in the CSF of patients and did not find elevated levels. The number of dopamine receptors did not appear to be elevated either. Initial experiments had suggested an overabundance of D_2 receptors, which could in theory lead to excess dopamine-mediated signaling. However, dopamine receptors were found to increase with antipsychotic treatment, likely as a response to prolonged receptor blockade. In support of this idea, treatment-naïve patients were not found to have significantly increased numbers of dopamine receptors (Farde et al. 1990).

Thus, the matter appeared more complex than simply too much dopamine or too many receptors. Perhaps dysregulation in dopamine signaling was to blame. Evidence for this began to appear in the 1990s when Laruelle et al. (1996) reported that patients with schizophrenia released more dopamine in the striatum when given amphetamine than did healthy subjects. Similarly, striatal neurons showed enhanced uptake of dopamine precursors. It seemed then that instead of having an elevated basal level of dopamine, the problem could lie with excess release.

Dopamine receptors vary in type across the brain. Subcortical structures, including the striatum and the accumbens, tend to have predominantly D_2 receptors; antipsychotic efficacy correlates strongly with blockade of this receptor type (see discussion earlier in this subsection). However, neuropsychological data indicate cognitive defects in schizophrenia such as working memory and executive dysfunction, which are associated with prefrontal regions. Prefrontal hypofunction has been seen on functional neuroimaging studies and has been linked to dysfunction in cortical dopamine signaling. The cerebral cortex has predominantly D_1 receptors, and dysfunction at the prefrontal D_1 receptors is indeed correlated with negative symptoms and some of the cognitive deficits of schizophrenia (Abi-Dargham and Moore 2003). Clozapine, an antipsychotic medication with superior efficacy in treatment-resistant schizophrenia, has a higher affinity for D_1 than for D_2 receptors.

Given this evidence, the emerging picture is that at least two dopaminergic systems are affected in schizophrenia. The first is the mesocortical system, which begins in the ventral tegmentum and extends to the PFC. Dopamine transmission is reduced here in schizophrenia and is associated with cognitive deficits and negative symptoms. Meanwhile, overactivity occurs in the mesolimbic system, which projects from the ventral tegmentum to the striatum, nucleus accumbens, amygdala, and hippocampus. Studies have reported locally specific D_1 receptor upregulation in prefrontal regions (Abi-Dargham and Moore 2003), which may be a compensatory response to chronic dopaminergic underactivity. This also may explain dopaminergic hyperactivity in the mesolimbic system, although this may arise independently (Howes and Kapur 2009). Overactivity in the mesolimbic system has already been associated with hallucinations and other positive symptoms of schizophrenia, but dysfunction here could additionally lead to inappropriate attribution of salience to cognitive and sensory processes; this in turn could lead to an idiosyncratic and disturbed understanding of reality (Davis et al. 1991; Howes and Kapur 2009). This model is attractive because it would tie both positive and negative symptoms to dysfunction in one neurotransmitter system. However, controversy remains on what the nature of the initial dysfunction is, how environmental effects exert their influence, and why symptoms first appear after adolescence.

The dopamine hypothesis has not been disproved. Indeed, any comprehensive explanation of schizophrenia would have to take into account the fact that D_2-blocking agents treat positive symptoms of psychosis, whereas dopamine-enhancing compounds provoke such symptoms. But despite clear evidence that dopaminergic dysregulation is present in schizophrenia, dopamine is not the whole story.

Glutamate Hypothesis of Schizophrenia

Recent attention has turned to the neurotransmitter glutamate. The primary excitatory neurotransmitter in the brain, glutamate is a ligand for both ionotropic NMDA receptors and the family of metabotropic glutamate (mGlu) receptors. Both types of receptors use glutamate as the primary ligand but are heavily modulated by many other ions and molecules. In turn, these receptors regulate complicated interconnected processes such as neuronal growth and development, as well as critical neuronal components of learning and memory such as long-term potentiation and synaptic plasticity (Li and Tsien 2009).

Although this area of research is relatively young, it has already given us a new potential treatment for schizophrenia. Specifically, the mGlu agonist LY404039 has shown anxiolytic and antipsychotic efficacy in preliminary animal experiments (Rorick-Kehn et al. 2007). One Phase II clinical trial showed promise in human subjects with schizophrenia (Mezler et al. 2010), but another was considered inconclusive because neither LY404039 nor an active comparator separated from placebo (Kinon et al. 2011). If LY404039 turns out to be a clinically useful compound, it would represent the first truly novel mechanism of action for antipsychotic drugs since the advent of chlorpromazine in the 1950s.

Just as the amphetamine model of psychosis was instrumental in the formation of the dopamine hypothesis, another drug of abuse illuminated the relation between glutamate and schizophrenia. Phencyclidine (PCP) is a noncompetitive NMDA receptor antagonist. Originally introduced as an anesthetic, it was soon withdrawn from use because of strange neuropsychiatric side effects, including hallucinations, delirium, disorientation, and a "schizophrenia-like" syndrome that included social withdrawal and negative symptoms (Munch 1974). Later research showed that PCP also worsened psychosis in individuals with schizophrenia and hastened relapse (Keshavan et al. 2008), much like amphetamine does. Furthermore, chronic NMDA receptor blockade leads to degeneration in the amygdala, hippocampus, anterior cingulate gyrus, and entorhinal cortex, mimicking some of the neuroimaging changes seen in schizophrenia (Olney and Farber 1995).

A glutamate hypothesis of schizophrenia is attractive for other reasons. One is that NMDA receptors are instrumental in normal brain development (Goff and Wine 1997). Glutamate plays a role in guiding young neurons to their targets, in synaptogenesis, and in the strengthening of neuronal synapses. Glutamatergic signals also guide synaptic pruning as the CNS matures, as well as regulate the programmed death of neurons that are not destined to survive. Glutamate thus helps direct the ebb and flow of the growing brain. Glutamate is also the main agent of excitotoxicity. When neurons are exposed to increased glutamate in the synaptic cleft for a long time, the cells die through apoptosis. This type of apoptotic cell death is not associated with the gliosis seen in degenerative brain diseases.

Glutamate is also an attractive target of schizophrenia research because it can tie together some of the findings seen in other neurotransmitter systems. For example, we have already seen that the activity of parvalbumin-containing GABAergic interneurons is reduced in schizophrenia. Cortical GABAergic interneurons help regulate the balance between inhibition and excitation (see subsection "Brain Cytology Is Different in Schizophrenia," earlier in this chapter), and in the face of decreased NMDA receptor activity, they decrease their own GABA-mediated inhibition of pyramidal cells. Indeed, such changes in GABA signaling can be induced through administration of NMDA receptor antagonists and provide evidence for the idea that hypofunction in NMDA-mediated glutamate signaling may underlie many of the neuronal and clinical aspects of schizophrenia (Belforte et al. 2010). Subcortical NMDA receptor hypoactivity on GABAergic interneurons, for example, could lead to hyperactivity in glutamatergic projections to the cortex, which could then experience apoptotic changes as a result of glutamatergic excitotoxicity (Stone et al. 2007).

Disruptions in NMDA signaling can produce neuropsychological and behavior changes like those seen in schizophrenia. Belforte et al. (2010) bred mice that lacked the NR1 subunit of the NMDA receptor. As predicted, they showed decreased activity in GABAergic neurons. The mice also showed deficits in executive function and in PPI. Similarly, the mouse analogue of the P50 suppression was impaired (Halene et al. 2009). Thus, NMDA dysfunction leads to objectively impaired sensory gating.

Necessarily, any hypothesis describing a defect in glutamate signaling would need to account for the wealth of evidence pointing toward dopamine dysregulation. To review, the clinical potency of antipsychotic medications correlates with their affinity for the D_2 receptor; amphetamine, which stimulates dopamine release, provokes psychotic symptoms; and the negative symptoms of schizophrenia are associated with reduced dopamine activity in the PFC. As is the case with GABA signaling, the dopamine and glutamate systems are tightly linked. For example, dopamine inhibits glutamate release in the cortex and hippocampus, whereas NMDA receptors modulate dopamine release in inhibitory, stimulatory, and phasic modes (David et al. 2005). One glutamatergic pathway extends from the PFC to the GABAergic interneurons in the ventral tegmental area. These inhibitory interneurons decrease the activity of dopaminergic neurons projecting to the mesolimbic system. Thus, decreased NMDA receptor activity would remove GABAergic inhibition, leading to limbic dopaminergic hyperactivity, which has been associated with the positive symptoms of psychosis. Additionally, NMDA receptors excite mesocortical dopaminergic neurons directly. Glutamatergic hypofunction here would lead to reduced activity in cortical dopamine neurons; this has been associated with cognitive and negative symptoms of schizophrenia. Note that once again, the picture of schizophrenia that emerges is of a disease extending far beyond one region of the brain into a network of interlinked neural circuits.

The glutamate hypothesis is therefore not incompatible with the dopamine hypothesis. In fact, if NMDA receptor hypoactivity were truly the hallmark of schizophrenia, it would extend the dopamine hypothesis and would explain the pathology of the illness at a more fundamental level. It would also explain many of the clinical, cognitive, and neuropsychological components of the illness. However, it still does not explain how the changes come about in the first place. To shed light on the origins of the pathology, we turn to the neurodevelopmental model of schizophrenia.

Neurodevelopmental Model and Dysconnection

Schizophrenia Phenotype

The schizophrenia phenotype is clearly complex. It begins with a propensity for psychotic symptoms, which are obviously the most easily observed outward signs of the illness. These intermittent manifestations are present to varying degrees in various individuals and thus are markers of an ill "state" rather than the underlying biological "trait." Many trait markers, however, do appear to be present at the beginning of the illness and, compared with the clinical symptoms, are much more stable over time. These include the structural neuroimaging findings described earlier, as well as characteristic cognitive deficits and neuropsychological phenomena such as sensory gating disturbances. Given the strong evidence for the genetic basis of schizophrenia (which we explore in the next subsection), it is worthwhile to examine other stable trait markers to see how they might inform about the origins of the illness.

First, researchers have consistently found the presence of mild neurological dysfunction in people with schizophrenia. The abnormalities include problems with sensory representation such as astereognosis, agraphesthesia, and right/left confusion. Motor coordination is also impaired in schizophrenia, with patients showing abnormalities in gait, repetitive motions, and tests of fine motor control and synchrony. People with schizophrenia also have subtle problems in carrying out complex sequential motor activities. These collected abnormalities have been called neurological *soft signs,* a term that probably stems from an erroneous belief that the abnormalities are "ambiguous, unreal, fleeting, nonreproducible, nonlocalizable, and uninterpretable" (Heinrichs and Buchanan 1988, p. 11). In reality, this characterization does not apply. These findings are consistently present in people with schizophrenia, and they are present regardless of the current burden of positive symptoms; they are reliably state-independent. The signs are present at the onset of psychosis. They are also present, to an intermediate degree, in healthy relatives of people with schizophrenia (Chan and Gottesman 2008). They are independent of the effects of antipsychotic treatment. Thus, far from being elusive and transitory, these signs are stable and well-recognized clinical features of the disease.

Several rating scales are available for quantifying the degree and specific types of neurological deficits that are present. This allows researchers to compare patients, to look for heterogeneity within the findings, and to explore structural, functional, and genetic correlations. For example, sensory integration and motor coordination abnormalities have been linked respectively to differences in cortical and subcortical gray matter changes. The degree of soft signs as a whole has been correlated with frontotemporal volume reductions. A research effort is ongoing to explore clinical and genetic correlations and to more fully integrate these findings with our understanding of the pathology of schizophrenia.

A constellation of minor physical anomalies is seen more frequently in patients with schizophrenia than in a healthy population (see Compton and Walker 2009 for a review; see Weinberg et al. 2007 for a meta-analysis). Minor physical anomalies are subtle differences in craniofacial and distal extremity morphology that are of no functional significance, and limited or no cosmetic importance, but are nevertheless informative developmental markers. The findings include differences in head circumference, skull length, eyebrows, ear position, ear shape, facial symmetry, and width of the mouth. Patients also have a more frequent incidence of low-set ears, small earlobes, hypertelorism, narrow V-shaped palate, and tongue furrows. Limb changes include the presence of palmar creases, abnormal nail morphometry, curved fifth fingers, partial fusion of middle toes, and an abnormally large gap between the first two toes. As a group, patients are also more likely than healthy control subjects to have a visible nail fold plexus (Curtis et al. 1999). Patients also tend to have changes in dermatoglyphics, the ridge-and-whorl patterns on their hands and feet.

The minor physical anomalies are fascinating because of what they might tell us about the pathology of schizophrenia and the timing in which it unfolds. The minor physical anomalies themselves take shape as the fetus develops in utero. Obviously, they are present long before any psychotic symptoms arise. They are also unaffected by any environmental, medical, or psychological stressors that might occur after birth. The craniofacial abnormalities are of particular interest because the structures of the face and head develop in synchrony with the underlying brain and nervous system. Insults striking at a critical time in embryogenesis are likely to affect both. Two possible etiologies are relevant to schizophrenia. First, minor physical anomalies may be a result of intrauterine events such as hypoxia, infection, or malnutrition. It is well known that prenatal stressors can cause physical anomalies; in the case of fetal alcohol syndrome, maternal alcohol consumption causes children to be born with intellectual disability, narrow eyes with large epicanthic folds, and a smooth upper lip. In twin pairs of differing birth weights, the smaller twin has a higher rate of minor physical anomalies (Compton and Walker 2009). The ultimate timing of the insults may vary, depending on the nature of the event and the system involved.

The second possible etiology is genetic. The velocardiofacial syndrome, described in detail in the next subsection, illustrates how genetic changes can lead to a combination of physical abnormalities and neuropsychiatric illness. No specific genetic locations have yet been implicated in minor physical anomalies and schizophrenia, but the field is young and explorations are ongoing. Still, much evidence exists for a genetic basis. For example, some studies report that minor physical anomalies are seen more frequently in healthy relatives of people with schizophrenia than in the general population. In particular, mouth and palate changes are increased in families in which schizophrenia is present. Not every study finds that minor physical anomalies are heritable, however, which is compatible both with the intrauterine explanation above and with the fact that some genetic transformations can arise in an individual de novo.

Genetic Factors

We have already seen evidence consistent with a genetic basis to schizophrenia: the schizophrenia phenotype includes physical abnormalities in addition to cognitive and sensory processing deficits, structural brain changes, and neuropsychological differences; trait markers of the illness are present in first-episode psychosis and thus are independent of the effects of medication or other treatment; and trait markers are seen to intermediate degrees in healthy relatives.

The disease also runs in families. Multiple studies agree that the heritability of schizophrenia is about 80%, with the concordance rate for monozygotic twins being about 40%. Concordance rates for dizygotic twins are between 5% and 15% (Cardno et al. 1999). In children who have been adopted away after birth, the risk of schizophrenia correlates to risk in the birth parents, not the adoptive parents. This shows that a vulnerability to schizophrenia is clearly heritable, although these statistics necessarily leave plenty of room for both spontaneous genetic events and environmental insults.

As compelling as the evidence is, unequivocal linkage to specific candidate genes is much harder to find. Many linkage studies have been done with the aim of determining which gene or genes might be at play. The emergent picture is that schizophrenia, with some rare exceptions, is more complicated than simple one-gene neuropsychiatric illnesses such as Huntington's disease or fragile X syndrome. In fact, multiple genes likely exert additive effects, with other genes conferring differing degrees of protection. Different individuals likely have various combinations of risk genes, with differing degrees of penetrance. Finally, variability is seen in the genetic literature, such that many linkage studies show conflicting results (Harrison and Weinberger 2005). This is certainly due in part to the difficulty in finding clear evidence linking a syndrome to genes that have only a small effect on the phenotype. Still, some genes do have a fair amount of evidence supporting their involvement, at least in some individuals.

The *COMT* gene, on band 22q11, codes for the protein catechol-*O*-methyltransferase. This is involved in methylating catecholamine neurotransmitters such as dopamine and rendering them inactive. Therefore, *COMT* plays a role in regulating neurotransmission. Deletion of one copy of *COMT* leads to velocardiofacial syndrome (also known as DiGeorge syndrome), which is associated with facial abnormalities such as cleft palate and hearing loss, cardiac abnormalities such as the tetralogy of Fallot, endocrine problems, intellectual disabilities, and a psychiatric syndrome reminiscent of schizophrenia. In fact, this is one of the rare instances in which a single genetic mutation can give rise to a schizophrenia-like illness. Although velocardiofacial syndrome increases one's risk of psychosis by 25 times, and up to 30% of people with the syndrome become psychotic, this deletion is present in only a small percentage of the total number of individuals with schizophrenia.

More commonly with *COMT*, a single nucleotide polymorphism (SNP) occurs in which valine is substituted for methionine at codon 158. This so-called Val158Met substitution produces a version of the COMT protein that alters the amount of dopamine in synapses and has been linked clinically to deficits in executive function and working memory. People with this SNP also show differences in neurophysiological markers such as the P300 evoked potential and antisaccades (Haraldsson et al. 2010). However, the role that the Val158Met polymorphism plays in schizophrenia is unclear, and evidence for linkage is conflicting. Most likely, Val158Met and other *COMT* polymorphisms contribute to the illness not as single causative agents but as members of a constellation of etiological risk factors (Harrison and Weinberger 2005).

Linkage analysis also has associated *NRG1*, a gene on chromosome 8 that codes for the protein neuregulin-1, with an increased risk for schizophrenia. Neuregulin-1 has many isoforms that are created through alternative splicing. These multiple gene products are involved in cell signaling, neuronal growth and migration, axon guidance, myelination, and synaptic plasticity. Mice bred to be missing one copy of *NRG1* have fewer functional NMDA receptors; they show schizophrenia-like behaviors and sensory gating deficits. Interestingly, these deficits can be reversed with clozapine (Stefansson et al. 2002). Many hundreds of SNPs in *NRG1* have been found, but no mutation of *NRG1* has been identified that confers unique risk for schizophrenia. It remains a compelling target and an area of very active research.

Another gene of interest is dystrobrevin binding protein 1 (*DTNBP1*), which codes for the protein dysbindin. This has been identified in several linkage and family studies and is associated with working memory deficits, episodic memory deficits, and lower IQ (Harrison and Weinberger 2005). Like *COMT*, it seems to be more closely linked to cognitive impairment in general than to schizophrenia per se. Similar to *NRG1*, no single genetic mutation in *DTNBP1* has yet been identified. Still, expression of dysbindin is decreased in schizophrenia. The mechanism by which changes in dysbindin might give rise to the clinical phenotype is unclear, but recent work has implicated dysbindin in the placement of dopamine receptors in cell membranes (Iizuka et al. 2007).

Famously, the gene *DISC1* codes for the protein disrupted in schizophrenia 1. A balanced translocation in *DISC1* was seen to segregate with schizophrenia, schizoaffective disorder, and bipolar disorder in a large Scottish family (Millar et al. 2000). The products of *DISC1* are complex and seem to be involved in both neural plasticity and the formation of cytoskeletal proteins. These gene products may help regulate the growth of dendritic spines (Hayashi-Takagi et al. 2010). Similar to *COMT,* the *DISC1* translocation may explain much of the risk for schizophrenia but only in a relatively small number of individuals. Furthermore, the risk that *DISC1* confers seems to be toward psychosis and major mental illness in general rather than being specific for schizophrenia.

Several studies have implicated regulator of G-protein signaling 4 (*RGS4*) in schizophrenia, but other studies have found no associations. Its protein is found throughout the brain and is involved in neuronal growth and signaling. This gene is under dopaminergic control, but it is otherwise unclear what the functional significance of the associations with schizophrenia might be. The gene *GRM3* codes for mGluR3, a metabotropic glutamate receptor that is involved in modulating both glutamatergic and dopaminergic signal transmission. Variants in mGluR3 have been associated with increased risk of schizophrenia (Ghose et al. 2008). *RGS4* and the other genes mentioned earlier regulate things such as cellular signaling and neural growth and plasticity; they have been in part linked to clinically relevant cognitive deficits. Although these genes confer risk, they probably do so in combination with several other genes, many of which have yet to be identified. In most cases, the degree of risk attributable to one mutation or SNP is likely to be small.

Copy number variations are another source of genetic differences between individuals. Copy number variations occur when regions of DNA are either duplicated or deleted from the genome and can be inherited or can arise de novo. The number of base pairs affected ranges from the low thousands to the millions, and the number of affected genes is quite variable, ranging from one to dozens. Increasingly, copy number variations are being associated with various forms of neuropsychiatric disease (Cook and Scherer 2008). Two regions are worth mentioning here. A deletion at 2p16.3 is most clearly associated with changes within a single gene, *NRXN1* (Duan et al. 2010); this gene codes for a synaptic neuronal adhesion molecule involved in synapse formation (Kirov et al. 2009). Similarly, duplication of a 600-kilobase region at 16p11.2 is associated with an increased risk of schizophrenia, whereas a deletion in the same area is associated with developmental delay and autism. The 16p11.2 copy number variation spans almost 30 genes, at least 9 of which are expressed in the brain and are plausibly involved in regulating processes associated with schizophrenia, such as synaptic plasticity and neurotransmission (Duan et al. 2010). So far, all copy number variations associated with schizophrenia are rare and collectively explain only about 2% of cases (Bassett et al. 2010). As more are discovered, they may come to explain significantly more instances of the illness.

Many genetic associations seem to confer more risk for cognitive disturbances in general than for schizophrenia in particular. Several genes, for example, including *COMT, DISC1,* and *NRG1,* are associated not just with schizophrenia but also with bipolar disorder and other major mental illnesses. *DTNBP1* appears to be associated with psychosis, whether with schizophrenia or with mania (Craddock et al. 2006).

The inability to locate a single, specific genetic defect responsible for schizophrenia has given rise to the concept of the "endophenotype" (Gottesman and Gould 2003). This idea suggests that it may not be possible to find a single gene for schizophrenia, but it may be possible to find genetic abnormalities that code for some of the cognitive or clinical features of the illness. As Gottesman and Gould describe it, an endophenotype is an intermediate step along the pathway from genes to a syndrome. As a phenotype becomes more complex and is seen as a product of multiple genetic contributions, it becomes less informative to label any particular gene as uniquely causative. Complex disorders like schizophrenia are considered polygenetic, and an endophenotype is a more simple (i.e., more basic) step along the pathway from genes toward illness. An endophenotype may be more traceable to a genetic anomaly than to the whole syndrome itself. For example, there may not be a "gene for schizophrenia," but there may be an identifiable collection of genes that correspond to working memory deficits subserved by circuitry linking the DLPFC to the mediodorsal nucleus of the thalamus. Working memory deficits thus become a candidate endophenotype of the illness.

Gottesman and Gould (2003) proposed helpful characteristics for endophenotypes in psychiatry research: they should be associated with the illness and state-independent; they should be heritable; they should segregate with the illness in families; and they should be found in unaffected family members at a higher rate than in the general population. Discovery of endophenotypes should point toward genetic protective and risk factors and should help increase our biological understanding of heterogeneity within the illness. Ideally, this will lead to treatments or preventive measures that are based on the specific functional deficits at play.

Environmental Factors

Although the genotype clearly plays a large role in the etiology of schizophrenia, several environmental factors also are strongly associated with increased risk for the illness. Evidence comes from multiple lines of study, including obstetrics, immunology, sociology, and the study of the effects of recreational drugs.

For many years, obstetric complications have been seen to increase one's risk for schizophrenia. Not every study has confirmed this, but most do; typically, investigators find that obstetric complications approximately double someone's chances for developing schizophrenia (Clarke et al. 2006). The obstetric complications with the highest risk of adverse fetal events, including preeclampsia, breech delivery, severe fetal distress, postnatal seizures, and life-threatening viral infections, may increase the risk of schizophrenia fivefold (Preti et al. 2000). Similarly, the incidence of obstetric complications is increased in people in their first episode of psychosis or who show a clinical syndrome suggestive of prodromal schizophrenia (Ballon et al. 2008).

The final common pathway for obstetric complications may be fetal hypoxia. Perinatal hypoxia could increase the risk for schizophrenia in at least two ways. First, it may preferentially damage certain areas of the brain, such as the hippocampus and frontotemporal regions, and this damage may then become clinically apparent as the underlying neural circuits mature in early adulthood. Second, several of the genes implicated in schizophrenia, including *NRG1, COMT, DTNBP1,* and *GRM3,* are more sensitive to hypoxia than are randomly selected genes (Fatemi and Folsom 2009), and thus their roles in regulating signal transduction, synaptogenesis, and plasticity may be impaired as a result of birth complications. In any event, up to 30% of infants experience some kind of obstetric complication, and the vast majority do not go on to develop schizophrenia; similarly, the vast majority of patients with schizophrenia have not had any birth trauma at all (Clarke et al. 2006). Therefore, although these events may increase risk, they are not likely to be causative in and of themselves, and they explain only a few cases.

Maternal infection also seems to increase one's risk for schizophrenia, with the influenza virus being the pathogen that has received the most attention. Initial efforts looked at the incidence of schizophrenia during periods of historic influenza epidemics; later studies asked mothers of schizophrenic patients to recall their history of infections during pregnancy. These investigations reported that prenatal influenza infection approximately doubled the odds of a child having schizophrenia, but the studies were subject to confounds and recall bias because maternal infection was not definitively confirmed. Much firmer support of these findings arrived from Brown et al. (2004), when maternal serum that had been prospectively frozen was later assayed for antibodies to influenza. This was long after their children had grown up to develop (or not develop) the illness. Maternal influenza infection in the first trimester, confirmed by serum assay and matched against control subjects, was found to increase the risk of schizophrenia by up to sevenfold, thus providing compelling evidence for a link.

Other infections also increase the risk. Prenatal rubella confers up to 20 times the risk. Maternal antibodies against toxoplasmosis predicted a 2.5 times increased risk of schizophrenia, as did polio, empyema, and various upper respiratory infections. Finally, retroviral infection also has been seen in both first-episode and chronic patients more than in healthy control subjects (Karlsson et al. 2001). Proposed mechanisms of action for these viruses include direct effects on the developing brain and through the release of inflammatory cytokines.

Some infections occur more frequently in winter months, and this has been put forward as an explanation for the curious fact that people born during the winter have an increased risk of developing schizophrenia. The effect is small, with a relative risk comparing winter birth with summer birth of about 1.2. Still, the effect was noticed as early as 1929 and has been seen consistently ever since (see Tochigi et al. 2004). The link between winter births and maternal infection is plausible but has not yet been definitively proven; other factors that might explain the increased incidence in winter births include lower ambient temperature, seasonal access to nutrition, seasonal environmental toxins, and maternal hormone balance. For now, the increased incidence in winter months remains unexplained.

The incidence of schizophrenia is also higher in urban areas, by about a factor of between 2 and 4. Worldwide, this has important public health implications because the percentage of people growing up in urban areas has been steadily increasing. As with birth in winter months, the mechanism may be through increased exposure to infections in the prenatal period. Increased pollution or the presence of industrial toxins may play a role. In any event, the effects of an urban environment persist after investigators controlled for socioeconomic status, the number of people in the household, and the number of older siblings. Interesting links are found between perceived social cohesion and schizophrenia: even when studies control for economic disparity, groups of people who report a tight and supportive sense of community have a lower risk of schizophrenia (and other mental illnesses as well). Large cities tend to disrupt social cohesion, and this may be one mechanism by which the risk for psychosis is enhanced (Kelly et al. 2010). Similarly, stress itself may increase the risk. In a recent review, Clarke et al. (2006) described studies showing that stressful events such as paternal death, family strife, prenatal experience of calamitous natural disaster or war, and unplanned pregnancy are all associated with about a twofold increase in the risk for schizophrenia.

Cannabis use is another suspected independent risk factor for the development of psychotic illness. Early observations linked marijuana use with the development of positive symptoms (hallucinations and delusions) in healthy people and with the worsening of symptoms in people with schizophrenia. Since then, some studies concluded independently that cannabis use increases the risk for schizophrenia by about threefold (Semple et al. 2005). This risk is even more pronounced in people who have an underlying genetic predisposition. For example, cannabis users with the Val158Met *COMT* mutation have a greatly increased risk for psychotic illness compared with nonusers (Müller-Vahl and Emrich 2008). There also seems to be a dose and age relation, with more frequent and younger use increasing the odds of developing psychotic symptoms. In addition, evidence suggests that marijuana use may worsen the course of schizophrenia, lead to more severe symptoms, and result in a greater number of hospitalizations over the course of a lifetime.

The biological basis for the psychoactive effects of cannabis has only recently been made clear. The main active ingredient in marijuana is tetrahydrocannabinol (THC), which binds cannabinoid receptors in the CNS. These receptors appear to be concentrated most densely in areas of the brain that are highly associated with the pathology of schizophrenia: the PFC, hippocampus, anterior cingulate cortex, and basal ganglia. Endogenous ligands bind these receptors to modulate appetite, muscle relaxation, pain perception, memory, learning, and synaptic plasticity. The CB_1 receptor is coded for by the *CNR1* gene, which has a copy number variation associated with schizophrenia. Evidence has emerged recently that schizophrenia might involve overactivity of the CB_1 receptor because stimulation with exogenous THC leads to symptoms of avolition, cognitive dysfunction, and blunted affect (Müller-Vahl and Emrich 2008). Additionally, the CB_1 receptor appears to modulate the dopamine system: after taking THC, human volunteers show decreased D_2 receptor binding in the striatum and increased plasma metabolites of dopamine. This has led to the speculation that cannabis use leads to increased dopaminergic activity. Interestingly, clozapine displaces ligands from the CB_1 receptor and has been shown to decrease cannabis use in people with schizophrenia and substance use disorders. By decreasing activity in the cannabinoid system, clozapine may promote enhanced stability in the dopamine system, and this could explain some of its increased relative efficacy compared with other antipsychotic agents. These findings have naturally led to speculation that pharmacological modification of the cannabinoid system may lead to novel therapies for schizophrenia. One candidate compound, cannabidiol, has been found in preliminary trials to have antipsychotic efficacy, with a side-effect profile similar to that of second-generation antipsychotics (Müller-Vahl and Emrich 2008).

To conclude, we must note that all of the environmental risk factors for schizophrenia that have been discovered so far are fairly common, and their individual contributions to the disorder are small. For example, the overwhelming majority of people who experience obstetric complications, maternal exposure to perinatal infections, urban living, and exposure to cannabis do not develop schizophrenia; likewise, many patients with schizophrenia have not had exposure to any of these risk factors. Rather than saying that cannabis, hypoxia, or any of the other environmental factors are causative, it is much more accurate to simply state that stressors in an individual's life interact in multiple and complex ways with an inherited predisposition to mold the final shape and severity of the illness.

Disconnection or Dysconnection?

It is clear that the phenomena that predispose an individual to schizophrenia occur early in life. With the exception of cannabis use, the meaningful risk events take place before birth (in the form of genetic liability) or in the fetal and perinatal periods. The timing of these events and the evidence of cytological differences and incomplete neuronal migration implicate a faulty neurodevelopmental process. Schizophrenia, it seems, is a disease not solely of disconnection—in which properly functioning neuronal connections are which some neuronal networks are assembled in a way that is ultimately unable to sustain proper cognition. How does this happen?

Schizophrenia is a neurodevelopmental disorder. A person is born with a certain amount of genetic liability for the illness in the form of SNPs, copy number variations, large deletions, or other genetic anomalies, either inherited or acquired de novo. On top of this genetic risk, the individual receives input from environmental moderators such as those discussed in the previous subsection. This combination of genetic liability and environmental interaction influences the ultimate expression of the illness.

Most of the environmental risk factors for schizophrenia exert their influence during embryonic neurogenesis. Signs that this disrupts normal neurodevelopment include the evidence that many neurons are arrested in white matter on their journey from the periventricular zones to the cortex. As opposed to a degenerative event in which neurons are destroyed, it seems that these particular neurons never quite reached their intended destinations. Migration occurs during the second trimester of pregnancy, the time in which prenatal insults are suspected to work their damage. The result is thought to be a functional misconnection between the cerebral cortex and deeper regions of the brain, which would lead to disrupted neurotransmission and impaired cognition.

Although frank psychosis does not develop until late adolescence or early adulthood, subclinical changes are seen earlier and often proceed in a recognized pattern. Cognitive deficits, especially attention issues, have been seen in children who go on to develop schizophrenia. These are present by at least age 9 and precede other symptoms by years. Depression, the most frequently reported prodromal symptom, often precedes psychosis by 5 years or more. Social isolation and functional disability appear as the prodrome progresses, also preceding psychosis by 2–4 years. Gray matter loss, beginning in frontal regions, takes place before psychotic symptoms emerge and progresses in synchrony with emerging impairments in executive functioning and sensory processing (Thompson et al. 2001). The signs of prodromal psychosis are nonspecific and therefore very difficult to interpret prospectively. Still, on a population basis, we see that schizophrenia is associated with a rolling progression of changes that begin in utero and develop through adolescence. The syndrome reaches its maximal expression in early adulthood as the final stages of neurodevelopment take place. Schizophrenia, tragically, seems to mature along with the developing brain.

This developmental narrative explains why psychotic symptoms do not show up until in early adulthood. Neural circuits may become insufficient for normal cognition only when brain maturation is complete. For example, circuits involving the DLPFC reach their functional maturity in adulthood: children perform poorly on neuropsychiatric tests for adult prefrontal functions, such as executive functioning and working memory (Weinberger 1987). The implication for schizophrenia is that the immature neural circuitry is appropriate for the cognitive demands of childhood, but at the time the brain should be developing into its most specialized functions, it actually matures beyond its capabilities. This is when the hallmarks of dysconnection become clinically evident: cognition breaks down, and the person's functional appreciation and integration of reality become impaired. Interesting evidence comes from psychopharmacology, in that the effects of ketamine in children are different from those in adults. Children are much less prone to psychotic experiences when taking ketamine than mature adults are (Müller 2008). Furthermore, NMDA receptor hypofunction is not nearly as neurotoxic in young animals as it is in adults (Olney and Farber 1995). Thus, the final steps in neurocognitive maturation may show preexisting cognitive incapacities that had been silent up until this point.

The clinical hallmarks appear to be problems with organized communication in the brain. This is supported by many of the lines of evidence described thus far. For example, many of the genes implicated in schizophrenia are related to signal transmission, neuronal migration, and synaptic plasticity. Evidence from both anatomical studies and neuroimaging points toward diffuse problems in schizophrenia instead of to one "broken" region of the brain. Interestingly, parallel changes are seen throughout interconnected regions, suggesting that problems might be distributed across functional networks. This has been called the "dysconnection hypothesis" (Friston and Frith 1995): the idea that the fundamental pathology in schizophrenia is faulty communication between brain regions. The neurons are there, but the functional connections between them are incorrect, and this leads to ineffective interregional communication. This would include impaired signal transmission between regions of cortex, affecting both cognition and processing of stimuli, and would lead to problems with salience, context, sensory integration, and memory. It also includes impaired signaling in corticothalamic networks. The thalamus, like the cortex, is rich in GABAergic interneurons. It receives all signals passing from sensory organs to the cortex, as well as signals passing from one region of the cortex to another. Thus, it is in an ideal position to coordinate the smooth flow of information, and so dysconnection of thalamocortical circuits may prevent orderly cognition. This could be experienced as poor mental coordination, what Andreasen (1997) described as "cognitive dysmetria." Clinical deficits would then be apparent in any cognitive function that relies on smooth interregional flow of information.

Conclusion

Schizophrenia is a developmental condition that proceeds from a background of increased genetic risk, through the cumulative effects of environmental stressors, into an adult syndrome of dysfunction and psychosis. The final common pathway of both early risk and later effects is the mechanism of neural connectivity and plasticity. The next generation of research is taking place in these areas because many unanswered questions remain. For example, the full clinical presentation of schizophrenia, particularly with regard to the multiplicity of positive symptoms, has yet to be satisfactorily explained. The relative contributions of genetic and environmental risk factors to the heterogeneity of the illness are not well understood.

Future directions for therapy include interventions that normalize neuronal signaling, including drugs that affect the NMDA/glutamate system and reduce glutamate-mediated excitotoxicity. Clinical trials are also in progress for medications that may improve some of the cognitive deficits in schizophrenia. Promising targets include alpha-7 nicotinic acetylcholine receptors, 5-HT$_6$ serotonin receptors, and H$_3$ histaminic receptors, all of which have reached Phase II (Wallace et al. 2011). Cognitive remediation exercises show promise in restoring functionality. Prevention may be much more difficult because in some cases, if not most, the seeds of adult pathology are planted before birth. Still, neuroprotective interventions may someday reduce the ultimate disease burden. Much investigation is indeed taking place around the schizophrenia prodrome, in the hopes of improving both early identification and early treatment. The specificity of much of this evidence needs further investigation; for example, many of the biological changes seen in schizophrenia are similar to changes found in other neurocognitive disorders. Researchers are also looking for biological heterogeneity in schizophrenia: the variety of clinical presentations suggests that several distinct or overlapping processes may be at work, each perhaps with its own separate risk factors and prognosis. In any case, the field is moving incrementally forward toward a time when major mental illnesses are redefined on the basis of biology and etiological risk factors rather than clinical presentation. The next generation of research promises to be exciting and enlightening.

References

Abi-Dargham A, Moore H: Prefrontal DA transmission at D1 receptors and the pathology of schizophrenia. Neuroscientist 9:404–416, 2003

Adler LE, Olincy A, Waldo M, et al: Schizophrenia, sensory gating, and nicotinic receptors. Schizophr Bull 24:189–202, 1998

Akbarian S, Bunney WE, Potkin SG, et al: Altered distribution of nicotinamide–adenine dinucleotide phosphate–diaphorase cells in frontal lobe of schizophrenics implies disturbances of cortical development. Arch Gen Psychiatry 50:169–177, 1993

Alho K, Sainio K, Sajaniemi N, et al: Event-related brain potential of human newborns to pitch change of an acoustic stimulus. Electroencephalogr Clin Neurophysiol 77:151–155, 1990

American Psychiatric Association: Diagnostic and Statistical Manual of Mental Disorders, 3rd Edition. Washington, DC, American Psychiatric Association, 1980

Andreasen NC: The role of the thalamus in schizophrenia.Can J Psychiatry 42:27–33, 1997

Andreasen NC, Olsen S: Negative v positive schizophrenia. Definition and validation. Arch Gen Psychiatry 39:789–794, 1982

Andreasen NC, O'Leary DS, Flaum M, et al: Hypofrontality in schizophrenia: distributed dysfunctional circuits in neuroleptic-naïve patients. Lancet 349:1730–1734, 1997

Ballon JS, Dean KA, Cadenhead KS: Obstetrical complications in people at risk for developing schizophrenia. Schizophr Res 98:307–311, 2008

Barger G, Dale HH: Chemical structure and sympathomimetic action of amines J Physiol 41:19–59, 1910

Bassett AS, Scherer SW, Brzustowicz LM: Copy number variations in schizophrenia: critical review and new perspectives on concepts of genetics and disease. Am J Psychiatry 167:899–914, 2010

Baumeister AA, Francis JL: Historical development of the dopamine hypothesis of schizophrenia. J Hist Neurosci 11:265–277, 2002

Belforte JE, Zsiros V, Sklar ER, et al: Postnatal NMDA receptor ablation in corticolimbic interneurons confers schizophrenia-like phenotypes. Nat Neurosci 13:76–83, 2010

Bhatt DH, Zhang S, Gan W-B: Dendritic spine dynamics. Annu Rev Physiol 71261–71282, 2009

Bogerts B, Meertz E, Schönfeldt-Bausch R: Basal ganglia and limbic system pathology in schizophrenia. A morphometric study of brain volume and shrinkage. Arch Gen Psychiatry 42:784–791, 1985

Brockhaus-Dumke A, Schultze-Lutter F, Mueller R, et al: Sensory gating in schizophrenia: P50 and N100 gating in antipsychotic-free subjects at risk, first-episode, and chronic patients. Biol Psychiatry 64:376–384, 2008

Brown AS, Begg MD, Gravenstein S, et al: Serologic evidence of prenatal influenza in the etiology of schizophrenia. Arch Gen Psychiatry 61:774–780, 2004

Buchanan RW, Vladar K, Barta PE, et al: Structural evaluation of the prefrontal cortex in schizophrenia. Am J Psychiatry 155:1049–1055, 1998

Bunney WE, Bunney BG: Evidence for a compromised dorsolateral prefrontal cortical parallel circuit in schizophrenia. Brain Res Brain Res Rev 31:138–146, 2000

Cardno AG, Marshall EJ, Coid B, et al: Heritability estimates for psychotic disorders: the Maudsley twin psychosis series. Arch Gen Psychiatry 56:162–168, 1999

Carlsson A: The occurrence, distribution and physiological role of catecholamines in the nervous system. Pharmacol Rev 11:490–493, 1959

Carlsson A: Antipsychotic drugs, neurotransmitters, and schizophrenia. Am J Psychiatry 135:165–173, 1978

Chan RC, Gottesman II: Neurological soft signs as candidate endophenotypes for schizophrenia: a shooting star or a Northern star? Neurosci Biobehav Rev 32:957–971, 2008

Clarke MC, Harley M, Cannon M: The role of obstetric events in schizophrenia. Schizophr Bull 32:3–8, 2006

Compton MT, Walker EF: Physical manifestations of neurodevelopmental disruption: are minor physical anomalies part of the syndrome of schizophrenia? Schizophr Bull 35:425–436, 2009

Cook EH, Scherer SW: Copy-number variations associated with neuropsychiatric conditions. Nature 455:919–923, 2008

Craddock N, O'Donovan MC, Owen MJ: Genes for schizophrenia and bipolar disorder? Implications for psychiatric nosology. Schizophr Bull 32:9–16, 2006

Csernansky JG, Schindler MK, Splinter NR, et al: Abnormalities of thalamic volume and shape in schizophrenia. Am J Psychiatry 161:896–902, 2004

Curtis CE, Iacono WG, Beiser M: Relationship between nailfold plexus visibility and clinical, neuropsychological, and brain structural measures in schizophrenia. Biol Psychiatry 46:102–109, 1999

David HN, Ansseau M, Abraini JH: Dopamine-glutamate reciprocal modulation of release and motor responses in the rat caudate-putamen and nucleus accumbens of "intact" animals. Brain Res Brain Res Rev 50:336–360, 2005

Davis KL, Kahn RS, Ko G, et al: Dopamine in schizophrenia: a review and reconceptualization. Am J Psychiatry 148:1474–1486, 1991

Duan J, Sanders AR, Gejman PV: Genome-wide approaches to schizophrenia. Brain Res Bull 30:93–102, 2010

Eastwood SL, Harrison PJ: Interstitial white matter neurons express less reelin and are abnormally distributed in schizophrenia: towards an integration of molecular and morphologic aspects of the neurodevelopmental hypothesis. Mol Psychiatry 8:769, 821–831, 2003

Ehrlichman RS, Luminais SN, White SL, et al: Neuregulin 1 transgenic mice display reduced mismatch negativity, contextual fear conditioning and social interactions. Brain Res 1294:116–127, 2009

Elston GN: Cortex, cognition and the cell: new insights into the pyramidal neuron and prefrontal function. Cereb Cortex 13:1124–1138, 2003

Falkai P, Schneider-Axmann T, Honer WG: Entorhinal cortex pre-alpha cell clusters in schizophrenia: quantitative evidence of a developmental abnormality. Biol Psychiatry 47:937–943, 2000

Farde L, Wiesel FA, Stone-Elander S, et al: D2 dopamine receptors in neuroleptic-naive schizophrenic patients: a positron emission tomography study with [11C]raclopride. Arch Gen Psychiatry 47:213–219, 1990

Farde L, Nordström AL, Wiesel FA, et al: Positron emission tomographic analysis of central D1 and D2 dopamine receptor occupancy in patients treated with classical neuroleptics and clozapine. Relation to extrapyramidal side effects. Arch Gen Psychiatry 49:538–544, 1992

Fatemi SH, Folsom TD: The neurodevelopmental hypothesis of schizophrenia, revisited. Schizophr Bull 35:528–548, 2009

Freedman R, Adler LE, Myles-Worsley M, et al: Inhibitory gating of an evoked response to repeated auditory stimuli in schizophrenic and normal subjects: human recordings, computer simulation, and an animal model. Arch Gen Psychiatry 53:1114–1121, 1996

Friston KJ, Frith CD: Schizophrenia: a disconnection syndrome? Clin Neurosci 3:89–97, 1995

Garey L: When cortical development goes wrong: schizophrenia as a neurodevelopmental disease of microcircuits. J Anat 217:324–333, 2010

Ghose S, Crook JM, Bartus CL, et al: Metabotropic glutamate receptor 2 and 3 gene expression in the human prefrontal cortex and mesencephalon in schizophrenia. Int J Neurosci 118:1609–1627, 2008

Goff DC, Wine L: Glutamate in schizophrenia: clinical and research implications. Schizophr Res 27:157–168, 1997

Goto Y, Yang CR, Otani S: Functional and dysfunctional synaptic plasticity in prefrontal cortex: roles in psychiatric disorders. Biol Psychiatry 67:199–207, 2010

Gottesman II, Gould TD: The endophenotype concept in psychiatry: etymology and strategic intentions. Am J Psychiatry 160:636–645, 2003

Halene TB, Ehrlichman RS, Liang Y, et al: Assessment of NMDA receptor NR1 subunit hypofunction in mice as a model for schizophrenia. Genes Brain Behav 8:661–675, 2009

Haraldsson HM, Ettinger U, Magnusdottir BB, et al: Catechol-O-methyltransferase Val 158 Met polymorphism and antisaccade eye movements in schizophrenia. Schizophr Bull 36:157–164, 2010

Harrison PJ, Weinberger DR: Schizophrenia genes, gene expression, and neuropathology: on the matter of their convergence. Mol Psychiatry 10:40–68, 2005

Hayashi-Takagi A, Takaki M, Graziane N, et al: Disrupted-in-Schizophrenia 1 (DISC1) regulates spines of the glutamate synapse via Rac1. Nat Neurosci 13:327–332, 2010

Healy D: The Creation of Psychopharmacology. Cambridge, MA, Harvard University Press, 2004

Heckers S: Neuropathology of schizophrenia: cortex, thalamus, basal ganglia, and neurotransmitter-specific projection systems. Schizophr Bull 23:403–421, 1997

Heinrichs DW, Buchanan RW: Significance and meaning of neurological signs in schizophrenia. Am J Psychiatry 145:11–18, 1988

Hickok G: The functional neuroanatomy of language. Phys Life Rev 6:121–143, 2009

Howes OD, Kapur S: The dopamine hypothesis of schizophrenia: version III—the final common pathway. Schizophr Bull 35:549–562, 2009

Iizuka Y, Sei Y, Weinberger DR, et al: Evidence that the BLOC-1 protein dysbindin modulates dopamine D2 receptor internalization and signaling but not D1 internalization. J Neurosci 27:12390–12395, 2007

Jacobi W, Winkler H: Encephalographische studien au chronisch schizophrenen, Arch Psychiatrie Nervenkr 81:299–332, 1927

Jacyna LS: Somatic theories of mind and the interests of medicine in Britain, 1850–1879. Med Hist 26:233–258, 1982

Johnstone EC, Crow TJ, Frith CD, et al: Cerebral ventricular size and cognitive impairment in chronic schizophrenia. Lancet 2(7992):924–926, 1976

Karlsson H, Bachmann S, Schröder J, et al: Retroviral RNA identified in the cerebrospinal fluids and brains of individuals with schizophrenia. Proc Natl Acad Sci U S A 98:4634–4639, 2001

Kelly BD, O'Callaghan E, Waddington JL, et al: Schizophrenia and the city: a review of literature and prospective study of psychosis and urbanicity in Ireland. Schizophr Res 116:75–89, 2010

Kerns JG, Nuechterlein KH, Braver TS, et al: Executive functioning component mechanisms and schizophrenia. Biol Psychiatry 64:26–33, 2008

Keshavan MS, Tandon R, Boutros NN, et al: Schizophrenia, "just the facts": what we know in 2008 part 3: neurobiology. Schizophr Res 106:89–107, 2008

Kinon BJ, Zhang L, Millen BA, et al: A multicenter, inpatient, phase 2, double-blind, placebo-controlled dose-ranging study of LY2140023 monohydrate in patients with DSM-IV schizophrenia. J Clin Psychopharmacol 31:349–355, 2011

Kirov G, Rujescu D, Ingason A, et al: Neurexin 1 (NRXN1) deletions in schizophrenia. Schizophr Bull 35:851–854, 2009

Konick LC, Friedman L: Meta-analysis of thalamic size in schizophrenia. Biol Psychiatry 49:28–38, 2001

Kovalenko S, Bergmann A, Schneider-Axmann T, et al: Regio entorhinalis in schizophrenia: more evidence for migrational disturbances and suggestions for a new biological hypothesis. Pharmacopsychiatry 36 (suppl 3):S158–S161, 2003

Kubicki M, McCarley RW, Shenton ME: Evidence for white matter abnormalities in schizophrenia. Curr Opin Psychiatry 18:121–134, 2005

Kubicki M, McCarley R, Westin C-F, et al: A review of diffusion tensor imaging studies in schizophrenia. J Psychiatr Res 41:15–30, 2007

Kurtz MM, Wexler BE, Fujimoto M, et al: Symptoms versus neurocognition as predictors of change in life skills in schizophrenia after outpatient rehabilitation. Schizophr Res 102:303–311, 2008

Laruelle M, Abi-Dargham A, van Dyck CH, et al: Single photon emission computerized tomography imaging of amphetamine-induced dopamine release in drug-free schizophrenic subjects. Proc Natl Acad Sci U S A 93:9235–9240, 1996

Lawrie S, Johnstone E, Weinberger D (eds): Schizophrenia: From Neuroimaging to Neuroscience. New York, Oxford University Press, 2004

Levy DL, Holzman PS, Matthysse S, et al: Eye tracking and schizophrenia: a selective review. Schizophr Bull 20:47–62, 1994

Lewis DA: GABAergic local circuit neurons and prefrontal cortical dysfunction in schizophrenia. Brain Res Brain Res Rev 31:270–276, 2000

Lewis DA, Lieberman JA: Catching up on schizophrenia: natural history and neurobiology. Neuron 28:325–334, 2000

Li F, Tsien JZ: Memory and the NMDA receptors. N Engl J Med 361:302–303, 2009

Lieberman JA, Kane JM, Alvir J: Provocative tests with psychostimulant drugs in schizophrenia. Psychopharmacology (Berl) 91:415–433, 1987

Mezler M, Geneste H, Gault L, et al: LY-2140023, a prodrug of the group II metabotropic glutamate receptor agonist LY-404039 for the potential treatment of schizophrenia. Curr Opin Investig Drugs 11:833–845, 2010

Milev P, Ho B-C, Arndt S, et al: Predictive values of neurocognition and negative symptoms on functional outcome in schizophrenia: a longitudinal first-episode study with 7-year follow-up. Am J Psychiatry 162:495–506, 2005

Millar JK, Wilson-Annan JC, Anderson S, et al: Disruption of two novel genes by a translocation co-segregating with schizophrenia. Hum Mol Genet 9:1415–1423, 2000

Morris BR: A theory as to the proximate cause of insanity. Prov Med Surg J 7:303–306, 1844

Müller N: Inflammation and the glutamate system in schizophrenia: implications for therapeutic targets and drug development. Expert Opin Ther Targets 12:1497–1507, 2008

Müller-Vahl KR, Emrich HM: Cannabis and schizophrenia: towards a cannabinoid hypothesis of schizophrenia. Expert Rev Neurother 8:1037–1048, 2008

Munch JC: Phencyclidine: pharmacology and toxicology. Bull Narc 26:9–17, 1974

Nieman D, Becker H, van de Fliert R, et al: Antisaccade task performance in patients at ultra high risk for developing psychosis. Schizophr Res 95:54–60, 2007

O'Driscoll GA, Callahan BL: Smooth pursuit in schizophrenia: a meta-analytic review of research since 1993. Brain Cogn 68:359–370, 2008

Olney JW, Farber NB: Glutamate receptor dysfunction and schizophrenia. Arch Gen Psychiatry 52:998–1007, 1995

Pakkenberg B: Post-mortem study of chronic schizophrenic brains. Br J Psychiatry 151:744–725, 1987

Pakkenberg B: Pronounced reduction of total neuron number in mediodorsal thalamic nucleus and nucleus accumbens in schizophrenics. Arch Gen Psychiatry 47:1023–1028, 1990

Pakkenberg B: Total nerve cell number in neocortex in chronic schizophrenics and controls estimated using optical dissectors. Biol Psychiatry 34:768–772, 1993

Palha AP, Esteves MF: The origin of dementia praecox. Schizophr Res 28:99–103, 1997

Peper JS, Brouwer RM, Boomsma DI, et al: Genetic influences on human brain structure: a review of brain imaging studies in twins. Hum Brain Mapp 28:464–473, 2007

Pierri JN, Chaudry AS, Woo TU, et al: Alterations in chandelier neuron axon terminals in the prefrontal cortex of schizophrenic subjects. Am J Psychiatry 156:1709–1719, 1999

Preti A, Cardascia L, Zen T, et al: Risk for obstetric complications and schizophrenia. Psychiatry Res 96:127–139, 2000

Rajkowska G, Selemon LD, Goldman-Rakic PS: Neuronal and glial somal size in the prefrontal cortex: a postmortem morphometric study of schizophrenia and Huntington disease. Arch Gen Psychiatry 55:215–224, 1998

Reichova I, Sherman SM: Somatosensory corticothalamic projections: distinguishing drivers from modulators. J Neurophysiol 92:2185–2197, 2004

Rorick-Kehn LM, Johnson BG, Knitowski KM, et al: In vivo pharmacological characterization of the structurally novel, potent, selective mGlu2/3 receptor agonist LY404039 in animal models of psychiatric disorders. Psychopharmacology (Berl) 193:121–136, 2007

Schmahmann JD: Vascular syndromes of the thalamus. Stroke 34:2264–2278, 2003

Schultz CC, Koch K, Wagner G, et al: Complex pattern of cortical thinning in schizophrenia: results from an automated surface based analysis of cortical thickness. Psychiatry Res 182:134–140, 2010

Seeman P, Lee T: Antipsychotic drugs: direct correlation between clinical potency and presynaptic action on dopamine neurons. Science 188:1217–1219, 1975

Seidman LJ: Schizophrenia and brain dysfunction: an integration of recent neurodiagnostic findings. Psychol Bull 94:195–238, 1983

Selemon LD, Rajkowska G, Goldman-Rakic PS: Abnormally high neuronal density in the schizophrenic cortex: a morphometric analysis of prefrontal area 9 and occipital area 17. Arch Gen Psychiatry 52:805–820, 1995

Semple DM, McIntosh AM, Lawrie SM: Cannabis as a risk factor for psychosis: systematic review. J Psychopharmacol 19:187–194, 2005

Shelley AM, Ward PB, Catts SV, et al: Mismatch negativity: an index of a preattentive processing deficit in schizophrenia. Biol Psychiatry 30:1059–1062, 1991

Shenton ME, Dickey CC, Frumin M, et al: A review of MRI findings in schizophrenia. Schizophr Res 49:1–52, 2001

Sherman SM, Guillery RW: On the actions that one nerve cell can have on another: distinguishing "drivers" from "modulators." Proc Natl Acad Sci U S A 95:7121–7126, 1998

Siegel BV, Buchsbaum MS, Bunney WE, et al: Cortical-striatal-thalamic circuits and brain glucose metabolic activity in 70 unmedicated male schizophrenic patients. Am J Psychiatry 150:1325–1336, 1993

Sim K, Cullen T, Ongur D, et al: Testing models of thalamic dysfunction in schizophrenia using neuroimaging. J Neural Transm 113:907–928, 2006

Smith RC, Calderon M, Ravichandran GK, et al: Nuclear magnetic resonance in schizophrenia: a preliminary study. Psychiatry Res 12:137–147, 1984

Stefansson H, Sigurdsson E, Steinthorsdottir V, et al: Neuregulin 1 and susceptibility to schizophrenia. Am J Hum Genet 71:877–892, 2002

Stone JM, Morrison PD, Pilowsky LS: Glutamate and dopamine dysregulation in schizophrenia—a synthesis and selective review. J Psychopharmacol 21:440–452, 2007

Sullivan EV, Lim KO, Mathalon D, et al: A profile of cortical gray matter volume deficits characteristic of schizophrenia. Cereb Cortex 8:117–124, 1998

Swerdlow NR, Weber M, Qu Y, et al: Realistic expectations of prepulse inhibition in translational models for schizophrenia research. Psychopharmacology (Berl) 199:331–388, 2008

Taylor SF: Cerebral blood flow activation and functional lesions in schizophrenia. Schizophr Res 19:129–140, 1996

Thompson PM, Vidal C, Giedd JN, et al: Mapping adolescent brain change reveals dynamic wave of accelerated gray matter loss in very early onset schizophrenia. Proc Natl Acad Sci U S A 98:11650–11655, 2001

Tochigi M, Okazaki Y, Kato N, et al: What causes seasonality of birth in schizophrenia? Neurosci Res 48:1–11, 2004

Turetsky BI, Calkins ME, Light GA, et al: Neurophysiological endophenotypes of schizophrenia: the viability of selected candidate measures. Schizophr Bull 33:69–94, 2007

Umbricht D, Koller R, Schmid L, et al: How specific are deficits in mismatch negativity generation to schizophrenia? Biol Psychiatry 53:1120–1131, 2003

van Rossum JM: The significance of dopamine-receptor blockade for the mechanism of action of neuroleptic drugs. Arch Int Pharmacodyn Ther 160:492–494, 1966

Wallace TL, Ballard TM, Pouzet B, et al: Drug targets for cognitive enhancement in neuropsychiatric disorders. Pharmacol Biochem Behav 99:130–145, 2011

Weinberg SM, Jenkins EA, Marazita ML, et al: Minor physical anomalies in schizophrenia: a meta-analysis. Schizophr Res 89:72–85, 2007

Weinberger DR: Implications of normal brain development for the pathogenesis of schizophrenia. Arch Gen Psychiatry 44:660–669, 1987

Weinberger DR: From neuropathology to neurodevelopment. Lancet 346:552–557, 1995

Wise RA: Neurobiology of addiction. Curr Opin Neurobiol 6:243–251, 1996

Zanelli J, MacCabe J, Toulopoulou T, et al: Neuropsychological correlates of eye movement abnormalities in schizophrenic patients and their unaffected relatives. Psychiatry Res 168:193–197, 2009

3

Prodromal Phase and First-Episode Schizophrenia

Barnaby Nelson, Ph.D.

Eóin Killackey, D.Psych.

Alison R. Yung, M.D.

Mario Álvarez-Jiménez, Ph.D.

Patrick D. McGorry, M.D., Ph.D.

Since the early 1990s, a stepwise body of evidence has emerged indicating that early diagnosis and expert early care have essentially the same fundamental value in psychotic disorders as in other branches of medicine. Although questions remain as to the optimal duration and mode of delivery of early

We acknowledge the assistance of Dr. Sherilyn Goldstone in preparing this manuscript.

intervention, the best available evidence strongly supports it as a "best buy" among competing investment options in the mental health field (Mihalopoulos et al. 2009). Along the way, international clinical practice guidelines and a consensus statement have been published (Bertolote and McGorry 2005; International Early Psychosis Association Writing Group 2005), and clinical practice guidelines for the treatment of schizophrenia now typically have a major section on early psychosis (American Psychiatric Association 1997).

Crucially, it has been recognized that people who develop schizophrenia and related psychoses usually manifest a need for clinical care long before the more diagnostically salient positive psychotic symptoms fully emerge and persist. This need for clinical care comprises subjective distress, typically reaching the threshold for other diagnostic syndromes such as depression and anxiety and resulting in psychosocial impairment during the developmentally sensitive period of emerging adulthood. The operational definition of a *clinical phenotype*, which connotes a risk of early transition to psychotic disorder of between 200 and 400 times higher than in the general population, has spurred the field of psychiatry to focus strongly on research and clinical care in young people with potentially serious mental disorders of this kind. Although several issues remain unresolved, much progress has been made over a relatively short time on matters related to definition, stigma reduction, and treatment options.

Once positive psychotic symptoms have crossed a threshold of severity and persistence, typically with other comorbid syndromes, we remain in early intervention territory, with clear objectives in view. These objectives include reduction of the duration of untreated (and unresponsive) psychosis to a minimum—because this is a key risk factor for poor outcome (Marshall et al. 2005; Perkins et al. 2005)—and consistent multimodal and evidence-based care of the early "critical period" of illness postdiagnosis. This critical period is defined as between 2 and 5 years after diagnosis, with recent data indicating that 5 years is a better definition, because some of the gains of early intervention are eroded if premature discharge to standard mental health care occurs earlier than this (Bertelsen et al. 2008).

This chapter therefore is written from the point of view that effective pharmacological, psychological, and psychosocial treatments exist for psychosis in the ultra-high-risk (UHR) (possibly prodromal) or early stage after onset and that the early stage of illness is a key window of opportunity to apply those treatments to prevent or ameliorate symptoms and to preserve or restore function in a range of domains. In this chapter, we concentrate on practical suggestions and principles for clinicians working with this patient population.

From the outset, it is important to note that although the title of the chapter includes "first-episode *schizophrenia,*" the focus of discussion is on the prevention of frank or full-blown psychotic disorder rather than on schizophrenia as a discrete illness. The first psychotic episode is the target, which is regarded as a more proximal and therapeutically salient target than schizophrenia. Schizophrenia is a subtype of psychotic disorder to which some individuals progress after a first psychotic episode but is not an inevitable result of this first episode.

The Prodrome and Ultra-High Risk for Psychosis

Although there have been slightly different definitions of the prodrome, the UHR criteria as developed at the PACE Clinic, Melbourne, Australia, are the most widely accepted (see Table 3–1). The possibility of treating psychotic disorders during the prodromal phase is an alluring prospect for several reasons. The prodromal phase is characterized by a considerable array of psychiatric symptoms and disability, including self-harming and other health-damaging behaviors. A substantial amount of the disability that develops in psychotic disorders accumulates prior to the appearance of the full positive psychotic syndrome and may even create a ceiling for eventual recovery (Yung et al. 2004). In addition, studies have indicated that at some point in the transition from the prodromal phase to full-blown psychotic disorder, alterations in brain structure (and presumably function) occur (Pantelis et al. 2003). If the prodrome can be recognized prospectively and treatment provided at this stage, then any existing disability could be minimized, and recovery may be possible before symptoms and poor functioning become entrenched; additionally, the possibility of preventing, delaying, or ameliorating the onset of diagnosable psychotic disorder arises (see Table 3–2).

Typical clinical characteristics of UHR patients are listed in Table 3–3. The following is an example of a UHR patient seen at the PACE Clinic:

> Lucia, a 17-year-old student in her final year at high school, was referred to the PACE Clinic by her school welfare counselor, who had spoken with Lucia at the request of her teachers because they were concerned about changes in her be-

Table 3–1. Ultra-high-risk criteria for psychosis

1. Must be age 15–25 years.

2. Must have been referred to a specialized service for help.

3. Must meet the criteria for one or more of the following three groups:

Group 1: attenuated positive psychotic symptoms	• Presence of at least one of the following symptoms: ideas of reference, odd beliefs or magical thinking, perceptual disturbance, paranoid ideation, odd thinking and speech, odd behavior and appearance
	• Frequency of symptoms: at least several times a week
	• Recency of symptoms: present within the last year
	• Duration of symptoms: present for at least 1 week and no longer than 5 years
Group 2: brief, limited, intermittent psychotic symptoms	• Transient psychotic symptoms; presence of at least one of the following symptoms: ideas of reference, magical thinking, perceptual disturbance, paranoid ideation, odd thinking or speech
	• Duration of episode: less than 1 week
	• Frequency of symptoms: at least several times per week
	• Symptoms resolve spontaneously
	• Recency of symptoms: must have occurred within the last year
Group 3: trait and state risk factors	• Schizotypal personality disorder in the identified individual, or a first-degree relative with a psychotic disorder
	• Significant decline in mental state or functioning, maintained for at least 1 month and not longer than 5 years
	• Recency of symptoms: decline in functioning must have occurred within the past year

Table 3–2.   Advantages of prepsychotic intervention

- Onset of frank psychosis may be delayed, ameliorated, or prevented.

- Prodromal individuals may engage more quickly with treatment compared with patients who present late when psychotic symptoms are entrenched, social networks are more disrupted, and functioning is further deteriorated.

- Prodromal individuals may be more likely to accept treatment if full-blown psychosis does emerge compared with patients who have been unwell for longer before assistance is sought.

- A therapeutic relationship is already established with a treating team if frank psychosis develops.

- Effective treatment can be provided rapidly if the person does develop psychosis, possibly avoiding the need for hospitalization and minimizing the deleterious effect of extended untreated psychosis.

- Prepsychotic intervention offers the chance to research the onset phase of psychotic illness, which may provide insight into the core features of the psychopathology and psychobiology of psychosis.

Table 3–3.   Typical clinical characteristics of ultra-high-risk patients

- Attenuated psychotic symptoms, such as overvalued ideas, perceptual abnormalities, and mild thought disorder

- Lowered or unstable mood

- Social withdrawal

- Interpersonal difficulties, such as conflict with others or social cognition problems

- Self-harming behavior

- Substance misuse

- Functional difficulties, such as deterioration in school or work performance havior. They had noticed that she had become distant from most of her friends and had uncharacteristically become verbally abusive with one friend, accusing her of talking about her behind her back. The school welfare counselor consulted with Lucia's parents, who indicated that Lucia was spending more time in her bedroom alone recently. Lucia said that over the past 3 months, she had developed ideas that her family and friends were conspiring to harm her in some way. She said that she knew that this could not be true but was avoiding contact with others because this reduced the frequency of these thoughts. She indicated that on about four occasions in the past month, she had had experiences of hearing mumbling voices outside her head. On two occasions, these experiences occurred as she was trying to get to sleep, and on another occasion, the voices were clearer and were speaking negatively about her. Lucia expressed concern about these experiences and relief that she was able to speak about them with somebody. Lucia was assessed at the PACE Clinic. She said that she had experienced similar symptoms on and off for the past 18 months, usually coinciding with increased stressors in her life. Indeed, she spoke of feeling anxious about her forthcoming examinations and concerns that she would not achieve high enough marks to be accepted to the university degree she was interested in the following year. Lucia noted that her symptoms usually abated as the stressor passed.

Interventions in the Prepsychotic Phase

Case Management

Most of the treatments described in this section are generally provided in the context of case management settings. A full discussion of case management is beyond the scope of this chapter, but several discussions of the pros and cons of different case management models are available in the literature. Irrespective of the model used, the key goals of case management in both stages of illness are defined in Table 3–4.

Crisis Management

Crises may be experienced by both the UHR and the first-episode psychosis populations. The need for care irrespective of stage of illness takes precedence over the presence of a clear psychotic diagnosis. Risk issues therefore need to be taken into account. Assessing the risk of harm to self and others is an essential component of case management. Risk assessment tends to focus on the risk of physical harm to the patient (especially suicide) or to others, but other aspects of risk, such as neglect of any dependents and victimization by others,

Table 3–4. Goals of case management in the prepsychotic phase

- Providing ongoing monitoring of the patient's mental state and risk
- Ensuring that the patient and family or caregivers are appropriately informed about the nature of the patient's mental health issues and their treatment
- Reducing the trauma or anxiety associated with any necessary inpatient admissions
- Facilitating adequate treatment for comorbid disorders
- Assisting in reducing any adverse effect of the illness on the patient's psychosocial environment (e.g., relationships, accommodations, education, employment, financial security)
- Fostering the recovery of the patient, reintegration into society, and restoration of a normal developmental trajectory
- Providing support and appropriate referrals to family members
- Fostering adherence with specialist services

also need to be considered. Prompt and regular formal risk assessments are required, and the results should be communicated to other staff and caregivers involved in treatment and supervision. Emergency and after-hours services must be available, and young people must know how to access after-hours support should they need it.

Psychological Treatment for Ultra-High-Risk Patients: Cognitive-Behavioral Therapy

Cognitive-behavioral therapy (CBT) was originally developed for the treatment of depression, although an article on CBT principles being used to treat psychotic symptoms was published as early as 1952 (Beck 1952). More recent studies that have applied CBT to UHR populations have reported encouraging results. There have been three key studies of CBT in the prepsychotic group (McGorry et al. 2002; Morrison et al. 2004; Yung et al. 2011). All three found that CBT was effective in reducing the rate of transition to psychosis. Importantly, CBT also was found to be well accepted and tolerated by high-risk patients in all studies. These studies provided preliminary evidence that CBT, incorporated within a broader case management approach, is a treatment of proven safety and efficacy in the UHR population.

It has been argued that CBT may have some advantages over antipsychotic medication for indicated prevention of psychosis in high-risk patients. These advantages include the following:

- Being more acceptable, more tolerable, and less stigmatizing to patients
- Having no risk of exposing false-positive case patients to pharmacological side effects
- Providing effective treatment for false-positive case patients, who despite not going on to develop psychosis, generally suffer from other disorders, such as mood and anxiety disorders.

Cognitive-Behavioral Therapy and the Stress-Vulnerability Model

The stress-vulnerability model of psychosis informs the CBT treatment approach. This model incorporates biological, psychological, and social factors in understanding the development of psychotic disorders. A central assumption of the model is that environmental stressors (such as relationship issues, substance use, lifestyle factors) are key factors in precipitating illness onset in vulnerable individuals. The more vulnerable an individual, the less stress is required to trigger the onset of symptoms. Consideration of biological, social, and psychological stressors; protective factors; and underlying biological vulnerability can guide the development of individualized treatment plans. This model implies that the implementation of appropriate coping strategies may ameliorate the influence of vulnerability. Therefore, strengthening the individual's coping resources forms a core component of cognitive therapy for the UHR group.

Assessment and Engagement in Cognitive-Behavioral Therapy

The assessment and engagement phase of CBT is crucial. Patients may be confused or distressed by their symptoms, and early sessions provide an opportunity for the therapist to develop a formulation for the patient that can provide the patient with some understanding of the symptoms, as well as guide the course of therapy. This early phase of therapy also provides an opportunity for the therapist to emphasize the collaborative nature of the therapy and to judge the appropriate nature of the interventions and therapeutic relationship on the basis of the patient's developmental level and symptomatic presentation.

CBT for the UHR group adapts strategies developed for the acute and recovery phases of psychotic illnesses. Cognitive models approach the core symptoms of psychosis as deriving from basic disturbances in information processing, which result in perceptual abnormalities and interpretive errors. Cognitive biases, inaccurate appraisals, and core self-schema further contribute to unusual beliefs (Garety et al. 2001). CBT aims to assist people to develop an understanding of the cognitive processes (including biases and maladaptive appraisals) that influence their thoughts and emotions and to develop more realistic and positive views of themselves and events around them.

In general, CBT aims to assist patients to monitor negative automatic thoughts; recognize the connections between cognitions, affect, and behavior; challenge dysfunctional beliefs; and promote more reality-oriented interpretations. Cognitive techniques involve eliciting or "catching" negative automatic thoughts and then "testing" these thoughts. "Testing" techniques include listing evidence for and against, uncovering logical inconsistencies, and using behavioral experiments. For example, in the case of Lucia presented earlier, this might include asking Lucia to list evidence for and against her impression that her friends and family were conspiring to harm her, drawing attention to interactions with her family and friends that were inconsistent with her paranoid thoughts, and behaviorally testing out whether increased contact with others did in fact increase her paranoid thoughts.

It is important for the therapist to form a strong, collaborative, and respectful relationship with the patient. Although CBT includes elements of challenging and testing, it is based on an empathic, supportive attitude in the therapist. The therapist aims to facilitate an environment in which the young person is accepted and cared for and in which he or she can discuss concerns and share experiences with the therapist.

Cognitive-Behavioral Therapy Treatment Modules

Although stress management forms the backbone of CBT for UHR patients, it is important to address the wide array of presenting symptoms in this population. To this end, the therapy includes a range of individual modules targeting specific symptom groups. However, it may not be appropriate to target one group of symptoms in isolation; that is, any course of therapy—or, indeed, any individual therapy session—may incorporate aspects of more than one module. The assessment of presenting problems and the patient's own perception of his or her functioning informs the selection of modules to be implemented during the course of therapy.

Stress Management module.   In keeping with the stress-vulnerability model of psychosis, elements of the stress management module should be provided to all UHR patients. This module has the added advantage of providing an easily understood introduction to CBT principles, which sets the direction of future sessions. The components of this module are drawn from traditional stress management approaches including relaxation training, education about stress and coping, and more specific cognitive strategies (Clark 1989). Strategies for improving stress management are listed in Table 3–5.

Attenuated Positive Symptoms module.   The strategies incorporated within the attenuated positive symptoms module are primarily drawn from cognitive approaches to managing full-blown positive symptoms (Drury et al. 2000; Lewis et al. 2001). The goal of this module is to enhance strategies for coping with positive symptoms when they occur, to recognize early warning signs of these symptoms, and to prevent their exacerbation through the implementation of preventive strategies. For example, the therapist might assess with the patient the relationship between feeling distressed and anxious and experiencing psychotic symptoms. The therapist and patient might then collaboratively brainstorm ways to alleviate stress that might also prevent or alleviate the experience of the distressing voices or unusual thoughts. The patient can then try these strategies between sessions to test if they are useful. The strategies then can be adjusted accordingly.

The fact that the experience of positive symptoms by UHR individuals is less intense and/or frequent than the experience of frank psychosis can assist in guiding UHR individuals to recognize and manage these symptoms. For example, unusual perceptual experiences may be more easily recognized as anomalous, and attenuated delusional thoughts (overvalued ideas) might be more easily dismissed or challenged than more entrenched delusional thoughts. Through CBT strategies, the therapist can use the patient's insight into symptoms or doubts about experiences as a means of assisting the patient to challenge these symptoms. Strategies for addressing positive symptoms are listed in Table 3–6.

Negative Symptoms/Depression module.   Negative symptoms include low motivation, emotional apathy, cognitive and motoric slowness, underactivity, lack of drive, poverty of speech, and social withdrawal. These symptoms can often be difficult to distinguish from depressive symptoms, although emo-

Table 3–5. Strategies for improving stress management

Psychoeducation about the nature of stress and anxiety	Psychoeducation involves a detailed discussion of the physical, behavioral, and cognitive signs of stress. The physiological reaction concomitant with "fight or flight" responses is described to assist in the process of distinguishing adaptive stress from unhealthy levels of stress. Personal signals of maladaptive levels of stress also may be identified.
Stress monitoring	Patients are encouraged to record varying stress levels over specific periods and to identify triggers and consequences of anxiety or stress.
Stress management techniques	Such techniques include relaxation, meditation, exercise, and distraction.
Maladaptive coping techniques	Maladaptive techniques are identified, such as excessive substance use and excessive social withdrawal. The psychoeducation provided is aimed at reducing health-damaging behaviors and promoting more adaptive responses to stress.
Cognitions associated with subjective feelings of stress or heightened anxiety	Cognitions are identified, including the completion of relevant inventories or questionnaires.
Cognitive restructuring	Dysfunctional thoughts that may be maintaining anxiety or stress are countered with a more functional cognitive style (e.g., more positive coping statements, positive reframing, and challenging).
Goal setting and time management	The therapist assists the patient with goal-setting and time management skills.
Assertiveness training	The therapist assists the patient in developing assertiveness skills.
Problem-solving strategies	Strategies may include assisting the patient to develop skills such as brainstorming responses to situations, role-playing possible solutions, goal setting, and time management.

Table 3–6.   Strategies for dealing with positive symptoms

Psychoeducation about symptoms	A biopsychosocial account of the origins of unusual experiences tailored to the individual patient is provided. This can serve to "normalize" these experiences and to enhance motivation for treatment. The therapist's language must be appropriately modified for this population. For instance, because these individuals have not been given a psychotic disorder diagnosis, it may not be helpful to use the term *psychosis*. Use of this term may depend on the individual's level of anxiety about the possibility of developing a psychotic disorder and his or her general cognitive level. Generally, it is most useful to adopt the language that the patient uses to refer to unusual experiences. Focusing discussion on dealing with current symptoms is often more productive than concentrating on potentially negative outcomes.
Verbal challenge and reality testing of delusional thoughts and hallucinations	An individualized, multidimensional model of beliefs relating to delusional thinking or perceptual abnormalities is developed. This model is based on issues such as the meaning that the individual attributes to the experiences, the conclusions he or she draws from the experiences, and how he or she explains the experiences. This model is then challenged by examining the supporting evidence and generating and empirically testing alternative interpretations of experiences.
Coping enhancement techniques	Techniques include distraction, withdrawal, eliminating maladaptive coping strategies, and stress reduction techniques.

Table 3–6. Strategies for dealing with positive symptoms *(continued)*

Normalizing psychotic experiences	This strategy involves suggesting to patients that their attenuated psychotic symptoms are not discontinuous from normality or unique to them, and this insight can serve to decrease some of the associated anxiety and self-stigma.
Reality testing of hallucinations or delusional thinking	In collaboration with the patient, the therapist devises specific experiments to test the beliefs that the patient holds.
Self-monitoring of symptoms to enhance the patient's understanding of the relation of the symptoms to other factors, such as environmental events and emotional states.	An important component of self-monitoring is for the patient to be alert to any worsening of symptoms, which could indicate the onset of frank psychosis. These strategies should be revisited toward the end of the therapy process (see "Cognitive-Behavioral Therapy Termination and 'Booster' Sessions" subsection).

tional flatness as opposed to depressed mood is often used as a key distinguishing feature. Treatment of these symptoms is incorporated into the therapy because evidence suggests that they have a significant effect on the future course of the disorder (Strauss 1989). Additionally, negative symptoms may be easier to treat in the UHR population than in individuals with established psychotic disorder because the symptoms are less firmly entrenched. Cognitive-behavioral strategies used to target depression and negative symptoms include the standard strategies developed for the treatment of depression, such as those listed in Table 3–7.

Negative symptoms can sometimes serve a protective function, in the sense of ensuring that the individual avoids potentially stressful situations, which may precipitate or exacerbate positive symptoms. If indications are that negative symptoms may be serving this protective function, then the patient should be encouraged to take a slow, graded approach to increasing activity levels and challenging tasks.

Comorbidity module. The comorbidity module includes cognitive-behavioral strategies for more severe anxiety and substance use symptoms experi

Table 3–7.   Strategies for dealing with depression or negative symptoms

Psychoeducation	Information should cover both biological and psychological aspects of depression. This aspect of treatment also should include working with the patient to recognize the effect depressive and negative symptoms may have on other symptoms.
Goal setting	Achievable goals should be identified based on the patient's current functioning.
Activity management	These should include both mastery and pleasure activities.
Problem solving	Problem-solving strategies are introduced.
Social skills training	Social skills training is provided.
Cognitive restructuring	Identification and challenging of negative automatic thoughts.
Physical exercise	A realistic physical exercise program is established.

enced by UHR patients. The most frequent comorbid problems experienced by UHR patients are social anxiety, generalized anxiety, panic disorder, obsessive-compulsive symptoms, posttraumatic symptoms, and substance use (Yung et al. 2004). Components of this module are listed in Table 3–8.

A thorough assessment of substance use should be conducted. This includes examination of triggers of use, changing patterns of use over time, perceived benefits and costs of use, and an evaluation of motivation to address substance use. This process may identify other underlying conditions, such as depression, positive psychotic symptoms, or anxiety, that have been contributing to problematic substance use. This formulation of substance use may guide the focus of therapeutic intervention. If substance use is seen as a response to stressors, the development of other coping strategies may assist in reducing substance use. One of the key roles for the therapist may be in providing patients with information about the substances they use and to encourage them to reduce associated harm.

Cognitive-Behavioral Therapy Termination and "Booster" Sessions

As the patient approaches the end of his or her therapy sessions, it may be useful to schedule the sessions further apart (e.g., change from weekly to every 2 weeks)

Table 3–8. Strategies for addressing comorbidity

- Psychoeducation about the comorbid symptoms and, in line with the stress-vulnerability model, the possibility of comorbid symptoms exacerbating attenuated psychotic symptoms.

- Developing an appropriate model to explain the patient's symptoms, informed by life experiences, coping strategies, developmental level, ongoing stressors, available supports, and so on. This model can be used to orient patients to the goals of therapy and as a springboard for other strategies.

- Presenting a cognitive-behavioral model of anxiety, including discussion of the relation between cognitions, affect, and behavior.

More specific strategies might be used, depending on the presenting problems, including

- Management of physiological symptoms of anxiety through relaxation, meditation, and other stress management techniques.

- Exposure techniques, both in vivo and imaginal.

- Behavioral strategies, such as thought stopping, distraction, and activity scheduling.

- Motivational interviewing in relation to substance use.

- Cognitive strategies, including stress inoculation training and cognitive restructuring.

to help the patient adjust to coping independently of the therapist. Over the last several sessions, the therapist should review with the patient the course of therapy, including the initial presenting problems and progress through treatment. This may include providing a verbal or written summary of the course of therapy. After discharge, one or two "booster" sessions may be scheduled to monitor how the patient is progressing following discharge and to reinforce strategies that have been introduced during therapy. The optimal period of treatment has not yet been determined, but we recommend at least 6 months of treatment because this initial 6-month period has been found to be the highest period of risk for transition to full-threshold psychosis for UHR patients.

Psychoeducation in Ultra-High-Risk Patients

Psychoeducation is a means whereby the consumer of mental health services (and/or his or her family) is educated about the illness and its treatment. So that the patient may participate in decisions about treatment to the fullest degree possible, psychoeducation is a necessary process.

Psychoeducation can be conducted separately, but it also can be included as part of other interventions, such as family interventions. Psychoeducation in the early phases tends to focus on supporting and educating the individual or family about psychosis and schizophrenia, generally from a biopsychosocial perspective. As the patient progresses in recovery, the subject matter may devolve to more general topics, such as life skills and adapting to the changes necessary to manage the illness. Examples of different areas of psychoeducation are included in all the treatment modules noted earlier in Tables 3–5 through 3–8.

Information also should be given to other people who may not be direct primary caregivers but who frequently come into contact with patients with schizophrenia. These may include workers at community agencies, local government employees, and workers at supported accommodation residences, as well as the general public. A more appropriate term for this process is *mental health literacy* rather than *psychoeducation*.

Pharmacological Treatment for Ultra-High-Risk Patients

Antipsychotic Medication

The use of antipsychotic medication with UHR patients is based on the established efficacy of this medication with psychotic populations. It is thought that this might translate to the prepsychotic phase—that is, that antipsychotic medication may be useful in treating existing attenuated psychotic symptoms and in preventing the emergence of frank psychosis.

The first PACE intervention trial used low-dose risperidone (1–2 mg/day) in combination with CBT (McGorry et al. 2002). Few side effects were reported. However, many patients were nonadherent (42%) or only partially adherent (13%) to medication. The conclusion from this trial was that it may be possible to delay the onset of psychosis, although the "active ingredient" in the treatment provided (antipsychotic medication or cognitively oriented therapy) was not clear. However, the fact that the rate of transition to psychosis remained significantly lower in the risperidone-adherent subgroup at the end of the posttreatment 6-month follow-up period compared with the control group provides some evidence for the potential efficacy of antipsychotic medication in this population. The Prevention Through Risk Identification,

Management, and Education (PRIME) team reported a similar pattern of results with olanzapine. This study also had problems with adherence, with 32% of the patients dropping out of treatment (McGlashan et al. 2006).

A second trial of antipsychotic medication (risperidone + CBT versus placebo + CBT versus placebo + supportive therapy) was recently completed at PACE. Low transition rates were reported in all three treatment groups at 6 months (4.7%, 9.1%, and 7.1%, respectively), which is in keeping with the reported reduction in transition rates in UHR clinics. The reasons for the reduced transition rates are unclear: they may be due to earlier detection and treatment of UHR samples, different referral patterns and sampling from referral sources, more effective psychosocial interventions, or a combination of these factors (Yung et al. 2007). The low transition rates in all three treatment groups in this trial make it difficult to interpret the differential efficacy of these treatments. Supportive therapy may be just as effective as antipsychotic medication, especially very early in the course of symptoms (see Yung et al. 2011 for further discussion).

In recognition of the need for further evaluation of the appropriateness and efficacy of antipsychotics in the UHR population, given their possible short- and long-term side effects, these medications should not be considered as a first treatment option for this group at present. Exceptions may include situations in which the patient has a rapid deterioration of mental state, hostility, and aggression that poses a risk to the patient or others; severe suicidality; or depression that does not respond to other treatments. Antipsychotics also may be tried for patients who have not responded to psychosocial interventions and who are still unwell and functioning poorly. If antipsychotic medication is considered, then low-dose atypical agents are recommended. They should be used on a trial basis for a limited time only and at the lowest dose possible to minimize the risk of extrapyramidal side effects. If clinical benefit and resolution of symptoms occur after 6 weeks, the medication may be continued for a further 6 months to 2 years, with the consent of the patient. The atypical antipsychotics are the agents of first choice for young patients because they have been shown to be associated with fewer extrapyramidal side effects than first-generation agents. Apart from the movement disorders, the major side effects reported for the atypical agents include significant weight gain and an increased risk of diabetes and metabolic disturbance.

Other common side effects include sedation, fatigue, and decreased libido; less common side effects include prolactinemia and cardiac arrhythmias. In the few studies involving first-episode and prodromal patients that have been published so far, apart from weight gain, the other side effects reported have been relatively mild and/or transient, and thus the atypical antipsychotics appear to be well tolerated in this vulnerable patient group (International Early Psychosis Association Writing Group 2005). However, firm recommendations for pharmacological treatment, including optimal dose and duration of treatment, will be forthcoming only after more research.

Other Pharmacological Agents

Although these studies indicate the possible benefit of antipsychotic medication in the UHR population, other interventions may be more appropriate for the early stages of illness. Conceptually, this is supported by the clinical staging model (McGorry et al. 2006), which proposes that the earlier in the course of illness that treatment is offered, the safer it should be and the more effective it may be in terms of remission and recovery rates. Neuroprotective agents and antidepressants have been suggested as alternatives to antipsychotic medication.

The rationale for neuroprotective agents is that dysfunctional regulation of generation and degeneration in some brain areas might explain neurodevelopmental abnormalities seen in early psychosis. Neuroprotective strategies counteracting the loss or supporting the generation of progenitor cells may therefore be a therapeutic avenue to explore. Candidate therapies include omega-3 fatty acids, lithium, and glycine.

A randomized, double-blind, placebo-controlled trial of omega-3 fatty acids in the UHR group was recently completed in Vienna, Austria. This study found that 1.2 g/day of omega-3 fatty acids (eicosapentaenoic acid [EPA] and docosahexaenoic acid [DHA]; "fish oil"), provided for 12 weeks, was effective in reducing the transition rate to first-episode psychosis in UHR adolescents (Amminger et al. 2010). Of 81 participants, 76 (93.8%) completed the intervention. By study end (12 months), 4.9% (2 of 41) of the individuals in the omega-3 group and 27.5% (11 of 40) in the placebo group made a transition to psychosis ($P=0.004$). Omega-3 also significantly reduced positive symptoms, negative symptoms, and global symptoms and improved functioning compared with placebo. Consistent with a preventive effect, group differences were sustained after cessation of interventions. This study is currently being replicated on a larger scale by an international consortium of UHR clinics.

Several studies have reported the possible benefit of antidepressants in reducing risk of psychosis in high-risk samples. Cornblatt et al. (2007) reported a naturalistic study of young people with prodromal symptoms treated with either antidepressants or antipsychotics. Of the 28 patients, 12 (42.9%) who had been prescribed antipsychotics went on to develop psychosis in the following 2 years, whereas none of the 20 patients taking antidepressants subsequently developed psychosis. Similar results were reported by Fusar-Poli et al. (2007) on the basis of a medical file audit. Antidepressants may reduce the risk of psychosis onset by improving mood and thereby reducing the faulty appraisal of anomalous experiences. Antidepressants also may modulate the individual's response to environmental stressors, which may indirectly reduce the risk of subsequent psychosis. However, the results to date need to be interpreted with caution because of the uncontrolled nature of the studies: there may have been differences in baseline symptoms, functioning, or other variables between treatment groups, and nonadherence was far more prominent among patients prescribed antipsychotics than among patients prescribed antidepressants. Also, some contradictory evidence indicates that antidepressant medication is not associated with decline in symptom severity in UHR cases (see Walker et al. 2009). These considerations point to the need for controlled trials of antidepressants in the UHR population.

Summary of Interventions in the Prepsychotic Phase

The understanding of optimal treatment of UHR patients is still in its infancy and therefore requires constant evaluation. Although some evidence exists for the efficacy of the treatments reviewed in this section, ongoing research will provide a clearer indication of the most effective types of psychological and pharmacological interventions and suggest avenues for refining these interventions. Intervention research with this population should continue in the context of methodologically sound and ethical clinical trials. Larger sample sizes with a higher proportion of "true-positive" cases are required to increase the validity of the findings.

Because of the early stage of research in this field, it is important to keep an open mind with regard to possible treatments and be responsive to developments in related areas of research, including the treatment of established psychosis. In addition to intervention research, it is also necessary to continue attempts to determine the most potent psychopathological, neurocognitive, neurological, and biological vulnerability markers and combinations thereof for transition from "at-risk" mental state to full psychosis. This will not only assist in increasing the accuracy of identification of truly prodromal individuals (i.e., minimize "false-positive" cases) but also guide the refinement of treatment interventions.

First Psychotic Episode

A first episode of psychosis is distinguished from the UHR phase by an increased intensity and/or frequency of positive psychotic symptoms. First-episode psychosis can be divided into the period before psychosis is detected and the period after detection. Unfortunately, the undetected (and therefore untreated) phase can be prolonged, even in developed countries. Even when psychosis is detected, the initiation of effective treatment still may be delayed. Postdetection, the intervention goals are engagement and the initiation of pharmacological and psychosocial treatments. Intensive interventions aimed at maximal symptomatic and functional recovery and the prevention of relapse are ideally delivered during the early weeks and months of treatment.

First-Episode Psychosis and Duration of Untreated Psychosis

Several recent studies have supported the view that longer duration of untreated psychosis (i.e., treatment delay) results in poorer outcome for patients (Marshall et al. 2005; Perkins et al. 2005). These studies indicate that longer duration of untreated psychosis is both a marker and an independent risk factor for poor outcome. The Scandinavian Early Treatment and Intervention in Psychosis Study (TIPS; Larsen et al. 2006) has shown that reducing duration of untreated psychosis leads to early benefits in reducing suicidal risk and severity of illness at initial treatment and sustained benefits in terms of negative symptoms and social functioning. Although it is a malleable risk factor, duration of untreated psychosis accounts for a relatively modest amount of outcome variance, underlining the importance of treatment access, retention, and quality during the early phases of illness. Good evidence indicates that with appropriate public and health provider awareness campaigns, and the existence of first-episode psychosis services, duration of untreated psychosis can be significantly reduced (Melle et al. 2009).

Treatment in First-Episode Psychosis

Psychopharmacology

Pharmacotherapy is a first-line treatment in psychotic disorders. Engagement in other forms of therapy, especially psychological therapy, may be difficult for many patients until some symptom relief is gained through the use of medication. Although some uncontrolled research suggests that intensive psychosocial treatment alone may be more effective than antipsychotic medication alone (Bola and Mosher 2003), the absence of controlled research in this area prevents recommendation of psychosocial treatment in the absence of pharmacotherapy, especially in the acute phase.

The evidence indicates some advantages of atypical or second-generation antipsychotics for first-episode psychosis over typical or first-generation antipsychotics. The large multicenter European First Episode Schizophrenia Trial (EUFEST) (Kahn et al. 2008) showed that although most patients responded well to both typical and atypical medications, with no significant differences in efficacy, the discontinuation rate and tolerability were clearly superior for the atypical agents. This was true even when contrasted with very-low-dose haloperidol. The EUFEST data support the recommendations in the "International Clinical Practice Guidelines for Early Psychosis," which favors the use of atypical agents as first-line therapy because of their better tolerability (a crucial issue in drug-naïve first-episode patients) and the reduced risk of tardive dyskinesia (International Early Psychosis Association Writing Group 2005).

Several qualities of the first-episode psychosis group suggest a specifically tailored approach to pharmacotherapy. The first-episode psychosis group appears to be particularly sensitive to several anticipated side effects of medications, such as weight gain (Alvarez-Jimenez et al. 2008), sedation, and extrapyramidal side effects. Patients in this group also generally show more rapid improvement in symptoms than do patients with established schizophrenia (McEvoy et al. 2007).

Despite this, the first experience of antipsychotic medication may have considerable influence on engagement in and subsequent adherence to treatment (Lambert et al. 2004). Psychoeducation for both the patient and the caregivers with regard to possible benefits of medication and potential side effects is important and may improve compliance. Involving the patient in the decision-making process if possible is good practice. The fast response and the fact that side effects are dose-dependent and are often caused by rapid titration mean that a "start low, go slow" prescribing approach is warranted. Finally, it is important to recognize that diagnostic instability in first-episode psychosis may require ongoing adaptation of pharmacological interventions.

Psychological and Psychosocial Interventions

Cognitive-Behavioral Therapy

The basic principle of CBT for psychotic illnesses is that faulty thinking about a perception, either real in the case of a delusion or perceived to be real in the case of a hallucination, causes distress. The distress reinforces the faulty thinking. The reduction of this distress through the challenging of the faulty thinking then becomes the target of the therapy rather than the removal of the symptom. A good example of how this may occur was in the 2001 movie *A Beautiful Mind*, in which the central character realizes that the people he sees in his hallucinations never age. A CBT therapist would use this to challenge the belief that the hallucination is real. Obviously, this requires good rapport and specialist skills in the provision of CBT. A full discussion of CBT for psychosis is beyond the scope of this chapter; several good manuals are available for the use of CBT for schizophrenia (Bendall et al. 2005; Chadwick et al. 1996; Fowler et al. 1995).

The key elements of CBT for psychosis, which are briefly considered here, include engagement and assessment, formulation, and thought challenging.

Engagement and assessment.   Although the more impressive work is done a little down the track in CBT for psychosis, much like building a house, the most important part is the foundation. CBT for psychosis requires a high degree of collaboration between therapist and patient. This collaboration requires a significant amount of trust. This is not surprising when one reflects that in some parts of CBT, the therapist is likely to advance the suggestion that what the patient believes to be real, or externally produced, is neither but is possibly a symptom of an illness. Therefore, the assessment and engagement are paramount. The assessment needs to cover a detailed history of the person. The purpose of this is to determine what about the patient and his or her life may be the basis for the delusions or hallucinations.

> Daniel heard voices that told him that he was a lousy father, that he would end up homeless and unemployed, and that his intelligence was wasted on him. Delving into the patient's history, the therapist determined that Daniel was a bright young man who had been achieving well at university prior to the onset of his illness. He had had a child with a partner whom he no longer saw, and despite his intelligence, he was unemployed. Daniel had had periods of work but only in very-low-end jobs, and he had been unemployed for the past 18 months. For most of this period, he had been living with various friends and acquaintances but was coming to a point when he knew they would not continue to offer him accommodation. When Daniel's history was further explored, it was revealed that throughout his childhood his father had often communicated to him that he would amount to nothing.

Although not usually so obvious, Daniel's example serves to illustrate the importance of obtaining a good history. The content of hallucinations and delusions has in the past been thought to be meaningless epiphenomena, but in CBT, the belief is that they are very meaningful.

Concurrent with the assessment, engagement needs to be occurring. It is difficult in any form of therapy to make progress without good engagement. This can be difficult when, for funding or policy reasons, therapy is advanced very quickly. Often, engagement is a process that takes time. In some CBT for psychosis manuals, up to six sessions are allocated for good assessment, but much of this time may actually be about good engagement—the development of rapport and trust. Good engagement may just be seeing what has been missing in the interaction of other staff with the patient or by empowering them to make a choice about their presence in therapy.

> Matthew, a young man who had been an inpatient for some time, was referred for CBT for psychosis. His admission had been a difficult experience for him, his family, and other staff on the ward, and he no longer spoke with family members or staff. Matthew was informed in the first session of CBT that he did not have to answer any questions. Furthermore, he was informed that if he was asked a question, he could ask why that question was being asked, and if he didn't like the answer or believe the reason justified the intrusion of his privacy, then he didn't have to answer that either. Matthew's participation was

necessary for successful therapy, but he was being empowered to voluntarily bring that participation to the therapy sessions. This led to him being an active participant and a successful therapeutic experience.

Formulation.   The formulation is a dynamic shifting collaborative understanding of where the individual is at and how he or she came to be there. It is a central element of CBT for psychosis. There may in fact be two formulations. The first might be the therapist's formulation about the patient. This may draw on the obtained history and the input of other staff, family, and other relevant persons and be based on a solid understanding of CBT theory. The second is the collaborative understanding between the patient and the therapist of how the patient got to be where he or she is. The formulation will suggest how the patient might make progress and where he or she wants to make that progress. These two formulations both may be discussed to highlight the differences and to show where there is room for hypothesis testing.

> Tamara, a 22-year-old international student, was living in a foreign city. She was isolated and alone. She started to hear six male and female voices. Initially, they were quite mean to her, but over time, they started to point out things she needed to do such as brush her teeth or gave her advice about what she should wear. The voices continued to evolve into a group of spies who would train her also to become a spy.

The formulation that Tamara's therapist arrived at was that the voices were maintained because they provided a role and a social life for her in the absence of either of those things, that the potential of being a spy for the country she was residing in would mean that she would not have to leave (a real issue because she was no longer studying because of her illness) to return to her home country, and that much of this was triggered by her isolation and some substance use. The shared formulation agreed about the triggering factors, was in partial agreement about the social life aspect, and was in disagreement about the prevention of leaving (the spy aspect of the delusion was the most strongly held). This formulation then provided scope for testing two competing hypotheses but with a shared set of understandings. Because the rapport and engagement were good, the difference in opinions was tolerated and respected by both parties.

Challenging psychotic thoughts.   Chadwick et al. (1996) explained that for the purpose of CBT in psychotic illness, delusions are delusions and hallucinations are delusions also because the important aspects of hallucinations are the thoughts and beliefs associated with them. That is, someone might hear a voice, but they are distressed only because they believe that it is the voice of the devil. As discussed earlier, the primary target of CBT for psychosis is to reduce the distress associated with symptoms. The two key ways of challenging delusions are through a Socratic dialogue and through an experiment. An example of the former is a patient who believed that everybody in the world was in a conspiracy to kill him, which, not surprisingly, was both distressing and debilitating because it meant that he basically hid inside his house. Two directions of Socratic questioning were used to challenge this belief. The first was to induce some doubt in the absoluteness of the belief. Significant engagement work had taken place, and a lot of trust existed in the therapeutic relationship. This allowed the therapist to ask why, if everyone in the world was in on the conspiracy, had she, the therapist, been left out? The patient was perplexed and had no easy answer. The second direction of questioning was to start with some distal elements and continue questioning closer and closer to the patient. Thus, he was asked about people in Somalia (which at the time was experiencing war and famine). Did they have time to meet to discuss this conspiracy? Had he met any Somalis? Was it possible that people in Somalia did not even know about him? It was easier for the patient to entertain these thoughts because they were very much removed from him. However, over several sessions, the location of the questions became closer to home. In the end, he was able to accept that maybe only 10 people in the world harbored any ill will toward him, which, given some incidents in his history, was much more realistic. His distress was considerably reduced, and the belief in the delusion was reduced to minimal levels.

The other method to challenge a belief is with an experiment. These can be hard to set up and require a lot of collaboration from the patient. In an experiment, the aim is to test two hypotheses against each other. This is usually the hypothesis of the therapist that a belief may have come about because of an illness versus the patient's hypothesis that there is a different explanation for the perception (in the case of a hallucination) or belief. In the case of Tamara, the international student mentioned earlier, an experiment was conducted. Along with her other beliefs about the voices, she believed that one of the voices, Travis, wanted to be in a romantic relationship with her. Over many sessions, her therapist questioned her about this relationship. She tried to ask

Tamara why it seemed to be entirely based on what Travis wanted and why he never showed up in person—was this any way to treat someone one purported to be romantically interested in? Eventually, an experiment was able to be set up. Tamara had indicated that Travis had finally agreed to meet her. A lot of work was put in to ensure that there could be no excuses for his absence if he did not show up. The therapist proposed to Tamara that if he did not show up, this might mean that he was not real. Again, this illustrates the level of trust, engagement, and collaboration needed in this therapy. Tamara was able to view this as an experiment. Travis did not show up, and Tamara and her therapist were able to discuss the implications, one of which was that Travis was not real. If he was not real, then maybe the rest of the voices were not real; although they had served the purpose of a social life, it might be better to make efforts to establish activities and friends outside of that group.

This has been a very brief look at some of the aspects of CBT for psychosis. Many other aspects, some of which are mentioned in the "Cognitive-Behavioral Therapy in Ultra-High-Risk Patients" subsection earlier in this chapter, can be read about in other useful therapy manuals of CBT for psychosis and schizophrenia (Bendall et al. 2005; Chadwick et al. 1996; Fowler et al. 1995; Kingdon and Turkington 1994).

Psychoeducation

Psychoeducation programs in patients with first-episode psychosis have had several positive results. These include improving adherence to treatment, better outcomes, better management of subsequent relapse, lower readmission rates, and a positive effect on patients' well-being (Pekkala and Merinder 2002). As mentioned earlier in this chapter in "Psychoeducation in Ultra-High-Risk Patients," psychoeducation is a process that both educates the individual and the family about psychosis and allows them an informed part in treatment decisions. It can be conducted individually or in groups, with or without family members, and in some cases with family and without the patients.

Family Interventions

Family, broadly defined as those who have an emotional and a practical relationship to the person with UHR/first-episode psychosis (e.g., parents, partner, siblings), often play an important role in both caring for the patient and helping the patient care for himself or herself. However, this role is often considerably stressful and has the potential to lead to strain in the relationship, if not alienation. Family interventions cover a wide variety of practices, which are conducted in a range of situations. They can be psychoeducational, therapeutic, skills based, conducted with or without the patient present and in multifamily groups or with one family alone, and brief in duration (e.g., single or few sessions) or conducted over an extended period. A recent review of 28 studies of family interventions in patients with schizophrenia found that family interventions have a range of positive effects, including decreasing relapse, reducing hospital admission, and encouraging medication compliance (Pharoah et al. 2010). The effect on families was to reduce the burden of illness, increase knowledge, and decrease expressed emotion. Evidence indicates that multifamily groups may be better than single family groups; however, families may have a preference for single family groups, and this should be respected when possible. Local and national support groups are also effective in supporting the family, and referrals to consumer and caregiver networks are recommended.

Family members of young people are often distressed and anxious about the changes they have noticed in their relative. Support for these family members is helpful. Psychoeducation regarding being at high risk for, or having, early psychosis should be provided to family members to deal with distress and to minimize the possible negative outcome of illness status on family functioning (e.g., pathologizing the UHR individual and stigmatization). Information should be provided to parents about their child's progress and treatment as appropriate. This process needs to be sensitive to the young person's confidentiality and privacy. Additionally, it may become apparent that systemic family issues are a factor in the young person's distress and symptoms. These issues may be addressed in the clinic or may require a referral to a more specialized family service.

Vocational Interventions

The onset of prodrome and/or psychosis most often falls in a key period of vocational development. Often the practical results of this are that education is either not completed or completed at a standard lower than may have otherwise been achieved or that employment is not gained or maintained. In the absence of a mental illness, not finishing high school and a lack of employment experience are two of the largest barriers to entering the competitive labor market. Despite wanting to work, more than 40% of people with first-episode psychosis are unemployed (Killackey et al. 2008), and even in the presence of a specialized mental health service, this does not improve. Rates of unemployment have been found to increase with longer duration of illness. Unemployment is associated with an increase in marginalization, poorer health outcomes, lower self-esteem, and increased substance use.

Employment is an important path back to other areas of functioning such as social and economic participation. Functional recovery is increasingly being recognized as equally important to symptomatic recovery. The opportunity to reduce functional disability is one of the most important elements of the early intervention paradigm. The method of vocational recovery that has the most evidence underpinning it is called supported employment, the most defined form of which is called Individual Placement and Support (IPS) (Becker and Drake 2003). Supported employment has been found to be superior in 16 randomized trials to date. Importantly for early psychosis, three randomized trials in this population found a significant advantage to IPS compared with community-based employment agencies (Killackey et al. 2008).

The key elements of IPS are as follows:

1. IPS is focused on competitive employment (i.e., jobs that are not set aside but open to anyone with the appropriate skills or qualifications to apply for) as an outcome.
2. IPS is open to any person with mental illness who chooses to look for work, and acceptance into the program is not determined by measures of work-readiness or illness variables.
3. Job searching commences directly on entry into the program.
4. The IPS program is integrated with the mental health treatment team.
5. Potential jobs are chosen on the basis of consumer preference.
6. Support provided in the program is time-unlimited, continuing after employment is obtained, and is adapted to the needs of the individual (Becker and Drake 2003).

A seventh principle, also sometimes considered as part of the model of IPS, is the provision of welfare benefits counseling (Bond 2004).

Weight Gain Interventions

One of the main side effects of some atypical antipsychotic medications is a particularly high risk of significant weight gain and metabolic problems, and these risks must be carefully managed and prevented whenever possible. Indeed, studies report that up to 80% of individuals taking atypical antipsychotics have significant gain in body weight (Green et al. 2000). This antipsychotic side effect has recently become a major concern in the treatment of psychosis because weight gain has been associated with reduced quality of life, social stigma, greater morbidity (cardiovascular disease, diabetes mellitus, osteoarthritis, and some types of cancer), and mortality.

Weight gain is arguably a greater problem for young people experiencing a first-episode psychosis. This group is considered to be especially susceptible to very rapid and pronounced weight gain, which could interfere with the early recovery process. First, younger populations are less disposed to adhering to medication regimens, and potential weight gain may exacerbate noncompliance. Second, the physical changes produced by weight gain may result in social discrimination and stigma because young patients are more sensitive to issues of body image and self-esteem than are their older counterparts.

As a result, there has been a growing interest in developing treatment alternatives to control or attenuate weight gain. A recent review of interventions to reduce weight gain in schizophrenia concluded that evidence was insufficient to support the general use of adjunctive pharmacological interventions (Faulkner et al. 2007). Conversely, nonpharmacological weight management interventions have been shown to be effective in reducing or attenuating antipsychotic-induced weight gain compared with treatment as usual (Alvarez-Jimenez et al. 2008). Interestingly, a recent randomized controlled trial has shown that it is possible to attenuate antipsychotic-induced weight gain in drug-naïve young patients with behavioral techniques (Alvarez-Jimenez et al. 2006). This latter study showed the effectiveness, feasibility, and acceptability of preventive strategies, which comprised dietary counseling, exercise increase, and behavioral techniques, for first-episode psychosis patients who commenced antipsychotic treatment.

Next Steps in First-Episode Intervention

CBT, family intervention, targeting of substance abuse and suicide risk, and vocational rehabilitation are the key psychosocial interventions in early psychosis and need to be much more intensively and widely deployed (Edwards and McGorry 2002). Assertive community treatment for the subset of poorly engaged patients is vital. Family interventions are also an essential element of care, as described earlier with regard to UHR treatment. They have been shown to lead to shorter periods of hospitalization in first-episode psychosis patients, assisting parents in supporting their children within the community (Lenior et al. 2001). A family psychosocial module was also an essential component in a relapse prevention intervention, which was more effective than standard care at preventing the occurrence of a second episode of psychosis (Gleeson et al. 2009). In patients with schizophrenia, the evidence indicates that the relapse rate can be reduced by 20% if relatives are included in treatment.

The Critical Period After Diagnosis and Treatment of First-Episode Psychosis

The years beyond the first psychotic episode have been referred to as the "critical period" (Birchwood 2000). Treatment goals in this phase are sustained engagement and tenure in specialized care; continuing effective medication management; and the use of effective psychosocial interventions to minimize the risk of relapse and the development of disability and to maximize social and functional recovery. Proof of concept is now established for these strategies at least in the short term (Bertelsen et al. 2008; Craig et al. 2004; Gleeson et al. 2009).

Beyond the first episode, we know that the first 2–5 years postdiagnosis are crucial in setting the parameters for longer-term recovery and outcome. This is the period of maximum risk for disengagement, relapse, and suicide, as well as coinciding with the major developmental challenges of forming a stable identity, peer network, vocational training, and intimate relationships. It makes sense that a stream of care specially focused on young people and on this stage of illness is required to maximize the chances of engagement, continuity of care, appropriate lifestyle changes, adherence to treatment, family support, and vocational recovery and progress. Indeed, the available evidence from naturalistic and randomized studies strongly supports the value of specialized early psychosis programs in improving outcome in the short term. If these programs are provided for only 1–2 years, then evidence also shows that some of the gains are eroded, suggesting that for a substantial subset at least, specialized early psychosis care needs to be provided for a longer period, probably up to 5 years in many cases (Bertelsen et al. 2008). At this point, persisting illness and disability may be present in a much smaller percentage of people whose needs subsequently may be well met by more traditional mental health services for older adults. This may be a much better point to transfer care.

Relapse Prevention

Naturalistic long-term follow-up studies have shown that the early course of psychosis is characterized by repeated relapses, and up to 80% of first-episode psychosis patients experience a relapse within 5 years remission from the initial episode (Gitlin et al. 2001; Robinson et al. 1999). This is significant because with each subsequent relapse, the risk of developing persistent psychotic symptoms increases. Recurrent psychotic episodes are associated with progressive loss of gray matter, which may reduce the effectiveness of antipsychotic medications (Ho et al. 2003). Relapse is also likely to interfere with the social and vocational development of young people with psychosis, which may have an effect on long-term outcomes. Moreover, economic analyses have indicated that the cost for treatment of relapsing psychosis is four times that of stable psychosis (Almond et al. 2004). It is, therefore, not surprising that reducing the number of relapses has become a major goal of interventions for first-episode psychosis (Robinson et al. 1999).

Treatment alternatives to prevent relapse in first-episode psychosis include both psychosocial interventions and pharmacological treatments. To date, three large randomized controlled trials have found specialist first-episode psychosis programs to be effective in preventing relapse in relation to the usual care provided by nonspecialist mental health services in the first 2 years after psychosis onset (Cullberg et al. 2002; Larsen et al. 2001; Penn et al. 2005). However, given that the available evidence indicates that some of the gains of specialist first-episode psychosis programs are eroded over longer periods (McGorry et al. 2008), future trials should investigate the long-term effect of first-episode psychosis programs in relapse prevention.

A recent clinical trial confirmed the short-term effectiveness of a novel 7-month multimodal CBT intervention, delivered to both the individual and the family, for relapse prevention in remitted first-episode psychosis patients compared with a specialist youth first-episode psychosis program (Gleeson et al. 2009). The relapse prevention therapy comprised five phases of therapy underpinned by a relapse prevention framework and focused on increasing awareness for the risk of setbacks and how to minimize them, identification of potential early warning signs of relapse, and formulation of an individualized relapse prevention plan. Family intervention also incorporated psychoeducation about relapse risk as well as a review of early warning signs and formulation of a relapse prevention plan. These results showed that relapse can be reduced to very low levels (5%) during this initial period of maintenance treatment for patients who have responded to acute phase treatments. Taken together, these data lend support to the contention that multimodal CBT interventions specifically designed to prevent relapse offered to remitted first-episode psychosis patients may improve further on relapse rates achieved by a high-quality specialist first-episode psychosis service. However, the long-term effectiveness of this intervention remains to be established.

Two controlled trials have examined the effectiveness of family interventions to reduce relapse in first-episode psychosis patients. One trial found that a family intervention consisting of group and individual counseling sessions for 18 months was effective in reducing relapse rates compared with treatment as usual (Zhang et al. 1994). The second trial, which showed no difference between treatment conditions, evaluated a brief individual intervention comprising seven sessions of psychoeducation (Leavey et al. 2004). Similarly, the extant literature consistently shows that longer-term family programs produce stronger clinical effects than do shorter interventions in multiepisode patients (Pitschel-Walz et al. 2001). These results indicate that longer family interventions may be needed to obtain clinical benefits in first-episode psychosis patients.

Further evidence indicated that families who received a cognitive-based relapse prevention intervention showed a significant and sustained benefit in terms of appraisals related to caregiving, including greater positive personal experiences of caring. This finding may be a result of an increased preparedness among the families for intervening early to prevent possible relapses. In other words, family relapse prevention interventions may increase the families' recognition of their potential to contribute to the care and well-being of their relative, thereby increasing their appraisals of the positive aspects of caregiving. Nonetheless, given the consistent evidence for relapse prevention for family interventions in the later phases of schizophrenia and the theoretical potential of these interventions to prevent psychotic relapse, it is surprising that so few randomized controlled trials have evaluated their effectiveness in first-episode psychosis patients. Further research is warranted to determine the effectiveness of family interventions in young people with first-episode psychosis.

Regarding pharmacological interventions, only three small and relatively old studies have tested the effectiveness of typical antipsychotics compared with placebo in first-episode psychosis patients. These studies showed that the former was more effective in preventing relapse. However, only typical antipsychotics were tested, and these trials had small samples, limiting the generalizability of the findings to clinical practice (Kane et al. 1982; McCreadie et al. 1989). Moreover, no clinical trial has been conducted to test the effectiveness of atypical antipsychotics compared with placebo in preventing relapse in first-episode psychosis.

Finally, only one trial examined the effectiveness of a guided discontinuation strategy compared with maintenance treatment in young patients with psychosis. The discontinuation strategy consisted of gradual symptom-guided tapering of dosage and discontinuation if feasible plus restoration of antipsychotic treatment if early warning signs of relapse emerged. Maintenance treatment was superior to the discontinuation strategy in preventing relapse during the first 18 months following clinical remission; however, no difference was seen between treatment groups in number of hospital days or social functioning (Wunderink et al. 2007). Given this, the effectiveness of discontinuation strategies in first-episode psychosis patients needs to be investigated in combination with intensive psychosocial treatments to determine the most cost-effective treatment approach.

Conclusion

The period from being at a noticeably increased risk for psychosis through the first 5 years after the onset of psychosis is increasingly being recognized as containing multiple points for intervention. A relation is now recognized between earlier intervention and the reduction or avoidance of disability in functional life domains. In both UHR and first-episode psychosis groups, the key to successful intervention is the use of a wide range of targeted pharmacological and psychosocial interventions, including CBT, family work, educational and vocational rehabilitation, and relapse prevention. Psychotic illness targets numerous life domains, and it makes sense that treatments for it would do no less. Several important issues require further research, such as the optimum period of intervention for the UHR and first-episode psychosis population, the relative efficacy of pharmacological and psychosocial interventions, the possibility of a staged approach to implementing these interventions, and the development of further interventions for managing treatment side effects and preventing relapse.

Suggested Readings

Books/Articles

Addington J, Francey SM, Morrison AP (eds): Working With People at High Risk of Developing Psychosis. Chichester, UK, Wiley, 2006

International Early Psychosis Association Writing Group: International clinical practice guidelines for early psychosis. Br J Psychiatry Suppl 48:S120–S124, 2005

Jackson H, McGorry PD (eds): The Recognition and Management of Early Psychosis: A Preventive Approach, 2nd Edition. New York, Cambridge University Press, 2009

McGorry PD, Yung AR, Phillips LJ, et al: Randomized controlled trial of interventions designed to reduce the risk of progression to first-episode psychosis in a clinical sample with subthreshold symptoms. Arch Gen Psychiatry 59:921–928, 2002

Phillips LJ, Francey SM: Changing PACE: psychological interventions in the prepsychotic phase, in Psychological Interventions in Early Psychosis: A Treatment Handbook. Edited by Gleeson JMF, McGorry PD. Chichester, UK, Wiley, 2004, pp 23–39

Yung AR, Phillips LJ, McGorry PD: Treating Schizophrenia in the Prodromal Phase. London, Taylor & Francis, 2004

Relevant Web Sites

Orygen Youth Health (http://oyh.org.au)

References

Almond S, Knapp M, Francois C, et al: Relapse in schizophrenia: costs, clinical outcomes and quality of life. Br J Psychiatry 184:346–351, 2004

Alvarez-Jimenez M, Gonzalez Blanch C, Vazquez-Barcueio JL, et al: Attenuation of antipsychotic-induced weight gain with early behavioral intervention in drug-naive first-episode psychosis patients: a randomized controlled trial. J Clin Psychiatry 67:1253–1260, 2006

Alvarez-Jimenez M, Gonzalez-Blanch C, Crespo-Facorro B, et al: Antipsychotic-induced weight gain in chronic and first-episode psychotic disorders: a systematic critical reappraisal. CNS Drugs 22:547–562, 2008

American Psychiatric Association: Practice Guidelines for the Treatment of Patients With Schizophrenia. Washington, DC, American Psychiatric Association, 1997

Amminger GP, Schafer MR, Papageorgiou K, et al: Long-chain omega-3 fatty acids for indicated prevention of psychotic disorders: a randomized, placebo-controlled trial. Arch Gen Psychiatry 67:146–154, 2010

Beck AT: Successful outpatient psychotherapy of a chronic schizophrenic with a delusion based on borrowed guilt. Psychiatry 15:305–312, 1952

Becker DR, Drake RE: A Working Life for People With Severe Mental Illness. New York, Oxford University Press, 2003

Bendall S, Killackey E, Marois MJ, et al: ACE Manual. Melbourne, Australia, Orygen Youth Health Research Centre, 2005

Bertelsen M, Jeppesen P, Petersen L, et al: Five-year follow-up of a randomized multicenter trial of intensive early intervention vs standard treatment for patients with a first episode of psychotic illness: the OPUS trial. Arch Gen Psychiatry 65:762–771, 2008

Bertolote J, McGorry P: Early intervention and recovery for young people with early psychosis: consensus statement. Br J Psychiatry Suppl 48:S116–S119, 2005

Birchwood M: Early intervention and sustaining the management of vulnerability. Aust N Z J Psychiatry 34 (suppl):S181–S184, 2000

Bola JR, Mosher LR: Treatment of acute psychosis without neuroleptics: two-year outcomes from the Soteria project. J Nerv Ment Dis 191:219–229, 2003

Bond GR: Supported employment: evidence for an evidence-based practice. Psychiatr Rehabil J 27:345–359, 2004

Chadwick P, Birchwood M, Trower P: Cognitive Therapy for Delusions, Voices and Paranoia. New York, Wiley, 1996

Clark DM: Anxiety states: panic and generalized anxiety, in Cognitive Behaviour Therapy for Psychiatric Problems: A Practical Guide. Edited by Hawton K, Salkovskis PM, Kirk J, et al. Oxford, UK, Oxford University Press, 1989, pp 52–96

Cornblatt BA, Lencz T, Smith CW, et al. Can antidepressants be used to treat the schizophrenia prodrome? Results of a prospective, naturalistic treatment study of adolescents. J Clin Psychiatry 68:546–557, 2007

Craig TK, Garety P, Power P, et al: The Lambeth Early Onset (LEO) Team: randomised controlled trial of the effectiveness of specialised care for early psychosis. BMJ 329:1067, 2004

Cullberg J, Levander S, Holmqvist R, et al: One-year outcome in first episode psychosis patients in the Swedish Parachute project. Acta Psychiatr Scand 106:276–285, 2002

Drury V, Birchwood M, Cochrane R: Cognitive therapy and recovery from acute psychosis: a controlled trial, III: five-year follow-up. Br J Psychiatry 177:8–14, 2000

Edwards J, McGorry PD: Implementing Early Intervention in Psychosis: A Guide to Establishing Early Psychosis Services. London, Dunitz, 2002

Faulkner G, Cohn T, Remington G: Interventions to reduce weight gain in schizophrenia. Cochrane Database of Systematic Reviews 2007, Issue 1. Art. No.: CD005148. DOI: 10.1002/14651858.CD005148.pub2.

Fowler D, Garety PA, Kuipers A: Cognitive Behaviour Therapy for Psychosis: Theory and Practice. Chichester, UK, Wiley, 1995

Fusar-Poli P, Valmaggia L, McGuire P: Can antidepressants prevent psychosis? Lancet 370:1746–1748, 2007

Garety PA, Kuipers E, Fowler D, et al: A cognitive model of the positive symptoms of psychosis. Psychol Med 31:189–195, 2001

Gitlin M, Nuechterlein K, Subotnik KL, et al: Clinical outcome following neuroleptic discontinuation in patients with remitted recent-onset schizophrenia. Am J Psychiatry 158:1835–1842, 2001

Gleeson JF, Cotton SM, Alvarez-Jimenez M, et al: A randomized controlled trial of relapse prevention therapy for first-episode psychosis patients. J Clin Psychiatry 70:477–486, 2009

Green AI, Patel JK, Goisman RM, et al: Weight gain from novel antipsychotic drugs: need for action. Gen Hosp Psychiatry 22:224–235, 2000

Ho BC, Andreasen NC, Nopoulos P, et al: Progressive structural brain abnormalities and their relationship to clinical outcome: a longitudinal magnetic resonance imaging study early in schizophrenia. Arch Gen Psychiatry 60:585–594, 2003

International Early Psychosis Association Writing Group: International clinical practice guidelines for early psychosis. Br J Psychiatry Suppl 48:S120–S124, 2005

Kahn RS, Fleischhacker WW, Boter H, et al: Effectiveness of antipsychotic drugs in first-episode schizophrenia and schizophreniform disorder: an open randomised clinical trial. Lancet 371:1085–1097, 2008

Kane JM, Rifkin A, Quitkin F, et al: Fluphenazine versus placebo in patients with remitted, acute first-episode schizophrenia. Arch Gen Psychiatry 39:70–73, 1982

Killackey E, Jackson HJ, McGorry PD: Vocational intervention in first-episode psychosis: individual placement and support v. treatment as usual. Br J Psychiatry 193:114–120, 2008

Kingdon D, Turkington D: Cognitive-Behavioural Therapy for Schizophrenia. Hove, UK, Lawrence Erlbaum, 1994

Lambert M, Conus P, Eide P, et al: Impact of present and past antipsychotic side effects on attitude toward typical antipsychotic treatment and adherence. Eur Psychiatry 19:415–422, 2004

Larsen TK, McGlashan TH, Johannessen JO, et al: Shortened duration of untreated first episode of psychosis: changes in patient characteristics at treatment. Am J Psychiatry 158:1917–1919, 2001

Larsen TK, Melle I, Auestad B, et al: Early detection of first-episode psychosis: the effect on 1-year outcome. Schizophr Bull 32:758–764, 2006

Leavey G, Gulamhussein S, Papadopoulos C, et al: A randomized controlled trial of a brief intervention for families of patients with a first episode of psychosis. Psychol Med 34:423–431, 2004

Lenior ME, Dingemans PM, Linszen DH, et al: Social functioning and the course of early onset schizophrenia: five-year follow-up of a psychosocial intervention. Br J Psychiatry 179:53–58, 2001

Lewis SW, Tarrier N, Haddock G, et al: A randomised controlled trial of cognitive behaviour therapy in early schizophrenia. Schizophr Res 49:263, 2001

Marshall M, Lewis S, Lockwood A, et al: Association between duration of untreated psychosis and outcome in cohorts of first-episode outcome patients: a systematic review. Arch Gen Psychiatry 62:975–983, 2005

McCreadie RG, Wiles D, Grant S, et al: The Scottish first episode schizophrenia study, VII: two-year follow-up. Scottish Schizophrenia Research Group. Acta Psychiatr Scand 80:597–602, 1989

McEvoy JP, Lieberman JA, Perkins DO, et al: Efficacy and tolerability of olanzapine, quetiapine, and risperidone in the treatment of early psychosis: a randomized, double-blind 52-week comparison. Am J Psychiatry 164:1050–1060, 2007

McGlashan TH, Zipursky RB, Perkins D, et al: Randomized, double-blind trial of olanzapine versus placebo in patients prodromally symptomatic for psychosis. Am J Psychiatry 163:790–799, 2006

McGorry PD, Yung AR, Phillips LJ, et al: Randomized controlled trial of interventions designed to reduce the risk of progression to first-episode psychosis in a clinical sample with subthreshold symptoms. Arch Gen Psychiatry 59:921–928, 2002

McGorry PD, Hickie IB, Yung AR, et al: Clinical staging of psychiatric disorders: a heuristic framework for choosing earlier, safer and more effective interventions. Aust N Z J Psychiatry 40:616–622, 2006

McGorry PD, Killackey E, Yung A: Early intervention in psychosis: concepts, evidence and future directions. World Psychiatry 7:148–156, 2008

Melle I, Larsen TK, Friis S, et al: Early detection of first psychosis: TIPS sample five year outcomes. Schizophr Bull 35 (suppl 1):330, 2009

Mihalopoulos C, Harris M, Henry L, et al: Is early intervention in psychosis cost-effective over the long term? Schizophr Bull 35:909–918, 2009

Morrison AP, French P, Walford L, et al: Cognitive therapy for the prevention of psychosis in people at ultra-high risk: randomised controlled trial. Br J Psychiatry 185:291–297, 2004

Pantelis C, Velakoulis D, McGorry PD, et al: Neuroanatomical abnormalities before and after onset of psychosis: a cross-sectional and longitudinal MRI comparison. Lancet 361:281–288, 2003

Pekkala ET, Merinder LB: Psychoeducation for schizophrenia. Cochrane Database of Systematic Reviews 2002, Issue 2. Art. No.: CD002831. DOI: 10.1002/14651858.CD002831.

Penn DL, Waldheter EJ, Perkins DO, et al: Psychosocial treatment for first-episode psychosis: a research update. Am J Psychiatry 162:2220–2232, 2005

Perkins DO, Gu H, Boteva K, et al: Relationship between duration of untreated psychosis and outcome in first-episode schizophrenia: a critical review and meta-analysis. Am J Psychiatry 162:1785–1804, 2005

Pharoah F, Mari J, Rathbone J, et al: Family intervention for schizophrenia. Cochrane Database of Systematic Reviews 2010, Issue 12. Art. No.: CD000088. DOI: 10.1002/14651858.CD000088.pub3.

Pitschel-Walz G, Leucht S, Bauml J, et al: The effect of family interventions on relapse and rehospitalization in schizophrenia—a meta-analysis. Schizophr Bull 27:73–92, 2001

Robinson D, Woerner MG, Alvir JM, et al: Predictors of relapse following response from a first episode of schizophrenia or schizoaffective disorder. Arch Gen Psychiatry 56:241–247, 1999

Strauss JS: Subjective experience of schizophrenia: toward a new dynamic psychiatry, II. Schizophr Bull 15:179–187, 1989

Walker EF, Cornblatt BA, Addington J, et al: The relation of antipsychotic and antidepressant medication with baseline symptoms and symptom progression: a naturalistic study of the North American Prodrome Longitudinal Sample. Schizophr Res 115:50–57, 2009

Wunderink L, Nienhuis FJ, Sytema S, et al: Guided discontinuation versus maintenance treatment in remitted first-episode psychosis: relapse rates and functional outcome. J Clin Psychiatry 68:654–661, 2007

Yung AR, Phillips LJ, McGorry PD: Treating Schizophrenia in the Prodromal Phase. London, Taylor & Francis, 2004

Yung AR, Yuen HP, Berger G, et al. Declining transition rate in ultra high risk (prodromal) services: dilution or reduction of risk? Schizophr Bull 33:673–681, 2007

Yung AR, Phillips LJ, Nelson B, et al: Randomized controlled trial of interventions for young people at ultra high risk for psychosis: 6-month analysis. J Clin Psychiatry 72:430–440, 2011

Zhang M, Wang M, Li J, et al: Randomised-control trial of family intervention for 78 first-episode male schizophrenic patients: an 18-month study in Suzhou, Jiangsu. Br J Psychiatry 24:96–102, 1994

4

Clinical Assessment in Schizophrenia

Stefano Pallanti, M.D.

Andrea Cantisani, M.D.

Clinical Diagnostic Assessment

Differential Diagnosis of Psychosis and Schizophrenia

Since the original Kraepelinian description of dementia praecox (Kraepelin 1919), clinical heterogeneity within schizophrenia has been recognized as an irreducible characteristic of the syndrome. Therefore, the search for "core" features has been incessant.

In DSM-5, still in progress, the most innovative aim is represented by the search for the so-called endophenotype (Gottesman and Gould 2003) of the disorder and the adoption of a translational approach, which would facilitate the integration of findings from neurobiological research and would lead to the eventual development of an "etiologically based, scientifically sound classification system" (Kupfer et al. 2002). This approach would replace the descriptive approach.

111

Although the debate around what should be considered primary and fundamental in schizophrenia is a central issue, clinical description remains the domain of the diagnostic definition.

Nevertheless, because no physical test currently confirms the presence of schizophrenia and because schizophrenia often shares a significant number of symptoms with other disorders (see Tables 4–1 and 4–2), misdiagnosis is a common problem. The average delay is 10 years from the first onset of symptoms to the correct diagnosis and treatment of psychiatric disorders.

Clinicians are aware that the phenotype is highly variable, that the symptomatological pattern does not define a specific syndrome (Cuesta et al. 2007), and that no clear and precise boundaries separate schizophrenia from other pathological entities such as bipolar disorder (Craddock and Owen 2010), both at the clinical level within the boundary category of schizoaffective disorders and at the genetic level (Lichtenstein et al. 2009).

Table 4–1.   DSM-IV-TR main diagnostic categories of psychotic disorders

Nonaffective psychotic disorders

    Schizophrenia

    Schizoaffective disorder

    Schizophreniform disorder

    Delusional disorder

    Brief psychotic disorder

    Psychotic disorder not otherwise specified

Affective psychoses

    Bipolar disorder with psychotic features

    Major depressive disorder with psychotic features

Substance-induced psychotic disorder

    Alcohol-induced

    Other substance-induced

Psychotic disorder due to a general medical condition

Source.   American Psychiatric Association 2000.

Table 4–2. Differential diagnosis and medical causes of psychosis

Neurological
  Trauma
  Multiple sclerosis
  Huntington's chorea
  Epilepsy
  Strokes
  Tumor
  Abscesses
  Normal pressure hydrocephalus
  Subarachnoid hemorrhage
  Intraparenchymal hemorrhage
  Auditory or optic nerve disease
  Fabry's disease
  Fahr's disease
  Wilson's disease
  Parkinson's disease

Metabolic and endocrine
  Cushing's syndrome
  Hyperthyroidism
  Hypothyroidism
  Acute intermittent porphyria
  Shock
  Renal failure
  Hepatic failure
  Electrolyte imbalance
  B_{12} deficiency
  Addison's disease
  Paraneoplastic syndrome
  Systemic lupus erythematosus

Pharmacological
  Antivirals
  Anticonvulsants
  Anticholinergics
  Baclofen
  β-Blockers
  Bromocriptine
  Cephalosporins
  Captopril
  Cimetidine
  Clonidine
  Corticosteroids
  Disulfiram
  Fluoroquinolones
  Methotrexate
  Nonsteroidal anti-inflammatory drugs
  Theophylline
  Vincristine

Substance abuse
  Alcohol
  Amphetamines
  Belladonna alkaloids
  Cannabis
  Cocaine
  Lysergic acid diethylamide
  Phencyclidine

Infections and toxins
  Syphilis
  Herpes encephalitis
  HIV/AIDS
  Creutzfeldt-Jakob disease
  Lyme disease
  Meningitis
  Malaria
  Heavy metal poisoning
  Carbon monoxide poisoning

Source. Adapted from Hilty et al. 1999.

Frequently, the risk of misdiagnosis concerns the so-called delusional hallucinatory illness, a disorder that no longer corresponds to the diagnosis of schizophrenia. Furthermore, a recent review of general population-based studies showed that psychotic symptoms such as paranoid delusional thinking and hallucinations are present in a mild form in 5%–8% of healthy people (Van Os et al. 2009).

Therefore, it is valuable to understand the difference between psychosis and schizophrenia. *Psychosis* is a general term used to describe psychotic symptoms. In contrast, *schizophrenia* represents an idiopathic form of psychosis. All forms of psychotic disorder due to a general medical condition must be preliminarily excluded. Several different brain disorders can lead to psychotic syndromes, including lesions in the brain resulting from head traumas; strokes; tumors; infections; and metabolic, genetic, or chromosomal disorders. Severe forms of depression may present psychotic symptoms, and bipolar disorder is often confused with schizophrenia and vice versa. In addition, several personality disorders and developmental disorders such as Asperger's syndrome must be excluded.

Whereas the "positive" component of the syndrome has become less central in the diagnostic assessment, the negative dimension, with the distinction between primary and secondary phenomena and cognitive disturbances, has been emphasized. In addition, increasing attention has been paid to the interpersonal dimension of the disorder in recent years because of the prevalence of outpatient therapeutic settings and subjective features such as coping strategies, subjective well-being, and psychosocial adjustment. These factors have been increasingly included in therapeutic planning. Moreover, the relevant effect of comorbidities—specifically, panic disorder, social anxiety, and substance-related disorders—is now widely investigated, as are metabolic and cardiovascular side effects.

People with schizophrenia are at greater risk for obesity, type 2 diabetes, dyslipidemia, and hypertension than is the general population. This increased susceptibility results in an increased incidence of cardiovascular disease (CVD) and reduced life expectancy, over and above that imposed by their mental illness. Metabolic syndrome vulnerability, described even in the preneuroleptic era, can be considered a feature of the schizophrenic disorder and should be included in the clinical targets. Therefore, the initial visit should include the evaluation of family and medical history, baseline weight and body mass index, visceral obesity (measured by waist circumference), blood pressure, fasting plasma glucose level, fasting lipid profiles, and electrocardiogram (ECG). Several of the antipsychotic medications, both typical and atypical, have been shown to prolong the QTc interval on the ECG. Prolongation of the QTc interval is of potential concern because the patient may be at risk for wave burst arrhythmia, a potentially serious ventricular arrhythmia. A QTc interval greater than 500 ms places the patient at a significantly increased risk for serious arrhythmia.

Lifestyle and unhealthy attitudes, specifically smoking (Kotov et al. 2010) and high intake of caffeinated beverages, should be assessed immediately and discussed with the patient and relatives to promote change and prevent complications such as the reduction of life expectancy and complicated comorbidities (e.g., smoking- and coffee-related increases in anxiety).

The assessment of sexual behavior also must be included in the diagnostic and therapeutic algorithm. The presence of at-risk behaviors and individual needs should be investigated at baseline. The latter may provide important information about the response to treatment and/or the impairment caused by the intake of antipsychotic medication (McCann 2003).

Neurological examination also should be part of the assessment (Heinrichs and Buchanan 1988) because subtle neurological impairments and soft neurological symptoms have been frequently reported in schizophrenic drug-naïve patients. The most reliable scale is the Neurological Evaluation Scale (NES; Buchanan and Heinrichs 1989), which is designed to standardize the assessment of neurological impairment in schizophrenia. The battery consists of 26 items. Studies of the specific adaptation of the neurological examination to schizophrenic patients reported three factors of interest: 1) a "coordination/Romberg" factor (including the fist-edge-palm test, finger-thumb opposition, rapid alternating movements, and Romberg test), 2) a "sensory integration" factor (including synkinesis, extinction, stereognosis, and audiovisual integration), and 3) an "eye movements/tandem walk/overflow movements" factor (including convergence, gaze impersistence, tandem walk, and adventitious overflow) (Sanders et al. 2005). In addition to the differential diagnostic utility, obtaining a comprehensive neurological history and performing a complete examination of patients with schizophrenia at the onset of their illness and before initiating pharmacotherapy may be useful for identifying clusters of neurodevelopmental indicators that are more specific for schizophrenia than for bipolar disorder. This examination also may help evaluate neurological function during the disease course and treatment compared with baseline. An electroencephalogram (EEG) also may be performed because the risk of epilepsy in schizophrenia is 11 times higher than in the general population, and some treatments may enhance this risk.

Neither computed tomography (CT) scans nor magnetic resonance images (MRIs) have diagnostic value; therefore, they may be performed only to address specific differential diagnostic questions.

The purpose of this chapter is to briefly clarify these important issues concerning the assessment of the schizophrenic patient during the entire course of illness, from first interview to remission.

Basic Assessment

In the last decade, increasing attention has been paid to the so-called prodromal phase of schizophrenia to identify high-risk subjects, and the inclusion of a psychosis risk syndrome or an attenuated psychotic symptoms syndrome in DSM-5 is now under debate. *High-risk prodromal subgroups* are defined as subjects who experience a brief or an intermittent psychotic state with attenuated positive symptoms and with genetic risk and functional decline (Yung and McGorry 1996). Although medical treatment shows no clear evidence of usefulness and efficacy in this population (De Koning et al. 2009), the clinician should be aware that this cohort of high-risk subjects needs to be constantly monitored and supported with treatment as early as possible to prevent a full-blown psychotic episode (see also Nelson et al., Chapter 3, "Prodromal Phase and First-Episode Schizophrenia"). The duration of untreated psychosis positively correlates with outcome, global functioning, and quality of life (Marshall et al. 2005). The Structured Interview for Prodromal Syndromes (SIPS; McGlashan et al. 2001) may be used to detect these syndromes. The SIPS includes the Scale of Prodromal Symptoms (SOPS; Miller et al. 1999), which is composed of 19 items grouped into four domains (positive, negative, disorganization, and general symptoms).

The possible presence of comorbidity also must be analyzed in this initial phase, particularly with panic, social anxiety, obsessive-compulsive disorder, or substance abuse, because they need prompt treatment (for further information, see Chapter 6, "Comorbidity in Schizophrenia," and Chapter 7, "Substance Use Disorders and Schizophrenia").

Moreover, these first-line assessments are relevant not only to investigate the psychopathology of the patient but also to build an appropriate therapeutic alliance, provide information about psychosis and mental disorders clearly and comprehensively, and educate family or caregivers about the nature of symptoms and the benefits of therapy to avoid the stigmatization and pessimism that are too often part of schizophrenia.

Diagnostic Issues

Whereas neurobiological research aims to deconstruct and reconceptualize schizophrenia by adopting the endophenotype strategy that offers powerful and exciting opportunities to understand the genetically conferred neurobiological vulnerabilities and to design molecularly based treatments for schizophrenia (Braff et al. 2007), clinicians continue to track the clinical phenotype and attempt to improve the outcome. Currently, the diagnosis is based on the DSM-IV-TR (American Psychiatric Association 2000) or ICD-10 (World Health Organization 1992) criteria, which are structured on a categorical approach. Major revisions in DSM-5 and ICD-11 will probably address the diagnostic procedure, including the evaluation of psychopathological dimensions in the diagnosis algorithm. Current research suggests that combining dimensional and categorical assessments of psychopathology provides more information about treatment issues and prognosis in the psychotic patient compared with either model alone (Dikeos et al. 2006).

Increasing evidence suggests that schizophrenic symptoms can be correlated and clustered into four different dimensions or factors:

1. The positive dimension (domain of reality distortion symptoms, including hallucinations and delusions)
2. The negative dimension (primary or secondary symptoms associated with the reduction of energy, motivation, and emotional reaction to stimuli)
3. The cognitive dimension (or disorganization dimension), including alterations in neurocognitive processes such as attention, memory, and executive functioning
4. The affective dimensions (both manic and depressive), which include clusters of affective symptoms that often can be observed in psychotic patients

The use of this complementary approach (including both categorical and dimensional representations) together with the quantification of symptoms

Table 4–3.   Strategies for diagnosis and assessment

- Consider the subjective experiences and psychosocial adaptations of the subjects at ultrahigh risk or diagnosed with attenuated psychotic syndrome.

- Assess cardiovascular functionality, metabolic status, and waist circumference; and perform electrocardiogram, specific neurological examination, and electroencephalogram.

- Combine categorical and dimensional assessment with particular attention to the cognitive and negative symptoms.

- Consider the presence of comorbid disorders to be included in the treatment plan.

- Carefully evaluate psychosocial functioning during the course of the illness.

- Distinguish primary (deficit syndrome) and secondary negative symptoms.

- Assess cognitive functioning and subjective complaints.

- Target and monitor treatment.

obtained with the appropriate rating scales could be very useful in evaluating the patient's course of illness and response to treatment.

We suggest this kind of diagnostic algorithm to allow the clinician to obtain a better and more useful characterization and assessment of every patient (Table 4–3).

The instruments to measure these dimensions are described in the following sections, except for those regarding the affective domain, which are described by Pallanti and Quercioli in Chapter 6, "Comorbidity in Schizophrenia."

Diagnostic Criteria

ICD-10 and DSM-IV-TR (Tables 4–4 and 4–5) are the most widely used diagnostic classifications. They are composed of different items and provide lists of distinctive symptoms that are required to formulate diagnoses. This kind of categorical approach is useful for clinical and research purposes because it provides a common ground on which to frame uniform constructs of psychiatric disorders. However, it has the important limitation of being specific only rarely and consequently includes more than one clinical entity in a single diagnostic category. This limitation is particularly relevant for schizophrenia and other psychotic disorders.

Table 4–4. ICD-10 diagnostic criteria for schizophrenia

I. At least one of the syndromes, symptoms and signs listed below under (1) or at least two of the symptoms and signs listed under (2) should be present for most of the time during an episode of psychotic illness lasting for at least one month (or at some time during most days).

1. At least one of the following:

    a) Thought echo, thought insertion or withdrawal, or thought broadcasting.

    b) Delusions of control, influence or passivity, clearly referred to body or limb movements or specific thoughts, actions, or sensations; delusional perception.

    c) Hallucinatory voices giving a running commentary on the patient's behavior, or discussing him between themselves, or other types of hallucinatory voices coming from some part of the body.

    d) Persistent delusions of other kinds that are culturally inappropriate and completely impossible (e.g., being able to control the weather or being in communication with aliens from another world).

2. Or at least two of the following:

    e) Persistent hallucinations in any modality, when occurring every day for at least one month, when accompanied by delusions (which may be fleeting or half-formed) without clear affective content, or when accompanied by persistent over-valued ideas.

    f) Neologisms, breaks or interpolations in the train of thought, resulting in incoherence or irrelevant speech.

    g) Catatonic behavior, such as excitement, posturing or waxy flexibility, negativism, mutism and stupor.

    h) "Negative" symptoms such as marked apathy, paucity of speech, and blunting or incongruity of emotional responses (it must be clear that these are not due to depression or to neuroleptic medication).

II. Most commonly used exclusion criteria: if the patient also meets criteria for manic episode (or depressive episode), the criteria listed under I.1 and I.2 above must have been met before the disturbance of mood developed.

The disorder is not attributable to organic brain disease or to alcohol- or drug-related intoxication, dependence or withdrawal.

Source. Reprinted from World Health Organization: *International Statistical Classification of Diseases and Related Health Problems,* 10th Revision. Geneva, World Health Organization, 1992. Used with permission.

Table 4–5.   DSM-IV-TR diagnostic criteria for schizophrenia

A. *Characteristic symptoms:*   Two (or more) of the following, each present for a significant portion of time during a 1-month period (or less if successfully treated):

    (1) delusions

    (2) hallucinations

    (3) disorganized speech (e.g., frequent derailment or incoherence)

    (4) grossly disorganized or catatonic behavior

    (5) negative symptoms, i.e., affective flattening, alogia, or avolition

  Note: Only one Criterion A symptom is required if delusions are bizarre or hallucinations consist of a voice keeping up a running commentary on the person's behavior or thoughts, or two or more voices conversing with each other.

B. *Social/occupational dysfunction:*   For a significant portion of the time since the onset of the disturbance, one or more major areas of functioning such as work, interpersonal relations, or self-care are markedly below the level achieved prior to the onset (or when the onset is in childhood or adolescence, failure to achieve expected level of interpersonal, academic, or occupational achievement).

C. *Duration:*   Continuous signs of the disturbance persist for at least 6 months. This 6-month period must include at least 1 month of symptoms (or less if successfully treated) that meet Criterion A (i.e., active-phase symptoms) and may include periods of prodromal or residual symptoms. During these prodromal or residual periods, the signs of the disturbance may be manifested by only negative symptoms or two or more symptoms listed in Criterion A present in an attenuated form (e.g., odd beliefs, unusual perceptual experiences).

D. *Schizoaffective and mood disorder exclusion:*   Schizoaffective disorder and mood disorder with psychotic features have been ruled out because either (1) no major depressive, manic, or mixed episodes have occurred concurrently with the active-phase symptoms; or (2) if mood episodes have occurred during active-phase symptoms, their total duration has been brief relative to the duration of the active and residual periods.

E. *Substance/general medical condition exclusion:*   The disturbance is not due to the direct physiological effects of a substance (e.g., a drug of abuse, a medication) or a general medical condition.

F. *Relationship to a pervasive developmental disorder:*   If there is a history of autistic disorder or another pervasive developmental disorder, the additional diagnosis of schizophrenia is made only if prominent delusions or hallucinations are also present for at least a month (or less if successfully treated).

Table 4–5. DSM-IV-TR diagnostic criteria for schizophrenia *(continued)*

Classification of longitudinal course (can be applied only after at least 1 year has elapsed since the initial onset of active-phase symptoms):

Episodic With Interepisode Residual Symptoms (episodes are defined by the reemergence of prominent psychotic symptoms); *also specify if:* **With Prominent Negative Symptoms**

Episodic With No Interepisode Residual Symptoms

Continuous (prominent psychotic symptoms are present throughout the period of observation); *also specify if:* **With Prominent Negative Symptoms**

Single Episode In Partial Remission; *also specify if:* **With Prominent Negative Symptoms**

Single Episode In Full Remission

Other or Unspecified Pattern

Source. Reprinted from the *Diagnostic and Statistical Manual of Mental Disorders, 4th Edition, Text Revision.* Washington, DC, American Psychiatric Association, 2000, pp. 312–313. Copyright © 2000 American Psychiatric Association. Used with permission.

Schizophrenia is defined in DSM-IV-TR as a syndrome characterized by long duration and presence of delusions and hallucinations, negative symptoms (alogia, blunted affect, avolition), and disorganized behavior or speech that causes consistent social or occupational dysfunction. In fact, psychosocial functioning is considered to play a central role in the definition of the diagnosis and therefore requires an accurate assessment. Thus, Morosini et al. (2000) developed a short and useful instrument (Personal and Social Performance Scale) to evaluate this aspect during the course of illness in a clinical setting. It consists of four main domains (socially useful activities, personal and social relationships, self-care, and disturbing and aggressive behavior) that the clinician rates in six degrees of severity (absent, mild, manifest, marked, severe, and very severe). The scale requires about 5 minutes to complete but provides accurate and relevant information about these diagnostic criteria and outcome parameters.

Alternatively, ICD-10 diagnostic criteria for schizophrenia have a cross-sectional approach and do not involve a social or functional decline measurement. The ICD-10 requires a shorter minimum duration for completion, a lower number of symptoms, and, with regard to positive symptoms, predominantly emphasizes Schneiderian first-rank symptoms.

The subtypes of schizophrenia in both classification systems are undifferentiated, paranoid, disorganized (or hebephrenic), catatonic, and residual.

Measurement of the Positive Dimension

Positive symptoms refer to a group of symptoms that involve impaired reality testing and reality distortion, including delusions or hallucinations. They can be more or less stable, and their severity can vary throughout the course of the illness. Their identification and assessment are usually easier than that required for negative symptoms. An accurate quantification of the positive dimension with a rating scale can be useful in monitoring the course of the disorder.

Brief Psychiatric Rating Scale

The Brief Psychiatric Rating Scale (BPRS; Overall and Gorham 1962) is one of the most used tools to evaluate clinical symptoms in psychiatric disorders. Many studies have highlighted the high reliability of this scale (Bech et al. 1993). Eighteen items measure general psychopathology and positive and affective symptoms, which are rated by the clinician after a brief nonstructured interview on a seven-point scale from "not present" (0) to "extremely severe" (6).

The items that provide information about the presence and severity of positive symptoms in schizophrenia are "conceptual disorganization," "grandiosity," "hallucinatory behavior," "unusual thought content," "uncooperativeness," "suspiciousness," and "hostility."

Scale for the Assessment of Positive Symptoms

The Scale for the Assessment of Positive Symptoms (SAPS) (together with the Scale for the Assessment of Negative Symptoms [SANS], discussed later in this chapter) was developed by Andreasen (1984) to explore and measure the positive dimension of schizophrenia. It is composed of 30 individual items and is divided into four main subscales (delusions, hallucinations, bizarre behavior, and formal thought disorders). Each subscale includes an item that measures the global domain score. The items are scored on a six-point scale from "absent" (0) to "severe" (5) and are rated by trained clinicians during a semistructured interview. Despite its high reliability and the quality of information provided, the SAPS is difficult to use during routine clinical assessment because of its extensiveness and complexity.

It is also important to establish the modality of emergence of the delu
sional hallucinatory syndrome and its correlation with environmental cueing,
anxiety, substances (such as caffeine), and circumstances as well as its personal
meaning (see discussion of comorbidity with panic disorder and social anxiety
in Chapter 6).

Positive and Negative Syndrome Scale

The Positive and Negative Syndrome Scale (PANSS; Kay et al. 1987) includes
18 items of the BPRS and 12 additional items from the Psychopathology Rating Schedule (Singh and Kay 1975). It is one of the most often used rating
tools for both research and clinical purposes because of its high reliability in
the assessment of symptoms and their changes during the course of the illness.
It consists of 30 items grouped into three major subscales: 7 items refer to the
negative dimension of the disorder, 7 to the positive dimension, and 16 to
general psychopathology. The items referring to the positive dimension of
schizophrenia are "delusions," "conceptual disorganization," "hallucinatory
behavior," "excitement," "grandiosity," "suspiciousness/persecution," and
"hostility." The clinician rates items during a semistructured interview, and
the scores range from "absent" (0) to "extreme" (7).

The PANSS offers a reliable and objective assessment of a broad variety of
symptoms in patients with schizophrenia, and it is considered a fine upgrade
of the BPRS, although it requires a long interview that is often difficult to perform during the daily clinical routine.

Measurement of the Negative Dimension

Negative symptoms are defined as a reduction or loss of normal behavioral, intellectual, and emotional functions, which are frequent and persistent characteristics of schizophrenia. Typical negative symptoms are apathy, anhedonia,
avolition, poor interpersonal rapport, passive social withdrawal, and blunted
affect. A common and often treatment-resistant symptom of schizophrenia is
anhedonia, the diminished capacity to experience pleasant emotions. One interpretation positions it between the negative and the cognitive dimension, defining it as the result of faulty memory functions such that patients are capable
of experiencing pleasure but underestimate it when recalling these experiences
(Horan et al. 2006a). Anhedonia can be reliably assessed and constitutes a distinctive, clinically relevant aspect of schizophrenia that should be included in a

comprehensive evaluation of negative symptoms (Horan et al. 2006b) to detect behavior changes and to assess the efficacy of rehabilitation treatments.

Negative symptoms can be classified as "primary" or "secondary" according to their etiology. Primary negative symptoms are thought to be a core feature of schizophrenia and are clinically expressed by avolitional characteristics. Therefore, they are persistent and less responsive to treatment. In contrast, secondary negative symptoms are transient and reversible and may represent, for example, the adverse effects of antipsychotic drugs, disorganization, psychotic or positive symptoms, or depression.

Carpenter et al. (1988) proposed the concept of "deficit syndrome," which refers to a schizophrenia subtype mainly characterized by persistent and disabling primary negative symptoms that last for at least 12 months. The deficit syndrome subtype of schizophrenia seems to be stable over time and differs in a variety of parameters such as risk and etiological factors, outcome, and treatment response (Kirkpatrick et al. 2001).

The relevance of negative symptoms in the course of schizophrenia is widely accepted. In particular, negative symptoms have an adverse effect on quality of life and outcome (Malla and Payne 2005; Moller et al. 2000), but their identification and quantification can be difficult because of the co-occurring positive symptoms and the possible confusion of these symptoms with signs of neurocognitive impairment.

Brief Psychiatric Rating Scale

The BPRS does not focus enough on the negative symptoms; therefore, its use may be not adequate to assess this dimension. The BPRS items related to negative symptoms are "emotional withdrawal," "motor retardation," and "blunted affect."

Positive and Negative Syndrome Scale

The general structure of the PANSS has been described in the preceding section. The following seven items analyze the negative dimension: "blunted affect," "emotional withdrawal," "poor rapport," "passive/apathetic social withdrawal," "difficulty in abstract thinking," "lack of spontaneity," and "flow of conversation and stereotyped thinking."

Scale for the Assessment of Negative Symptoms

The SANS was developed by Andreasen (1982) together with the SAPS to accurately evaluate the severity of negative symptoms. Nineteen items are grouped into five main clusters that include affective blunting, alogia, avoli-tion/apathy, anhedonia/asociality, and disturbance of attention.

Despite the precision and reliability of the scale, its use in the clinical routine can be difficult because of its complexity.

Schedule for the Deficit Syndrome

The gold standard for the diagnosis of deficit schizophrenia (Galderisi and Maj 2009) is represented by the operational criteria of the Schedule for the Deficit Syndrome (SDS), a semistructured interview that can be carried out by psychiatrists, psychologists, or social workers who have extensive clinical experience with schizophrenic patients.

The deficit or nondeficit categorization is based on the interview with the patient and the information provided by clinical records, relatives, and health professionals well acquainted with the patient's past and present psychopathological state. All information should focus on times of clinical stability because the categorization has no validity when made during acute psychotic states. The use of the SDS requires specific training.

Although the diagnosis of deficit schizophrenia is difficult, especially when ascertaining whether negative symptoms are primary or secondary, the interrater agreement is reported to be good, ranging from 0.73 to 1 for the overall classification into the deficit or nondeficit subtype and from 0.60 to 0.81 for each of the six negative symptoms that must be assessed for the categorization.

Kirkpatrick et al. (1989) provided data supporting the possibility of using the Proxy for the Deficit Syndrome (PDS) to diagnose deficit schizophrenia. The PDS is based on the subtraction of the BPRS scores on the affective items of anxiety, guilty feelings, depressive mood, and hostility from the item of blunted affect. When this method is compared with the gold standard evaluation method, it shows sensitivity and specificity rates of 79% and 89%, respectively. More recently, two proxy measures for the deficit syndrome based on the PANSS have been evaluated: the PDS1, based on an algorithm in which the score for the PANSS Affective Scale (anxiety, guilt, depression, and hostility) is subtracted from the score for blunted affect, and the PDS2, in which only the depression score is subtracted from blunted affect. The two measures had good specificity (78.6% and 79.5%, respectively) and moderate to very good sensitivity (61.4% and 86.4%, respectively).

The PDS was developed by Kirkpatrick et al. (1989) to identify deficit or nondeficit subgroups of schizophrenic patients. Six negative items are defined, including poverty of speech, diminished emotional range, diminished social drive, restricted affect, curbing of interest, and diminished sense of purpose. The rater has to discern whether the symptoms are primary or secondary.

The PDS does not provide any information about the variation of the symptoms over the course of illness but does allow the clinician to distinguish between primary and secondary symptoms. This feature has considerable relevance because several findings support the claim that they may represent two separate disease entities.

Measurement of the Neurocognitive Dimension

Neurocognitive dysfunctions are not part of the diagnostic criteria in DSM-IV-TR, even if it is now fully accepted that they represent not only a core aspect of the disorder but also candidate endophenotype features. Cognitive disturbances are highly prevalent and clinically severe in individuals with a diagnosis of schizophrenia (Keefe et al. 2005) and include difficulties concerning concentration and memory. These symptoms may be evident as follows:

- Slow thinking
- Difficulty in understanding
- Poor concentration
- Poor memory
- Difficulty in expressing thoughts
- Difficulty in integrating thoughts, feelings, and behavior
- Language communication difficulties
- Difficulty in decision-making processes

Generally, the performances of these patients are 1.5–2 standard deviations below the normal average, and the impairment involves several cognitive domains such as vigilance and attention, visual and verbal learning, working and long-term memory, reasoning and problem solving, speed of processing, verbal fluency, and social cognition (Nuechterlein et al. 2004).

The MATRICS Consensus (Measurement and Treatment Research to Improve Cognition in Schizophrenia) reviewed numerous studies focused on this topic and developed a battery of tests to assess all of the mentioned areas of the cognitive dimension in schizophrenia. These alterations seem to exist prior to the onset of disease, are manifest by the time of the first episode, and are not related to antipsychotic medication (Saykin et al. 1994).

What is actually more relevant from a clinical point of view is that neurocognitive impairment seems to predict poor social and functional outcome (Bowie and Harvey 2008; Green et al. 2000) and consequently should be carefully assessed, even if the search for more effective therapeutic interventions for these symptoms is still in progress (see Strik et al., Chapter 5, "Cognition and Schizophrenia"). In fact, it has been suggested that the treatment of cognitive deficits could improve the insight and coping strategies of schizophrenic patients, although debate is ongoing about this hypothesis. Difficulties related to the administration of complex test batteries and the scarcity of specifically trained personnel limit this assessment in daily practice. Furthermore, cognitive evaluation can be conducted only during a stable clinical phase and not in the course of an acute episode.

Interview-based measures, which consist of a few questions addressed directly to the patient and to his or her caregivers, might serve to briefly assess cognitive deficit. Keefe et al. (2006) developed the Schizophrenia Cognition Rating Scale, which allows the psychiatrist to rapidly evaluate cognitive impairment and its effect on everyday functioning. It is composed of 18 items, including the cognitive domains of memory and working memory, attention, reasoning, and motor and language skills, and it uses information recorded from the patient and his or her relatives or caregivers. For example, they are asked to determine if the subject seems able to remember the names of people that he or she knows or to follow a television show or other day-to-day tasks, and the psychiatrist then formulates a global rating.

A first-person account of cognitive complaints also can be used to investigate the cognitive domains. Subjective experiences of cognitive disturbances are assessed through a self-rated questionnaire, the Frankfurter Beschwerde-Fragebogen (Süllwold 1986). This instrument is composed of 98 yes/no questions assessing 10 phenomenological areas in four dimensions of subjective experience: automatic skills, perceptual disturbances, anhedonia, and overstimulation. The Frankfurter Beschwerde-Fragebogen evaluates a wide range of cognitive deficits and was developed from the spontaneous complaints of schizophrenic patients in a review of hundreds of clinical records. In a previous study (Pallanti et al. 1999), we reported that subjective cognitive disturbances, more than objective symptoms, are correlated to cognitively evoked potential (P300) alterations in schizophrenia and that the use of a questionnaire (in that case, the Frankfurter Beschwerde-Fragebogen) may appropriately cover the domain of schizophrenic cognitive disorders.

Despite their simple structure, these kinds of instruments provide very useful and reliable data that may allow the clinician to quickly assess cognitive deficits in a clinical environment and include them in the treatment plan.

Toward a Person-Oriented Clinical Evaluation of the Schizophrenic (Out)Patient

Because of the convergence of several theoretical changes in psychiatry in recent years—particularly the reduction of institutionalization for schizophrenic patients—a more person-centered outpatient path to recovery has emerged that points directly to rehabilitation and to the retrieval of lost cognitive and psychosocial functions (Remington et al. 2010). A specific type of assessment is required for this goal, and some important aspects of the disease (specifically emerging from the first-person experiences of the single subject) must be taken into account by the clinician with regard to their effect on the individual.

A comprehensive anamnesis is required to build the therapeutic alliance and to determine the age at onset of the appearance of the disorder and the premorbid, social, and educational characteristics of the subjects and the family environment.

The multidimensional evaluation of the patient's awareness of and reaction to the disintegrating experience of psychosis, in addition to the inspection and interpretation of the patient's coping resources and strategies, is critical to understanding the severity of the illness and to setting up a treatment plan.

Following this evaluation, the psychiatrist has to focus on assessing the attitude toward medication in both the patient and his or her relatives. If improvement has occurred under previous treatments, the patient's singular perspective on this improvement is relevant for the clinician in terms of compliance.

To develop such a comprehensive intervention, it is necessary to reach a very good communication level with both the patient and the family and to

Table 4–6. Strategies for person-centered clinical evaluation

- Assess insight level and its variations during the course of the disorder.

- Pay attention to biographical and anamnestic aspects.

- Evaluate the risk of suicidality.

- Reinforce the adaptive insight.

- Analyze and improve coping resources.

- Identify risk factors for nonadherence and assess patient's attitude toward medication.

- Pay attention to and try to improve patient's subjective well-being while reducing symptoms.

- Include family relationships in the assessment as well as how the family members cope with the ill subject.

- Reinforce the adaptive coping.

maintain an attitude that is open-minded and ready to dialogue at the critical moment of the diagnosis and during all therapeutic processes (Table 4–6).

Early Childhood Trauma, Stressful Life Events, and Importance of Biography

Early childhood trauma refers to a series of negative experiences such as physical or sexual abuse, neglect, and physical or emotional events during childhood or early adolescence. The effect of these events on schizophrenia is still under debate (Morgan and Fisher 2007), but some recently published large-scale, population-based studies (see review by Larkin and Read 2008) have suggested a dose-effect relation between the number of traumas during childhood and the risk of psychotic episodes in adulthood. Furthermore, compelling evidence exists for early trauma-related poor psychosocial functioning among schizophrenic patients. Increased exposure to trauma in childhood also correlates with suicidality (Lipschitz et al. 1996), hospital admission, use of medical services, general health problems, homelessness, and involvement in the criminal justice system (Rosenberg et al. 2007).

Another dimension to assess is the vulnerability of the subject (objectively and subjectively reported) to stressful events. The "behavioral sensitization" represents a possible mechanism by which previous exposures to severe stress could facilitate behavioral and biological responses to the same type of traumatic event in the future, even if milder in intensity (Collip et al. 2008). A recent study has shown that adolescents with a diagnosis of schizotypal personality disorder report a higher number of stressful events in everyday life than do healthy control subjects. At the 1-year follow-up, the number of stressful events correlated with an increase in prodromal symptoms (Tessner et al. 2011).

Awareness, Suicidality, and Coping

Insight has been defined as the patient's awareness of having a mental disorder, of symptoms, and of the social consequences and the need for treatment (Amador et al. 1996). It is a dynamic and multidimensional phenomenon rather than a categorical one, and it is characterized by a high variability among all psychiatric diseases, changing from one patient to another and across the course of the illness.

A lack of awareness of illness or insight has been considered a hallmark of schizophrenic illness and has become an increasingly important area of investigation. Various measurement scales have been proposed to assess insight in schizophrenia (see Lincoln et al. 2007), with the goal of exploring different components, such as the awareness of illness, the capacity to relabel psychotic experiences as abnormal, treatment compliance (Schedule for Assessing the Three Components of Insight), insight into the mental disorder (both present and past), awareness of the social consequences, the need for treatment, the perception of each symptom, and the attribution of symptoms to a disorder (Scale to Assess Unawareness of Mental Disorder).

It is well established that the awareness of disorder in schizophrenia is very low compared with all other major psychiatric conditions (Masson et al. 2001; Pini et al. 2001).

These deficits in insight have received particular attention in both clinical and research fields because of their possible interactions with social and clinical outcomes, course of symptoms, adherence to medication, depression, and suicide. However, no clear and strong evidence in any direction is found for most of these interactions (Lincoln et al. 2007).

Insight might be a necessary factor for better compliance, recovery, and faster rehabilitation, but it has been suggested that it might also be traumatizing and stigmatizing for the patient and related to lower self-esteem, hopelessness, depression, and suicide.

When focusing on the "worst case scenario," it is fundamental to prevent the downward spiral that leads to a high suicide risk; the correlation with schizophrenia has been documented (Cohen et al. 1990; Gupta et al. 1998). In considering the link between awareness and suicidality, from a clinical expert-based point of view (because empirical research has not yet succeeded in settling the debate), significant attention should be paid to the characteristics and fluctuations of each individual case. Some people with schizophrenia are more able to cope with the issues that such a diagnosis poses and to develop a positive attitude toward treatment. In other cases, denial and lack of insight do not interfere with therapy and do not increase the risk of self-harm. Careful and constant monitoring is crucially important, and any change in patient insight during the progression of the disorder must be appropriately decoded.

Moreover, two other elements seem to play important roles: hope and self-stigmatization. Hope (and hopelessness), together with depression, is considered a crucial emotion in the mediation between insight into mental illness and suicide. High levels of hope in conjunction with a remarkable awareness of illness correlate with an active coping inclination in schizophrenic subjects, whereas high levels of insight with low levels of hope are associated with an avoidant type of coping (Lysaker et al. 2005). Hope has a direct positive relation to many aspects of quality of life, even if it is negatively correlated to insight into illness (Hasson-Ohayon et al. 2009). Whether insight is considered a resource or a burden is obviously affected by the meanings that the patient attributes to schizophrenia as well as the effect of the disorder on social outcome. Assimilating the stigma of society about mental disease will more likely cause hopelessness or low self-esteem, whereas good insight with minimal levels of internalized stigma correlate with less impaired social function (Lysaker et al. 2007).

Therefore, it is essential to understand how the patient copes with the symptoms of the disorder and cognitive dysfunctions independently from the level of insight. Coping efforts represent an important process by which the affected individual can influence the effect of the illness on his or her life (Roe et al. 2006). Natural coping strategies seem to be very common in schizophrenic patients (about 70%) to manage psychotic symptoms (Farhall et al.

Table 4–7. Classification of coping strategies in schizophrenia

Problem centered	Compensatory activities of the subject directly aimed to modify or eliminate the sources of distress
Non–problem centered	Compensatory activities of the subject characterized by keeping distance, passive avoidance, or suppression
	Ineffective and not focused on the true stress source or on improvement of the subject's stress response
Behavioral	Characterized by observable behavior
Cognitive	Characterized by inner adaptation or compensatory cognitive processes
Emotional	Characterized by affective adaptation

2007). Various mechanisms are involved, such as asking for help, adjusting medication, accepting, fighting back, or acting in accordance with the symptoms (Farhall et al. 2007). The repertoire of these strategies varies from one individual to another (see Tables 4–7 and 4–8), but subjects with a broader range of coping behaviors tend to achieve better outcomes. Therefore, the clinical importance of assessing coping procedures is clear. The psychiatrist can improve the coping ability of the patient by teaching him or her new strategies, helping him or her focus on the most successful strategies, and motivating him or her to search for and discover new strategies.

In conclusion, a good clinical approach must reduce the insight-related risk of depression and suicide with the goal of improving social and functional outcome. It could be useful for increasing the so-called usable insight of the schizophrenic patient, distinguishing the symptoms of the disorder from reality and the illness itself from the identity of the patient while strengthening functional coping strategies and better treatment compliance (Lewis 2004).

(Non)adherence, Drug Attitude, and Subjective Well-Being

(Non)adherence plays a very important role in determining the success or failure of the treatment of psychiatric disorders, particularly schizophrenia. The individual's attitude toward medication and subjective evaluation of his or her own health status are extremely important. As reported in two comprehensive reviews, the average rate of unsatisfactory adherence in schizophrenic patients

Table 4–8. Examples of coping strategies: behavioral (B), cognitive (C), and emotional (E)

Problem centered

B—"I try to speak slower, looking for a point to anchor the thoughts that are blowing in my mind."

C—"I talk to myself, trying to find a way to deal with the problem."

E—"To begin with, I try to calm myself."

Non–problem centered

B—"I don't talk about the problem, but I try to look normal or friendly."

C—"I try to distract myself, thinking of other things."

E—"The only thing I can do is become very sad."

is about 40% (Cramer and Rosenheck 1998; Lacro et al. 2002), which represents one of the main causes of partial remission. Furthermore, an increased risk of relapse and rehospitalization is strongly associated with noncompliance.

Nonadherence is commonly described as the "failure or refusal to comply with treatment recommendations" (Haynes et al. 1979). Although the topic of compliance has been widely investigated in all medical fields, there is no exhaustive definition of it. The adherence to treatment is considered a difficult variable to measure and quantify. Instead of viewing (non)adherence as a single dichotomous variable, it may be more appropriate to consider it a complex group of different aspects that vary across individuals and fluctuate over the course of illness (Day et al. 2005), making it impossible to identify a unique intervention to address it.

What seems to be essential in determining behavior toward pharmacological treatment is the patient's personal assessment of his or her individual goals and priorities, the perceived severity of the symptoms and susceptibility to illness, and the global cost-benefit ratio of receiving antipsychotic treatment. Other variables, such as socioeconomic status, cultural issues, previous experiences, degree of insight, past or current substance abuse, duration of illness, quality of discharge planning, aftercare environment, and therapeutic alliance, all contribute to patient compliance to varying degrees (for a complete list, see Table 4–9) (Lacro et al. 2002).

Table 4–9.   Risk factors for nonadherence

Patient-related risk factors

    Poor insight

    Negative attitude toward medication

    History of nonadherence

    Past or current comorbid substance abuse

    Short duration of illness

Treatment-related risk factors

    Higher antipsychotic dose

    Complexity of treatment regimen

    Use of first-generation antipsychotics vs. second-generation antipsychotics

Environment-related risk factors

    Poor therapeutic alliance

    Poor outpatient-clinician relationship

    Family belief about medications

    Inadequate discharge planning and follow-up care

    Practical issues such as lack of money

    Stigmatization

A person-centered approach to the schizophrenic (out)patient must include an accurate assessment of all of these variables to plan the most flexible and successful long-term intervention. From the patient's point of view, compliance with a medication regimen is a means to reach important objectives in life, such as remission of psychosis or better social functioning. However, psychiatrists sometimes attribute an outcome status to adherence and are more concerned with compliance itself rather than the patient's feelings and well-being, thus spoiling the therapeutic alliance (Weiden 2007). The clinician should be aware that the costs and benefits of the treatment are more closely related to the patient's perceptions than to what the medical staff may think. This means that the cost-benefit balance may be different if evaluated from the two different points of view, leading to assessment inaccuracies (Weiden 2007).

Several scales have been developed to assess patient drug attitudes, such as the schizophrenia-specific Drug Attitude Inventory (Hogan et al. 1983) and Subjective Well-Being Under Neuroleptics scale (Naber 1995; Naber et al. 2001), and, less specifically, the Heinrichs-Carpenter Quality of Life Scale (Heinrichs et al. 1984) and the Quality of Life Enjoyment and Satisfaction Questionnaire (Endicott et al. 1993), which measure patients' quality of life.

In fact, psychiatrists should view (non)adherence as a core component of the disease that can vary over time and during the course of the illness, and they should be prepared to act via different approaches and educate the patients and their families to incorporate the therapy into their lives (Weiden 2007).

Assessment of Disturbed Processing of "Self" and "Other" and Phenomenological Principles of Cognitive-Behavioral Intervention

Any assessment implies an interaction with the schizophrenic patient and offers an opportunity for a therapeutic intervention, which begins during the first contact. Helping patients improve their self-perception is an essential component and aim of the therapeutic process. The uncoupling of assessment procedures and therapy is an untenable principle for practicing clinical psychiatry. The clinician should avoid using two separate sets of instruments for diagnosing and for treating patients and instead should use only one. This strategy will help enforce the patient's intentionality (i.e., the capacity to communicate the feel of his or her experiences and to make better sense of them) (Mundt 2005).

Therefore, including first-person inner experience in the evaluation process completes the clinical investigation (Lysaker and Lysaker 2010). The literature has widely suggested that schizophrenia involves alterations in self-experience (i.e., in how people experience themselves in the course of their many pursuits and relationships). Schematically, several areas of anomalous self-experience are potentially involved: disorders of the self and identity (most patients report persisting identity void or feelings of self-transformation) and perceptual disorders (hearing voices). A recollection of these experiences requires a specific modality of appraisal. *Phenomenology* can be defined as the science of the subjective. It concerns the investigation of what it is like to be in a certain state of mind and the patient's subjective attempt to organize this experience into a meaningful narrative understanding.

Narrative understanding brings together and gives sense to disparate experiences, creating connections between perceptions, emotions, beliefs, and cognitive "distortions" (the quotation marks represent the suspension of any presupposition or judgment as a preliminary act in this further in-depth investigation).

The symptoms that fall under the terms *transitivism* (recognition of alien identity pieces in the self) and *appersonation* (perception of external parts of the self dispersed in others) (Modestin et al. 2003) were first described by Eugen Bleuler and have long been considered the exclusive domain of philosophical or psychodynamic investigation. The disturbed processing that is at the origin of a confused recognition of "self" and "other" has only recently been reported to be related to the (dis)ability of patients to identify facial and vocal emotion, such as prosody. Prosody is the rhythm, stress, and intonation of speech that conveys important information about the sense of what is said (Fisher et al. 2008). A common substrate, the medial prefrontal cortex, is recruited during both social cognition tasks and self-referential processing (Ochsner et al. 2004). These impairments in source monitoring have been reported in patients without acute positive symptoms and in first-degree relatives. They may represent a trait marker for schizophrenia above and beyond the external response bias that has been described as a state marker in earlier studies, providing a cognitive neuroscientific interpretation of self-other disturbances (Brunelin et al. 2007). The results of phenomenological investigations suggest that the "loss of self" in schizophrenia involves compromised first- and second-person awareness, and affected individuals seem to have the residual ability to view themselves only from the "outside." A reduction of immediate self-awareness, specifically of the "feeling of agency" (the awareness that I am the source of this thought or movement), represents a fundamental constitutional fragility in schizophrenia.

Individuals may perceive themselves as a mechanism that thinks, perceives, and acts but experiences no meaningful selfhood (Lysaker and Lysaker 2001). These experiences are often so strange to the patient that he or she has never communicated them to anyone else, and the patient may lack words to express them or may adopt salient metaphors. To transmit the type of experience investigated here to another person requires a certain intimacy. The interviewer should adopt a neutral yet caring posture, rather than a curious one, and the interviewer should ideally provide the patient with the option of acting as a partner in a shared, mutually interactive investigation (a patient doc tor mutually interactive reflection) (Parnas et al. 2005).

Acutely ill, severely psychotic patients with globally disordered attention and cognition should not be interviewed in this stage. The interview should be semistructured, and it is recommended that the process begin with a social interview.

On the basis of these assumptions, in recent years some semistructured interviews have been proposed, including the Examination of Anomalous Self-Experience (EASE; Parnas et al. 2005). The EASE is largely based on clinical and phenomenological aspects derived from many interviews with incipient schizophrenia spectrum patients. However, it was also inspired and informed by the classic psychopathological descriptions of these subtle pathological phenomena (e.g., in the work of Pierre Janet, Hans Gruhle, Joseph Berze, Eugène Minkowski, and Wolfgang Blankenburg) and the German research group of Gerd Huber, Gisela Gross, Joachim Klosterkötter, Frauke Schultze-Lutter, and their colleagues, who were the few modern psychiatric scientists who took the patient's subjective experience seriously and studied it systematically (for a brief review, see Lysaker and Lysaker 2010). These readings are useful for learning the specific terminology to build the interview, even if some of these terms may seem redundant or lacking in content validity or even appear to overlap.

The EASE was developed on the basis of self-description to assess cognition, stream of consciousness, and self-awareness. This scale can be used in a partially open manner or as a checklist, but its correct application requires specific training and an accurate knowledge of both the instrument and the underpinning theories. It may be very useful in monitoring the course of the treatment and in improving the self-esteem of the patient by reinforcing the fragmented identity (Thewissen et al. 2008).

Although considerable debate continues about the significance beyond the proximal outcomes, a cognitive-behavioral approach should be considered worthy of recommendation. In addition to social skills training and cognitive remediation, this approach should be considered a useful adjunct to pharmacotherapy (Hogan 2010).

Many patients continue to experience occasional or persistent symptoms that interfere with their everyday functioning (Kane 1999) during pharmacological treatment. Cognitive-behavioral therapy (CBT) has emerged as a valuable adjuvant to pharmacological treatment in schizophrenia, and this combination has been found to increase the probability of recovery (Lieberman et al. 2001). Moreover, from the patient's point of view, this individual psychotherapeutic approach has been shown, in most cases, to improve quality of life (Coursey et al. 1995).

The CBT intervention in psychotic patients should follow some basic but necessary principles. Because the patient may be expressing very private, sometimes peculiar thoughts and feelings, the clinician's first task is to support him or her: to not make the patient feel judged and to help him or her perceive that he or she is being understood. This goal is important for reinforcing the therapeutic alliance and helping the patient regain self-esteem.

The delusional experiences reported by the patient might be bizarre, but the clinician should maintain a "phenomenological attitude" and suspend judgment on these issues. Instead, he or she should look "back to the things themselves," to use philosopher Edmund Husserl's famous saying. That is, phenomenology is concerned with how the person actually experiences the world, not with theories that try to account for that experience (Wiggins et al. 1990). Thus, it might be possible to reformulate the meanings of such experiences from misperception and delusion to "disturbing belief." These goals could be considered the starting point of a CBT-oriented intervention in schizophrenia.

In the case of a schizophrenic patient, CBT intervention must be brief because psychotic patients seem to prefer problem-centered, short, and less-frequent sessions (Coursey et al. 1995). The intervention has to be clear, concise, and specific. Assessing the individual's cognitive, emotional, and language capabilities should be mandatory to better achieve the therapeutic goals. For example, if the patient has a significant language deficit, the clinician should focus primarily on nonverbal communication. The psychiatrist should appear open-minded and sincere, focusing the questions on the central matter and basing the intervention on the individual characteristics of the patient, such as coping capabilities or awareness of delusional experience. Any modifications to these phenomena should be promptly recognized, and the therapeutic approach should vary in accordance with them.

The clinical assessment, both at baseline and at follow-up, is an appropriate time to conduct a brief CBT intervention, which then should be performed at every monitoring visit.

A brief targeted CBT intervention in an outpatient monitoring setting should be focused on the main dysfunctional aspects. The psychiatrist should prioritize the intervention because the timing of an outpatient monitoring visit does not allow a wider intervention (Pinninti et al. 2005). Appropriate targets of the therapy could be the prevention of crisis exacerbation or hospitalization, the management of nonadherence issues, the reinforcement of the therapeutic alliance, and the improvement of coping strategies.

For example, patients who manifested a higher rate of disturbing basic symptoms 1 month before relapse showed less effective self-generated coping strategies, enhanced susceptibility to stressful events, and more severe cognitive impairment in comparison with patients who did not complain of these symptoms (Pallanti et al. 1997). This kind of patient in this phase of the disorder may represent an appropriate target for CBT crisis intervention and may benefit from learning about more functional coping strategies.

The cost-effectiveness of this approach is still under assessment, but recent results indicate that it varies according to the outcome (Fowler et al. 2009; Garety et al. 2008; Granholm et al. 2005, 2007; Lynch et al. 2010) and according to the characteristics of the sample included. The approach seems to be more indicated for patients at high risk of developing schizophrenia or those in the prodromal phase (Eack et al. 2010; Rietdijk et al. 2010).

Communication of the Diagnosis to Patients, Relatives, and Peers

Clinicians have a duty to give patients information in a way that is understandable to them. Therefore, the psychiatrist may decide how much information to give and how and when to give it but should not avoid the issue or presume that the patients do not want to know. Information about their illness is recommended in good practice statements and offers potential benefits, including better engagement with services (Bebbington and Ramana 1995; Foulks et al. 1986), improved knowledge (Smith et al. 1992), higher quality of life (Atkinson et al. 1996), and reduced negative symptoms (Goodman and Quinn 1988).

Uninformed patients may discover their diagnosis in a distressing way, such as on a form, at court, or when accessing their records (Atkinson 1984).

There can be risks and difficulties in informing patients who have schizophrenia. The risk of suicide, which is thought to be highest in the early phases of the illness and associated with insight (Amador et al. 1996; King 1994), must be assessed for each patient.

Table 4–10. Remission criteria for schizophrenia

Positive and Negative Syndrome Scale items (score 3 or less on all items for 6 months)

P1	Delusions
P2	Conceptual disorganization
P3	Hallucinatory behavior
G5	Mannerisms/posturing
G9	Unusual thought content
N1	Blunted affect
N4	Passive/apathetic social withdrawal
N6	Lack of spontaneity and flow of conversation

It is also important to consider that caring relatives and friends eventually need to know about the diagnosis, when possible, according to the clinical situation. This decision should be made in consideration of the patient's wishes and specific needs. Patients may be concerned about being labeled by relatives and friends. In this case, it may be useful to suggest that they keep the diagnosis private and discuss it only with the person involved in the prevention and treatment plan.

Finally, because the clinical assessment of the psychotic patient also includes an evaluation of the family setting in which he or she usually lives, the psychiatrist should take this opportunity to begin an intervention inspired by the same principles to give the family an active role in the therapeutic project. The task for the clinician is to identify and promote effective and functional behaviors or coping strategies that reinforce the patient and help keep the recovery process as straightforward as possible.

It is mandatory to provide a concept of schizophrenia (Süllwold and Herrlich 1992) and to assess the first-person experiences of the subjects involved while also conveying the important message that a state of remission can be achieved in a certain percentage of cases. This statement is based on the recent evidence that led to the development of specific operational criteria for remission (Andreasen et al. 2005) (see Table 4–10). This may help patients and their relatives to be more positive about the disorder and may provide the clinician with a more objective perspective of the course of the disorder. This information should be provided to both patients and relatives at the very beginning of treatment to develop common strategies to deal with this very painful human adversity.

References

Amador XF, Friedman JH, Kasapis C: Suicidal behavior in schizophrenia and its relationship to awareness of illness. Am J Psychiatry 153:1185–1188, 1996

American Psychiatric Association: Diagnostic and Statistical Manual of Mental Disorders, 4th Edition, Text Revision. Washington, DC, American Psychiatric Association, 2000

Andreasen NC: Negative symptoms in schizophrenia: definition and reliability. Arch Gen Psychiatry 39:784–788, 1982

Andreasen NC: The Scale for the Assessment of Positive Symptoms. Iowa City, University of Iowa, 1984

Andreasen NC, Carpenter WT Jr, Kane JM, et al: Remission in schizophrenia: proposed criteria and rationale for consensus. Am J Psychiatry 162:441–449, 2005

Atkinson JM: To tell or not to tell the diagnosis of schizophrenia. J Med Ethics 2:1–24, 1984

Atkinson JM, Coia DA, Gilmour WH, et al: The impact of education groups for people with schizophrenia on social functioning and quality of life. Br J Psychiatry 168:199–204, 1996

Bebbington P, Ramana R: The epidemiology of bipolar affective disorder. Soc Psychiatry Psychiatr Epidemiol 30:279–292, 1995

Bech P, Malt VF, Dencker SJ, et al: Scales for assessment of diagnosis and severity of mental disorders. Acta Psychiatr Scand 87 (suppl 372):35–40, 1993

Bowie CR, Harvey PD: Communication abnormalities predict functional outcomes in chronic schizophrenia: differential associations with social and adaptive functions. Schizophr Res 103:240–247, 2008

Braff DL, Freedman R, Schork NJ, et al: Deconstructing schizophrenia: an overview of the use of endophenotypes in order to understand a complex disorder. Schizophr Bull 33:21–32, 2007

Brunelin J, d'Amato T, Brun P, et al: Impaired verbal source monitoring in schizophrenia: an intermediate trait vulnerability marker? Schizophr Res 89:287–292, 2007

Buchanan RW, Heinrichs DW: The Neurological Evaluation Scale (NES): a structured instrument for the assessment of neurological signs in schizophrenia. Psychiatry Res 27:335–350, 1989

Carpenter WT Jr, Heinrichs DW, Wagman AM: Deficit and nondeficit forms of schizophrenia: the concept. Am J Psychiatry 145:578–583, 1988

Cohen LJ, Test MA, Brown RL: Suicide and schizophrenia: data from a prospective community treatment study. Am J Psychiatry 147:602–607, 1990

Collip D, Myin-Germeys I, Van Os J: Does the concept of "sensitization" provide a plausible mechanism for the putative link between the environment and schizophrenia? Schizophr Bull 34:220–225, 2008

Coursey RD, Keller AB, Farrell EW: Individual psychotherapy and persons with serious mental illness: the client's perspective. Schizophr Bull 21:283–301, 1995

Craddock N, Owen MJ: The Kraepelinian dichotomy—going, going…but still not gone. Br J Psychiatry 196:92–95, 2010

Cramer JA, Rosenheck R: Compliance with medication regimens for mental and physical disorders. Psychiatr Serv 49:196–201, 1998

Cuesta MJ, Ugarte MD, Goicoa T, et al: A taxometric analysis of schizophrenia symptoms. Psychiatry Res 150:245–253, 2007

Day JC, Bentall RP, Roberts C, et al: Attitudes toward antipsychotic medication: the impact of clinical variables and relationships with health professionals. Arch Gen Psychiatry 62:717–724, 2005

De Koning MB, Bloemen OJ, van Amelsvoort TA, et al: Early intervention in patients at ultra high risk of psychosis: benefits and risks. Acta Psychiatr Scand 119:426–442, 2009

Dikeos DG, Wickham H, McDonald C, et al: Distribution of symptom dimensions across Kraepelinian divisions. Br J Psychiatry 189:346–353, 2006

Eack SM, Hogarty GE, Cho RY, et al: Neuroprotective effects of cognitive enhancement therapy against gray matter loss in early schizophrenia: results from a 2-year randomized controlled trial. Arch Gen Psychiatry 67:674–682, 2010

Endicott J, Nee J, Harrison W, et al: Quality of Life Enjoyment and Satisfaction Questionnaire: a new measure. Psychopharmacol Bull 29:321–326, 1993

Farhall J, Greenwood KM, Jackson HJ: Coping with hallucinated voices in schizophrenia: a review of self-initiated strategies and therapeutic interventions. Clin Psychol Rev 27:476–493, 2007

Fisher M, McCoy K, Poole JH, et al: Self and other in schizophrenia: a cognitive neuroscience perspective. Am J Psychiatry 165:1465–1472, 2008

Foulks EF, Persons JB, Merkel RL: The effect of patients' beliefs about their illnesses on compliance in psychotherapy. Am J Psychiatry 143:340–344, 1986

Fowler D, Hodgekins J, Painter M, et al: Cognitive behaviour therapy for improving social recovery in psychosis: a report from the ISREP MRC Trial Platform Study (Improving Social Recovery in Early Psychosis). Psychol Med 39:1627–1636, 2009

Galderisi S, Maj M: Deficit schizophrenia: an overview of clinical, biological and treatment aspects. Eur Psychiatry 24:493–500, 2009

Garety PA, Fowler DG, Freeman D, et al: Cognitive behavioural therapy and family intervention for relapse prevention and symptom reduction in psychosis: randomised controlled trial. Br J Psychiatry 192:412–423, 2008

Goodman CR, Quinn FL: Effects of a patient education program in the treatment of schizophrenia. Hosp Community Psychiatry 39:282–286, 1988

Gottesman II, Gould TD: The endophenotype concept in psychiatry: etymology and strategic intentions. Am J Psychiatry 160:636–645, 2003

Granholm E, McQuaid JR, McClure FS, et al: A randomized, controlled trial of cognitive behavioral social skills training for middle-aged and older outpatients with chronic schizophrenia Am J Psychiatry 162:520–529, 2005

Granholm E, McQuaid JR, McClure FS, et al: Randomized controlled trial of cognitive behavioral social skills training for older people with schizophrenia: 12-month follow-up. J Clin Psychiatry 68:730–737, 2007

Green MF, Kern RS, Braff DL, et al: Neurocognitive deficits and functional outcome in schizophrenia: are we measuring the "right stuff"? Schizophr Bull 26:119–136, 2000

Gupta S, Black DW, Arndt S, et al: Factors associated with suicide attempts among patients with schizophrenia. Psychiatr Serv 49:1353–1355, 1998

Hasson-Ohayon I, Kravetz S, Meir T, et al: Insight into severe mental illness, hope, and quality of life of persons with schizophrenia and schizoaffective disorder. Psychiatry Res 167:231–238, 2009

Haynes RB, Taylor DW, Sackett DL: Compliance in Health Care. Baltimore, MD, Johns Hopkins University Press, 1979

Heinrichs DW, Buchanan RW: Significance and meaning of neurological signs in schizophrenia. Am J Psychiatry 145:11–18, 1988

Heinrichs DW, Hanlon TE, Carpenter WT: The Quality of Life Scale: an instrument for rating the schizophrenic deficit scale. Schizophr Bull 10:388–398, 1984

Hilty DM, Lim RF, Hales RE: The psychotic patient. Prim Care 26:327–348, 1999

Hogan M: Updated schizophrenia PORT treatment recommendations: a commentary. Schizophr Bull 36:104–106, 2010

Hogan TP, Awad AG, Eastwood R: A self report scale predictive of drug compliance in schizophrenics: reliability and discriminative validity. Psychol Med 13:177–183, 1983

Horan WP, Green MF, Kring AM, et al: Does anhedonia in schizophrenia reflect faulty memory for subjectively experienced emotions? J Abnorm Psychol 115:496–508, 2006a

Horan WP, Kring AM, Blanchard JJ: Anhedonia in schizophrenia: a review of assessment strategies. Schizophr Bull 32:259–273, 2006b

Kane M: Management strategies for the treatment of schizophrenia. J Clin Psychiatry 60:13–17, 1999

Kay SR, Fiszbein A, Opler LA: The Positive and Negative Syndrome Scale (PANSS) for schizophrenia. Schizophr Bull 13:261–276, 1987

Keefe RS, Eesley CE, Poe MP: Defining a cognitive function decrement in schizophrenia. Biol Psychiatry 57:688–691, 2005

Keefe RS, Poe M, Walker TM, et al: The Schizophrenia Cognition Rating Scale: interview-based assessment and its relationship to cognition, real-world functioning and functional capacity. Am J Psychiatry 163:426–432, 2006

King JG: Building a legacy for the future: creating an integrated health care system. Manag Care Q 2:35–49, 1994

Kirkpatrick B, Buchanan RW, McKenney PD, et al: The Schedule for the Deficit Syndrome: an instrument for research in schizophrenia. Psychiatry Res 30:119–123, 1989

Kirkpatrick B, Buchanan RW, Ross DE, et al: A separate disease within the syndrome of schizophrenia. Arch Gen Psychiatry 58:165–171, 2001

Kotov R, Guey LT, Bromet EJ, et al: Smoking in schizophrenia: diagnostic specificity, symptom correlates and illness severity. Schizophr Bull 36:173–181, 2010

Kraepelin E: Dementia Praecox and Paraphrenia. Translated by Barclay RM. Edited by Robertson GM. Edinburgh, Scotland, E & S Livingstone, 1919

Kupfer DJ, First MB, Regier DA: A Research Agenda for DSM-V. Washington, DC, American Psychiatric Association, 2002

Lacro JP, Dunn LB, Dolder CR, et al: Prevalence of and risk factors for medication nonadherence in patients with schizophrenia: a comprehensive review of recent literature. J Clin Psychiatry 63:892–909, 2002

Larkin W, Read J: Childhood trauma and psychosis: evidence, pathways, and implications. J Postgrad Med 54:287–293, 2008

Lewis L: Mourning, insight, and reduction of suicide risk in schizophrenia. Bull Menninger Clin 68:231–244, 2004

Lichtenstein P, Yip BH, Bjork C, et al: Common genetic determinants of schizophrenia and bipolar disorder in Swedish families: a population-based study. Lancet 373:234–239, 2009

Lieberman RP, Kopelowicz A, Ventura J, et al: Operational criteria and factors related to recovery from schizophrenia. Int Rev Psychiatry 14:256–272, 2001

Lincoln TM, Lullman E, Rief W: Correlates and long term consequences of poor insight in patients with schizophrenia: a systematic review. Schizophr Bull 33:1324–1342, 2007

Lipschitz DS, Kaplan ML, Sorkenn JB, et al: Prevalence and characteristics of physical and sexual abuse among psychiatric outpatients. Psychiatr Serv 47:189–191, 1996

Lynch D, Laws KR, McKenna PJ: Cognitive behavioural therapy for major psychiatric disorder: does it really work? A meta-analytical review of well-controlled trials. Psych Med 40:1–16, 2010

Lysaker PH, Lysaker JT: Psychosis and the disintegration of dialogical self-structure: problems posed by schizophrenia for the maintenance of dialogue. Br J Med Psychol 74:23–33, 2001

Lysaker PH, Lysaker JT: Schizophrenia and alterations in self-experience: a comparison of 6 perspectives. Schizophr Bull 36:331–340, 2010

Lysaker PH, Campbell K, Johannesen JK: Hope, awareness of illness, and coping in schizophrenia spectrum disorders: evidence of an interaction. J Nerv Ment Dis 193:287–292, 2005

Lysaker PH, Roe D, Yanos PT: Toward understanding the insight paradox: internalized stigma moderates the association between insight and social functioning, hope and self-esteem among people with schizophrenia spectrum disorders. Schizophr Bull 33:192–199, 2007

Malla A, Payne J: First-episode psychosis: psychopathology, quality of life, and functional outcome. Schizophr Bull 31:650–671, 2005

Marshall M, Lewis S, Lockwood A, et al: Association between duration of untreated psychosis and outcome in cohorts of first-episode patients: a systematic review. Arch Gen Psychiatry 62:975–983, 2005

Masson M, Azorin JM, Bourgeois ML: Awareness of illness in schizophrenic, schizoaffective, bipolar and unipolar mood disorders: results of a comparative study of 90 hospitalized patients. Ann Med Psychol 159:369–374, 2001

McCann E: Exploring sexual and relationship possibilities for people with psychosis—a review of the literature. J Psychiatr Ment Health Nurs 10:640–649, 2003

McGlashan TH, Miller TJ, Woods SW, et al: A scale for the assessment of prodromal symptoms and states, in Early Intervention in Psychotic Disorders. Edited by Miller TJ, Mednick SA, McGlashan TH, et al. Dordrecht, The Netherlands, Kluwer Academic, 2001, pp 135–150

Miller TJ, McGlashan TH, Woods SW, et al: Symptom assessment in schizophrenic prodromal states. Psychiatr Q 70:273–287, 1999

Modestin J, Huber A, Satirli E, et al: Long-term course of schizophrenic illness: Bleuler's study reconsidered. Am J Psychiatry 160:2202–2208, 2003

Moller HJ, Bottlender R, Wegner U, et al: Long-term course of schizophrenic, affective and schizoaffective psychosis: focus on negative symptoms and their impact on global indicators of outcome. Acta Psychiatr Scand Suppl 407:54–57, 2000

Morgan C, Fisher H: Environmental factors in schizophrenia: childhood trauma—a critical review. Schizophr Bull 33:3–10, 2007

Morosini PL, Magliano L, Brambilla L, et al: Development, reliability and acceptability of a new version of the DSM-IV Social and Occupational Functioning Assessment Scale (SOFAS) to assess routine social functioning. Acta Psychiatr Scand 101:323–329, 2000

Mundt C: Anomalous self-experience: a plea for phenomenology. Psychopathology 38:231–235, 2005

Naber D: A self-rating to measure subjective effects of neuroleptic drugs, relationships to objective psychopathology, quality of life, compliance and other clinical variables. Int Clin Psychopharmacol 10:133–138, 1995

Naber D, Moritz S, Lambert M, et al: Improvement of schizophrenic patients' subjective well-being under atypical antipsychotic drugs. Schizophr Res 50:79–88, 2001

Nuechterlein KH, Barch DM, Gold JM, et al: Identification of separable cognitive factors in schizophrenia. Schizophr Res 72:29–39, 2004

Ochsner KN, Knierim K, Ludlow DH, et al: Reflecting upon feelings: an fMRI study of neural systems supporting the attribution of emotion to self and other. J Cogn Neurosci 16:1746–1772, 2004

Overall JE, Gorham DR: The Brief Psychiatric Rating Scale. Psychol Rep 10:790–812, 1962

Pallanti S, Quercioli L, Pazzagli A: Relapse in young paranoid schizophrenic patients: a prospective study of stressful life events, P300 measures, and coping. Am J Psychiatry 154:792–798, 1997

Pallanti S, Quercioli L, Pazzagli A: Basic symptoms and P300 abnormalities in young schizophrenic patients. Compr Psychiatry 40:363–371, 1999

Parnas J, Møller P, Kircher T, et al: EASE: Examination of Anomalous Self-Experience. Psychopathology 38:236–258, 2005

Pini S, Cassano GB, Dell'Osso L, et al: Insight into illness in schizophrenia, schizoaffective disorder, and mood disorders with psychotic features. Am J Psychiatry 158:122–125, 2001

Pinninti NR, Stolar N, Temple S: 5-minute first aid for psychosis. Curr Psychiatry 1:36–48, 2005

Remington G, Foussias G, Agid O: Progress in defining optimal treatment outcome in schizophrenia. CNS Drugs 24:9–20, 2010

Rietdijk J, Dragt S, Klaassen R, et al: A single blind randomized controlled trial of cognitive behavioural therapy in a help-seeking population with an at risk mental state for psychosis: the Dutch Early Detection and Intervention Evaluation (EDIE-NL) trial. Trials 11:30, 2010

Roe D, Yanos PT, Lysaker PH: Coping with psychosis: an integrative developmental framework. J Nerv Ment Dis 194:917–924, 2006

Rosenberg SD, Lu W, Meuser KT, et al: Correlates of adverse childhood events among adults with schizophrenia spectrum disorders. Psychiatr Serv 58:245–253, 2007

Sanders RD, Allen DN, Forman SD, et al: Confirmatory factor analysis of the Neurological Evaluation Scale in unmedicated schizophrenia. Psychiatry Res 133:65–71, 2005

Saykin AJ, Shtasel DL, Gur RE, et al: Neuropsychological deficits in neuroleptic naive patients with first-episode schizophrenia. Arch Gen Psychiatry 51:124–131, 1994

Singh MM, Kay SR: A comparative study of haloperidol and chlorpromazine in terms of clinical effects and therapeutic reversal with benztropine in schizophrenia: theoretical implications for potency differences among neuroleptics. Psychopharmacologia 43:103–113, 1975

Smith J, Birchwood M, Haddrell A: Informing people with schizophrenia about their illness: the effect of residual symptoms. J Ment Health 1:61–70, 1992

Süllwold L: Frankfurter Beschwerde-Fragebogen, in Schizophrene Basisstoerungen. Edited by Suellwold L, Huber G. Berlin, Germany, Springer, 1986, pp 145–159

Süllwold L, Herrlich J: Providing schizophrenic patients with a concept of illness: an essential element of therapy. Br J Psychiatry Suppl 18:129–132, 1992

Tessner KD, Mittal V, Walker EF: Longitudinal study of stressful life events and daily stressors among adolescents at high risk for psychotic disorders. Schizophr Bull 37:432–431, 2011

Thewissen V, Bentall RP, Lecomte T, et al: Fluctuations in self-esteem and paranoia in the context of daily life. J Abnorm Psychol 117:143–153, 2008

Van Os J, Linscott RJ, Myin-Germeys I, et al: A systematic review and meta-analysis of the psychosis continuum: evidence for a psychosis proneness-persistence-impairment model of psychotic disorder. Psychol Med 39:179–195, 2009

Weiden PJ: Understanding and addressing adherence issues in schizophrenia: from theory to practice. J Clin Psychiatry 68 (suppl 14):14–19, 2007

Wiggins OP, Schwartz MA, Northoff G: Toward a Husserlian phenomenology of the initial stages of schizophrenia, in Philosophy and Psychopathology. Edited by Spitzer M, Maher BA. New York, Springer-Verlag, 1990, pp 19–34

World Health Organization: International Statistical Classification of Diseases and Related Health Problems, 10th Revision. Geneva, World Health Organization, 1992

Yung AR, McGorry PD: The initial prodrome in psychosis: descriptive and qualitative aspects. Aust N Z J Psychiatry 30:587–599, 1996

5

Cognition and Schizophrenia

Werner Strik, M.D.

Stephanie Schmidt, M.Sc.

Volker Roder, Ph.D.

It is difficult to define schizophrenia as a clinical disorder. The constituting signs and symptoms are heterogeneous with regard to their phenomenology and their frame of reference. They include phenomena as varied as errors of judgment, affective distortions (e.g., suspiciousness), semantic and associative errors, false perceptions, and psychomotor blockades. In some cases, the level of description is interpretative rather than descriptive (e.g., ego disturbances) and more or less implicitly refers to genetics, neurotransmitter biology, and brain plasticity after live events or to dysfunctional reactions, including cerebral hyperarousal.

Over a century of schizophrenia research, there have been many attempts to identify *core symptoms*—that is, basic phenomena that can be linked to a possible biological or psychological pathophysiology and at the same time account for the emergent clinical properties of the disorder. In this context, the concept of cognitive disorders in schizophrenia is broadly accepted, even if—or perhaps just for the reason that—it is very inclusive and lacks a unique theory and definition, as shown in the following chapters.

To understand the importance of cognitive disorders in schizophrenia, we briefly describe the history and definition of the concept of cognition. The roots of the concept can be found in St. Thomas Aquinas's theory of knowledge. He delimited the domain of cognition, describing truth and deception of perception, understanding, and knowledge of objects, and contrasted them to the phenomena of the emotional world (*passiones animae*). In early psychology and psychiatry, however, the term *cognition* was not used to describe functional or dysfunctional phenomena. The related psychological processes were attributed to the classical symptom domains of thought, judgment, or memory. Rather than cognition, the subjective sense of consciousness of a psychological process was considered to be relevant for the understanding of the pathophysiology of a psychiatric disorder.

We can identify some major steps in the theoretical development of psychology and psychiatry leading to what we may call the *cognitive paradigm,* which today is the dominating framework for psychotic disorders. In European psychiatry, the seminal work of Karl Jaspers moved the focus of interest from descriptive psychopathology and brain pathology to the understanding of intrapsychic, conscious phenomena. One of the landmarks of his phenomenological approach was the criterion of comprehensibility, which distinguished "primary" from "secondary" psychotic symptoms. According to his definitions, a delusion or hallucination is comprehensible and therefore "secondary" if it is congruent with the explicit affective state. "Primary" delusions, on the other hand, cannot be empathically understood by intra- or extrapsychic circumstances and qualify as typical for schizophrenia. Although this criterion is time-honored and still used in current international classifications, it includes an implicit, unproven assumption: if the content of a delusion is not congruent with the affective state, then Jaspers assumes that the primary disorder is an error of judgment (i.e., a cognitive dysfunction). The alternative hypothesis—that a primary, incomprehensible affective state (e.g., psychotic anxiety) can generate cognitive distortions in terms of delusions of existential threat—is not considered. This focus on a presumptive primary disorder of cognition at the basis of central schizophrenic psychopathology may have pioneered the cognitive paradigm.

In the early twentieth century, many theories and descriptions focused on conscious experience; the leading methods were psychoanalysis and phenomenological psychopathology. Skinner's radical critique of the current methodologies in the 1950s, however, described these approaches as nonscientific. In response, research methods were developed to allow empirical experiments, including controlled experimental conditions and objective measurements of behavior. Consequently, the object of research and the entire concept of cognition shifted essentially: studies were focused on objectively observable stimuli and reactions, while intrapsychic, conscious experiences referred by the subject (psychoanalysis) or empathized by an observer (phenomenological psychopathology) were understood as metaphysical phenomena (i.e., as the product of an immaterial mind) and considered to be inaccessible to empirical methods. This excessively technical and reductionistic conception of brain function was later replaced by the concept of information processing, in which neural activity was envisaged as the carrier of the information and objects were defined in terms of the contents and formats of the information, events and scopes relative to the process, and measurable inputs and outputs. This paradigmatic shift in psychology was also called "the cognitive revolution" (Pinker 2003).

Since then, a variety of research methods have been developed to study cognition in normal and dysfunctional psychology, and the theoretical frameworks have been adapted to the insights from computational science, artificial intelligence, and neuroscience. This diversification has opened a wide range of possible research strategies but, on the other hand, makes it more and more difficult to find a unique definition for cognition and the related disorders. Furthermore, the classical contraposition between cognition and emotions has been challenged in recent years. The term *cognition* today suffers from being used as a jumble of everything that can be approximately understood as information processing in the brain.

To understand what is known about cognition and schizophrenia, the concept of cognition must be approached from different levels of observation. In the following sections, we define and describe some of these levels, focusing on their clinical relevance and their importance to understand the pathophysiology of schizophrenia symptoms. Instead of referring to a unique definition, the frame of reference can be different according to the methodological and theoretical context and is specified respectively.

Importance of Cognition in Schizophrenia

Research on cognitive dysfunctions in schizophrenia has increased in the last three decades (Wykes and Reeder 2005). In the early period of this growth in research, experimental psychopathology identified a wide array of cognitive abnormalities associated with schizophrenia, ranging from elemental visual feature processing to attention, social judgment, and attribution (Chapman and Chapman 1973; Frith 1979, 1992; Hemsley 1977; Ruckstuhl 1981). The recognition of cognitive functions as core symptoms of schizophrenia is not new and dates back to Kraepelin (1913) and Bleuler (1911/1950), but the renewed interest in the 1970s and 1980s seemed to be driven by a shift in the understanding of schizophrenia, in which it was no longer seen as a neurodegenerative disorder but as a neurodevelopmental one. According to this model, cognitive impairments in schizophrenia reflect pre- or perinatally acquired structural and functional brain abnormalities. Another reason for the heightened interest in research on cognitive dysfunction was that new, widely accessible, noninvasive tools for measuring cognition were becoming available in the form of neuropsychological tests and functional methods, especially functional imaging (Murray et al. 1992; Wykes and Reeder 2005).

A central empirical finding in schizophrenia is that 75%–85% of all patients show long-lasting cognitive impairments in relation to healthy control subjects as well as to people with mood disorders (Bowie et al. 2008; Gray and Roth 2007). These impairments seem to be relatively independent of antipsychotic medication, duration of hospitalization, and clinical symptoms (Green and Nuechterlein 2004). The cognitive and affective impairments in schizophrenia have consistently been conceptualized as representing two distinct dimensions of the disorder (Strik et al. 1989). Despite the prevalence and severity of cognitive impairment in schizophrenia, no single type or profile characterizes the illness. Heterogeneity in both quality and severity of impairments is the rule. There is sufficient variability that cognitive measures can predict within-group differences on other dimensions, such as treatment compliance and risk of relapse in first-episode patients (Chen et al. 2005) and longer-term outcome in more chronically ill patients (e.g., Brekke et al. 2005; Norman et al. 1999; Peer and Spaulding 2007; M.L. Silverstein et al. 1994, 2002; Straube 1993). This means, for clinical purposes, that the assessment must be able to identify and characterize individual cognitive differences in people with schizophrenia and that treatment must be flexible enough to accommodate these differences (Roder et al. 2010).

Furthermore, systemic vulnerability models (e.g., Nuechterlein and Dawson 1984; Nuechterlein et al. 1994) stimulated new hypotheses about the etiological roles of these cognitive abnormalities as markers, endophenotypes, and expressions of the disease. The results of research in high-risk populations corresponded well with the postulations of these models: cognitive abnormalities were found in children at risk (e.g., Niendam et al. 2003; Osler et al. 2007) and in unaffected first-degree relatives (Dollfus et al. 2002). In longitudinal studies, in support of the vulnerability hypothesis, impaired attention and related information-processing deficits in children at risk for schizophrenia were related to eventual onset (Erlenmeyer-Kimling et al. 2000). Such abnormalities were also associated with impairments in social functioning in adulthood (Cornblatt et al. 1992). These deficits remain relatively stable during the course of the illness and hardly fluctuate with positive symptoms (Kurtz 2005; Rund et al. 2007; Wykes and van der Gaag 2001).

Cognition Research

Neurocognition

Neurocognition can be defined as information processing that entails processes of attributing, linking, and appraising information underlying human behavior. Figure 5–1 shows a general model of information processing.

Neurocognition describes how the stream of information is perceived, processed, and finally translated into observable behavior and explains where disturbances can occur. The sensory input is first held as an exact copy in the sensory memory (sensory register) for a few milliseconds and decoded into brain electrical signals. Selective attention determines which information is considered as relevant for the decision and consequently transferred to the short-term, also called working, memory. The information in the short-term memory is then compared with previous experiences and knowledge retrieved from long-term memory. Finally, the criteria for the goal attainment are set, and the selected response is carried out. The first information-processing steps on the left side of the model require perceptive and attentive functions, whereas executive functions are needed for planning and realizing a behavioral

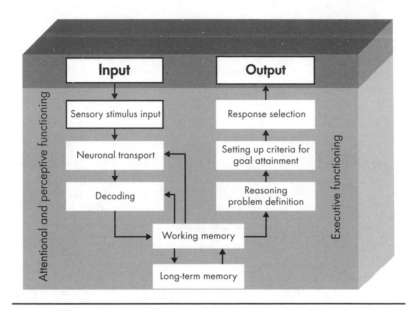

Figure 5–1.   General model of information processing.
Source.   Adapted from Roder et al. 2008.

response (Roder et al. 2008). A wide array of studies have shown that people with schizophrenia often experience impairments in several of the model components: in selective attention and vigilance (Birkett et al. 2007; Harris et al. 2007), working memory and explicit long-term memory (Aleman et al. 1999; Al-Uzri et al. 2006; Piskulic et al. 2007; Vance et al. 2007), and executive functions such as cognitive flexibility (Brüne et al. 2007), planning and problem solving (Huddy et al. 2007), and monitoring of behavior (Silver and Goodman 2007).

The lack of consensus about the relevant cognitive domains in schizophrenia and their assessment hampered the standardized evaluation of new treatments targeting cognitive deficits in schizophrenia. Therefore, the National Institute of Mental Health (NIMH) designed the Measurement and Treatment Research to Improve Cognition in Schizophrenia (MATRICS) Initiative to achieve a broad academic and industry consensus regarding the definition of the most important cognitive domains and to develop a reliable and valid cog-

nitive battery for use in clinical trials, especially for the evaluation of new pharmacological agents (Green and Nuechterlein 2004; Kern and Horan 2010;
Nuechterlein et al. 2004). Six separable neurocognitive areas or cognitive domains were consensually identified based on considerable deliberation of the
expert team and factor analyses (Green et al. 2005; Nuechterlein et al. 2004)
(see Figure 5–2).

1. **Speed of processing:** This domain emphasizes the speed of performance, including perceptual and motor components with which information is processed.
2. **Attention/vigilance:** Selective attention works as a filter, with the function of selecting information, prior to its further treatment, according
   to its importance. Insufficient filtering of the mass of information and a
   lack of inhibition of irrelevant stimuli, respectively, lead to an overflow
   of stimulation and a functional breakdown of thinking and feeling according to the context. The maintenance of attention over a longer time
   is referred to as *vigilance.*
3. **Working memory:** The verbal and nonverbal (visual and spatial) components of working memory are classified as executive functions and
   form the prerequisite for complex cognitive processes such as planning
   actions. Under an elevated level of stress or strain, schizophrenia patients
   experience an increasing limitation of working memory functions.
4/5. **Verbal and visual learning and memory:** In contrast to the short-term
   (working) memory, verbal and visual learning and memory—separately
   presented in the MATRICS Initiative—can be defined as the reception
   and long-term storage of verbal and nonverbal information in the long-
   term memory.
6. **Reasoning and problem solving:** In the literature, these domains are
   also subsumed as executive functions. It is helpful to distinguish between the working memory and complex strategies of planning and decision making.

The domain of social cognition (see Figure 5–2) was added despite a lack
of factor analytic support because of its theoretical meaning and increased importance in cognitive schizophrenia research (Nuechterlein et al. 2004).

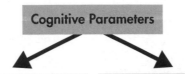

Neurocognition

- Speed of processing
- Attention/vigilance
- Working memory
- Verbal learning and memory
- Visual learning and memory
- Reasoning and problem solving

Social Cognition

- Emotion processing
- Social perception
- Theory of Mind (ToM)
- Social schemas
- Social attributions

Figure 5–2.   Cognitive parameters identified by the National Institute of Mental Health (NIMH) Measurement and Treatment Research to Improve Cognition in Schizophrenia (MATRICS) Initiative.
Source.   Adapted from Green et al. 2005; Nuechterlein et al. 2004.

Social Cognition

Schizophrenia is inherently seen as an interpersonal disorder in which difficulties result from the faulty construction of the social environment and one's role in it. Consequently, social cognitive processes of patients with schizophrenia have received increasing interest in the scientific community (Penn et al. 1997, 2006). The term *social cognition* is defined in various ways but generally refers to the mental operations that underlie social interactions, including the ability to perceive intentions and dispositions of others. In contrast to neurocognition, social cognition includes only information with social content (Brothers 1990; Green et al. 2005, 2008a).

A discussion group of researchers associated with the MATRICS Initiative established consensus on five relatively distinct types of social cognition (Green et al. 2005) (see Figure 5–2):

1. **Emotion processing:** Emotion perception or affect recognition is one domain of emotion processing, the process of perceiving and using emotions.

Impairments include slower and less accurate recognition of emotional stimuli and deficient regulation of emotional responses. Impairments tend to be more severe when the emotional content of processed information is more intense (e.g., Edwards et al. 2002; Hoekert et al. 2007).

2. **Social perception:** Patients show apprehension of key features of social situations and interactions. Impairments include deficient recognition of social cues and deficient processing of contextual information (e.g., Leonhard and Corrigan 2001).

3. **Theory of mind:** Patients have the ability to apprehend the mental and emotional states, perspectives, and intentions of others. Schizophrenic patients show difficulties understanding false beliefs, deception, irony, metaphors, or hints (e.g., Sprong et al. 2007).

4. **Social schemas:** Also called social knowledge, these bodies of declarative and procedural information guide social behavior. Scripts are particular types of schemas that contain information on social behavior appropriate to specific situations or circumstances. Impairments may represent deficient informational structures or deficient access to or execution of the information they contain (e.g., Corrigan and Penn 2001; Matsui et al. 2006).

5. **Social attributions:** A person formulates these causal explanations to understand social events and behaviors. Impairments may involve disproportionate or perseverative use of external personal attributions (causes attributed to other people), external situational attributions (causes attributed to situational factors), or internal attributions (causes attributed to oneself) (e.g., Bentall and Corcoran 2001; Martin and Penn 2002). Attributional impairments may overlap with emotion processing, social perception, and theory of mind impairments.

Today, investigators show increasing interest in social cognition, yet its history dates back much earlier when other terms were used. For example, in the 1950s to the 1980s, the role of the experimental and the social context on task performance (Cromwell and Spaulding 1978), the perception of stressful pictures (Buss and Lang 1965), social concept building (Whiteman 1954), and social reasoning processes (Gillis 1969) were investigated in schizophrenia. Although these early studies laid the groundwork, the results are questionable because of the lack of consensus on operational definitions of constructs and the lack of reliable tests (Penn et al. 1997).

Social cognition is relevant to current schizophrenia research in large part because social cognition is linked to basic neurocognition, clinical symptoms, and functional outcome and therefore may help shed light on the heterogeneity of symptoms and functional impairments in schizophrenia (Couture et al. 2006; Sergi et al. 2007; Green et al. 2008b). However, the notion that social cognition can be distinguished from basic neurocognitive functions and is best understood as a related but separate construct has gained increasing support (Couture et al. 2006; Green et al. 2008b), for the following reasons: 1) the correlations are only in the medium range (Wykes and Reeder 2005); 2) a specialized social cognitive network seems to exist (Brunet-Gouet and Decety 2006; Pinkham et al. 2008); 3) differential impairments in neurocognitive or social cognitive functions are possible (Pinkham et al. 2003); and 4) social cognition could explain the additional amount of variance in functional outcome that remains after control for neurocognitive functions (Addington et al. 2005; Pinkham and Penn 2006). Another reason for the importance of social cognition is that studies employing structural equation modeling suggest that social cognitive processes act as mediators between neurocognitive functions and functional outcome (e.g., Bell et al. 2008a; Brekke et al. 2005; Gard et al. 2009; Roder and Schmidt 2009; Schmidt et al. 2010; Sergi et al. 2006; Vauth et al. 2004). Therefore, integrated treatment programs are very promising (see subsection "Integrated Neurocognitive Treatments," later in this chapter).

Cognitive Assessment

Traditionally, the most important and concept-shaping method to study cognitive dysfunctions is neuropsychology. This method relies on experimental tests, which allow testing of performance in specific domains of psychic functions that can be attributed to the activity of definite brain regions. Validation of the tests was usually done in patients with circumscribed brain lesions. The advances in functional imaging allowed additional validations on the basis of activation experiments (Spring et al. 1991; Strauss et al. 2006).

Neuropsychological tests are essential for research and for clinical practice because they provide detailed information about type and degree of neurocognitive and social cognitive impairments. This is a prerequisite for the development of an individual profile of impairments, for indication to cognitive remediation therapy, and for therapy evaluation (Roder et al. 2008).

Table 5–1. MATRICS Consensus Cognitive Battery (MCCB)

Subdomain	Instrument(s)
Speed of processing	Brief Assessment of Cognition in Schizophrenia (BACS): Symbol-Coding
	Category Fluency: Animal Naming
	Trail Making Test: Part A
Attention/vigilance	Continuous Performance Test—Identical Pairs (CPT-IP)
Working memory	Wechsler Memory Scale—3rd Edition (WMS-III): Spatial Span (nonverbal)
	Letter-Number Span (verbal)
Verbal learning	Hopkins Verbal Learning Test—Revised (HVLT-R)
Visual learning	Brief Visuospatial Memory Test—Revised (BVMT-R)
Reasoning and problem solving	Neuropsychological Assessment Battery (NAB): Mazes
Social cognition	Mayer-Salovey-Caruso Emotional Intelligence Test (MSCEIT): Managing Emotions

Note. MATRICS = Measurement and Treatment Research to Improve Cognition in Schizophrenia.
Source. Adapted from Green et al. 2008a; Nuechterlein et al. 2008.

A major intention of the MATRICS Initiative was to choose specific neuropsychological tests for the cognitive domains mentioned earlier. An expert panel evaluated the degree to which each proposed test met specific selection criteria such as test-retest reliability and practicality (Green et al. 2008a; Nuechterlein et al. 2008). This led to the commercial availability of a standardized test battery, consisting of 10 instruments covering the seven measurement domains (MATRICS Consensus Cognitive Battery [MCCB], MATRICS Assessment, Inc.; see www.matricsinc.org/MCCB.htm). The domains and specific instruments in the consensus battery are shown in Table 5–1.

As research on social cognition in schizophrenia accelerates and expands, the need for systematic and standardized assessment of all defined social cognitive domains will intensify. Moreover, the MCCB also must show its practical value in clinical work and in different cultures in the future. Therefore, we provide an overview of some neuropsychological tests that are very often used for the assessment of neurocognitive and social cognitive impairments and may be a helpful complement to the MCCB.

- **Trail Making Test Parts A and B** (Reitan 1992): This paper-and-pencil test can be administered very easily and assesses speed of processing. The participant has to connect circled numbers and/or letters in ascending order as fast as possible.

- The most prominent measures of attention/vigilance are various (mainly computerized) versions of the **Continuous Performance Test (CPT)**. This sustained attention task was originally developed by Rosvold et al. (1956) and refined for schizophrenia research (Nuechterlein 1983). Every time a given target appears, the subject must immediately press a response button without getting distracted by other symbols.

- Cognitive flexibility as well as reasoning and problem solving are often measured by the **Wisconsin Card Sorting Test (WCST;** Heaton et al. 1993). The computerized version (Loong 1989) asks the subjects to match a maximum of 128 stimulus cards to 4 key cards. Cards can be matched according to three rules (color, number, form). The rule is changed without the patient's knowledge after 10 consecutive cards.

- The **Pictures of Facial Affect Test (PFA;** Ekman and Friesen 1976; Wölwer et al. 1996) entails 24 black-and-white photos of faces demonstrating different emotions on a screen. Each of the basic emotions (happiness, anger, fear, disgust, surprise, sadness, neutral) appears twice in the test. The participant has to mark the correct emotion by a mouse click.

- The **Schema Component Sequencing Task—Revised (SCST-R;** Corrigan and Addis 1995; German version: Vauth et al. 2004) is a computerized measure for social schema. It examines the recognition of temporal sequences of component actions in 12 specific social situations (e.g., asking for a salary increase, going to the movies). Subjects are asked to arrange them in the right order.

- To assess social attributions and social reasoning, the **Ambiguous Intentions Hostility Questionnaire** (Combs et al. 2007b) is a suitable test. Five social situations are described, and the participant needs to put himself or herself in each situation and to infer the other's intentions.

As for neurocognition, the definition of social cognition and the necessary contributing skills is a compromise between different psychological concepts. Furthermore, it depends on the coverage of the available tests. For example, a test measuring the recognition of emotional facial expression will suggest mimic recognition as a domain of social cognition. The presented examples of consensus-oriented domains are an interesting approach to focus the variety of psychological tests and theories on cognition onto the demands of schizophrenia research. A critique from the clinical point of view is the scarce evidence of how the cognitive impairments are psychologically related to the typical schizophrenic symptoms and of their diagnostic value. Neuroscience, on the other hand, has contributed to visualize possible related networks that are characteristically activated during specific cognitive tasks. It appears necessary, however, to collect further data that allow formulation of unifying theories of the underlying anatomy and brain system dynamics.

Electrophysiology

Electrophysiology was the first technique that allowed measuring biological correlates of the working brain, including cognitive processing. The early electroencephalogram (EEG) methods gave fascinating real-time patterns of electrical activity, modulated by brain pathology but also by mental operations. Many of the main principles of brain electric activity were already shown in the pioneer years of the method (e.g., that focal slow-wave activity was related to damaged brain tissue, spikes and spike-wave activity to epilepsy, 8–12 Hz alpha activity to closed-eye resting state, and fast beta activity to cognitive activity).

The value of the real-time measurements of brain activity and its modulation by cognition was, however, severely reduced by two limitations of the method: the physical impossibility of calculating the unique source of surface potentials in the brain space (i.e., the inverse problem) and the low signal-to-noise ratio in cognitive experiments. Both problems could be successfully addressed only when computer technologies became available. The methodological breakthroughs allowed by computer processing of digitized EEG signals were obtained by averaging repeated measurements related to sensory stimulations or cognitive operations (evoked potentials), the two dimensional representation of the brain electrical field distributions (brain mapping) (Lehmann 1989) and its temporal segmentation, the functional coupling of distant brain regions (coherence and 40 Hz activity) (Engel et al. 2001; Pfurtscheller and Andrew 1999; Rappelsberger et al. 1994; Singer and Gray 1995), the temporal segmentation of EEG into periods with stable topography (microstates) (Lehmann et al. 1987), and the modeling of the possible electrical source localizations in the three-dimensional brain space (Pascual-Marqui et al. 2002). In the following subsections, we summarize the value of each of the most important electrophysiological methods in cognition research.

Electroencephalography

The ongoing EEG has been consolidated as a valid instrument for the assessment of functional brain pathology and is currently used routinely for the diagnosis and monitoring of epileptic and functional organic brain disease. Furthermore, it is a low-cost screening instrument for local brain pathologies and for the functional changes related to degenerative brain diseases.

In cognition research, electroencephalography has contributed interesting insights. Progressive cognitive decline in dementia correlates with a general increase of slow-wave activity, an anteriorization of the alpha waves from the physiological occipital to central and frontal areas, and a shortening of the brain electrical microstates (Chiaramonti et al. 1997). In normal psychology, the EEG frequencies reflect different states of consciousness, although no precise boundaries exist. Delta and theta rhythms are associated with sleep and drowsiness, and alpha rhythms are associated with relaxed wakefulness; beta and higher frequencies appear during mental concentration and arousal.

Evoked and Event-Related Potentials

Information processing, including external stimuli, mental operations, or task execution, can cause measurable, systematic changes in the EEG signal. These changes are superimposed on the main frequencies. Time-locked averaging of the EEG periods related to the stimulus or to mental or behavioral events allows enhancement of the signal-to-noise ratio and generation of evoked (after simple sensory stimulation) or event-related (before or after mental or behavioral events) potentials.

According to the stimulation paradigm and the brain electrical response, several specific types of evoked potentials have gained importance in cognition research and have contributed interesting insights into schizophrenic pathophysiology. With a few exceptions, evoked and event-related potentials are classified according to the polarity of the averaged signal and to the time in milliseconds after the sensory stimulation or task presentation, respectively. Interestingly, this classification reliably distinguishes most conditions of the potentials in terms of cognitive processing speed and load and the implied sensory modality. In general, short latencies up to approximately 150 ms have been reliably related to simple sensory processing in the thalamus and in primary sensory cortex regions. Longer latencies up to approximately 350 ms, like the P300 potential, are associated with the cognitive discrimination of simple stimuli. Later potentials, like the N400 potential, appear during the cognitive processing of complex information.

In the following discussion, we introduce the most important evoked and event-related potentials and their significance for cognition. The P50 potential has very short latency. It is evoked by simple auditory clicks. Paired presentation of the clicks reduces the amplitude of the P50 response to the second click. This inhibition of an early neurophysiological response is interpreted as an expression of sensory gating, presumably involving the thalamus. Consistent abnormalities of this evoked potential have been found, which are thought to reflect a sensory filter deficit (Light and Braff 2003).

About 100 ms after auditory or visual stimulation, higher-amplitude potentials appear in temporal (N100) or occipital (P100) regions, which are related to the activity of the respective primary cortex. In particular, the amplitudes of auditory N100 have been investigated as a marker of attention and of early discrimination between different sensory stimuli. The latter is usually investigated, relying on a subtraction procedure between the reaction to a regular tone and the reaction to a deviant tone, which results in a difference wave called *mismatch negativity* (Naatanen et al. 2005).

Conscious discrimination tasks of simple auditory or visual stimuli evoke a characteristic potential with large amplitudes in the central region after about 300 ms, called P300. This potential has been extensively studied because it is influenced by the stimulus modality, the particular discrimination task, the required mental (e.g., silent counting) or behavioral (e.g., a button press) response, and several organic and functional brain disorders. In contrast to the earlier evoked potentials, not only latencies and amplitudes but also the spatial distribution of the related brain electrical field are significantly influenced by different cognitive aspects of the paradigm. In schizophrenia, typical findings are spatial distortions with left hemispheric deficits (Strik et al. 1994), linked to language-related deficits (Heidrich and Strik 1997) and signs of a generalized hyperarousal in acute remitting psychoses (cycloid psychoses) (Strik et al. 1997, 1998).

Among the long-latency event-related potentials, the N400 has gained particular interest in the study of language-related cognition and of disorders of higher-order brain functions. The N400 potential is evoked by verbal nonsense (i.e., a semantic error). A typical example is the sentence "The sky is green" where the N400 potential appears after the word "green." The potential is distributed broadly over the scalp and is modulated by a series of different experimental and clinical conditions. In schizophrenia, studies have indicated that N400 abnormalities are related to semantic processing (Mathalon et al. 2002) and thought disorders (Kostova et al. 2005).

For a review of the experimental settings and some of the clinical implications of mismatch negativity, P300, and N400, the reader is referred to Duncan et al. (2009).

Two types of slow brain electrical potentials that precede an event have a particular role in cognition research. The *contingent negative variation (CNV)* appears after a warning stimulus that precedes a second, imperative stimulus requiring a specific action (e.g., button press). The CNV is therefore a correlate of the mental preparation to a preannounced prompt for action—the mental state of a sprinter waiting for the starter's gun (Tecce 1971).

The second well-studied brain electrical phenomenon measurable before a motor action is the *readiness potential.* The difference from the CNV is that the readiness potential does not appear before a preannounced trigger stimulus but before a self-initiated movement. This potential has gained particular new interest in the context of the debate on the existence of a free will. In the 1980s, Libet et al. (1983) showed that the readiness potential preceded not only the motor action itself but also the subjective moment of decision to perform the action. This was interpreted as an indication that the neuronal activity is determining the will, and not vice versa. Consequently, the subject would have only the subjective sensation of having the freedom to decide but in reality would be a slave of his or her neuronal activity. Even if this reasoning appears somewhat tautological and circular, and is based on the unproven assumption that the readiness potential is the equivalent of the decision to act, it has initiated a fruitful public debate on determinism of human behavior, which involves neuroscience, law, humanities, education, and theology. The argument substitutes in modern terms the eternal yet irresolvable questions of the existence of an immaterial soul and of the legal and moral responsibility of one's own actions.

Electroencephalogram Microstates

The segmentation of the EEG into periods with similar topography has shown that the 2-dimensional activation patterns do not change continuously but remain stable for an average of 140 ms, up to several hundred milliseconds. These periods have been called *brain electrical microstates*. The changes from one pattern to the following, however, are very rapid. The continuous spatial stability of a brain electrical field strongly indicates that it is generated by the activity of the same network. Furthermore, the average time of stability of the fields is similar to the times known by psychological experiments (e.g., Sternberg paradigm) about the duration of basic cognitive operations. The brain electrical microstates therefore have been proposed to be the "atoms of thought"—that is, to reflect the dynamic network activity during information processing, which probably consists of the sequential activity of different brain systems (cognitive modules) with variable processing times that generate the alternating characteristic spatial activation patterns (Lehmann et al. 1987, 2006; Strik and Lehmann 1993).

Experimental studies have supported this hypothesis. It has been shown that the spatial configuration of the related brain electrical microstates differed between various internal modalities of cognition, particularly between abstract (i.e., dominantly language related) and visual contents of thought (Lehmann et al. 2006).

Coherence, Neuronal Coupling, and the Gamma Band

Higher brain activities such as cognitive processing are believed to rely on networks involving the contemporaneous activation of distant brain regions. The only physiological neural mechanism suitable to orchestrate such an activity with the pace necessary to bridge several centimeters in a millisecond is electrical signal transmission through axons and dendrites. This simple consideration explains basic conditions and mechanisms for large-scale functional networks. It must be assumed that such networks can be assembled only if the necessary axonal "hardwiring" (i.e., direct or indirect fiber connections) is present. These connections should be traceable with adequate methods in the white matter of the brain. Furthermore, for every specific cognitive task, the electrical signal selectively couples appropriate specialized brain regions; information is then transferred in the form of electrical signal patterns. To simplify, the radio paradigm can be applied for this process. The functional coupling is induced by a specific carrier frequency, and the information is exchanged by patterns of frequency modulation.

The described functional features of large-scale networks help to understand some of the relative constraints of the available brain imaging techniques. Positron emission tomography (PET), single-photon emission computed tomography (SPECT), and functional magnetic resonance imaging (fMRI) detect metabolic transmitter changes, secondary to the network activity; they are biased by general fluctuations of the metabolic state and, because of their relatively slow reaction times, by temporal overlaps of activity. Electrophysiology is able to detect the real-time information transduction within the brain; however, the measured signals are summary for big volumes and therefore ambiguous with regard to the origin and composition (direction and polarity) of the contributing brain electrical potentials (i.e., action potentials; excitatory and inhibitory presynaptic potentials).

Despite these constraints, modern electrophysiology has contributed to the understanding of the dynamics of large-scale functional networks in terms of possible mechanisms of synchronizing distant brain regions. Two methods deserve particular attention. The first is the *coherence measurement* of traditional EEG frequencies, which investigates so-called phase-locked frequencies. It measures the EEG frequencies with several electrodes at the scalp and detects phase synchrony of traditional frequency bands between distant brain regions. The assumption is that the underlying neuronal processes are functionally coupled if they oscillate synchronously. Such a pattern of cross-correlations should allow inferences about the active large-scale networks (Pfurtscheller and Andrew 1999). Many studies show the coherence patterns during normal and pathological cognition. A particularly interesting question for schizophrenia research addressed by this method is *corollary discharge* (i.e., the equivalent of a universal neural mechanism to monitor the individual's own actions). This phenomenon has been described in animals and consists of functional coupling of motor with sensory regions. Furthermore, it is assumed to prepare the sensory regions to receive inputs from stimuli generated by the individual's own actions. In other words, the cortical motor regions instantaneously inform the sensory regions about their current outputs so that these can be immediately expected and perceived as intentional by the system. The relevance in schizophrenia research is evident, because corollary discharge offers a possible mechanism for the disorder's self-monitoring and ego disturbances; that is, the fact that patients experience their own thoughts and actions as alien, resulting in phenomena such delusions and hallucinations (Ford and Mathalon 2008).

The second method of neuronal coupling that has received particular attention is the *gamma band* (i.e., high EEG frequencies around 40 Hz). Much more than the traditional EEG frequencies, this has become accepted as a possible mechanism for functionally harnessing neurons to networks. The gamma band has been an important breakthrough in reasoning about how neurons can cooperate at a higher order of complexity. Gamma band abnormalities have been proposed as possible endophenotypes of schizophrenia (Light et al. 2006; Salisbury et al. 2008).

Source Localization

The major problem of brain electrical source localization is irresolvable. The electrical signals of the neurons add up to the potentials measurable at the scalp. The way back is mathematically ambiguous because a potentially infinite combination of events can generate the same result. In physics, this limitation is known as the *inverse problem*, which indicates that it is mathematically impossible to calculate the single components from a sum of events.

However, methods allow valid calculations for the constituting sources of brain electrical events. These methods restrict the possible solutions based on a priori knowledge of the events. These constraints can be as trivial as the assumption that the source is localized in the brain space; they can be based on physiological facts (e.g., that neighboring neurons tend to fire synchronously); or they may use information from other methods about the involved brain structures during specific tasks. Although the calculated source locations cannot be definitely confirmed by these methods alone, they may be validated with other functional imaging methods. This has been extensively and successfully done in particular for the low-resolution brain electromagnetic tomography (LORETA) source modeling method (Pascual-Marqui et al. 2002).

Functional Imaging

Functional imaging is today the leading method for the investigation of cognition. Very different measurement methods allow imaging of functional changes during cognitive brain events. Among these are SPECT and PET, electrophysiological brain mapping and 3-dimensional source modeling, and near-infrared spectroscopy, and there have even been attempts to visualize cognitive performance by mapping the results of comprehensive neuropsychological test batteries on the cortex. The most accessible and at the same time exceptionally variable method is MRI. Many techniques allow measuring: for example, local blood oxygenation changes in real time (blood oxygen level–dependent changes; BOLD), the local perfusion (arterial spin labeling), the degree of directedness of white matter including fiber tracking (diffusion tensor imaging; DTI), and the local concentrations of specific molecules and transmitters (magnetic resonance spectroscopy).

Single-Photon Emission Computed Tomography

SPECT relies on the direct gamma irradiation of a radionuclide. In brain imaging, technetium (^{99m}Tc) hexamethylpropyleneamine oxime (HMPAO) is the most used because it is taken up by brain tissue proportional to brain blood flow. SPECT has a rather low spatial resolution of about 1 cm but is less expensive than PET and relies on less expensive machines, and the radioisotope generation is longer-lasting and less expensive. For the study of cognition, SPECT is very limited by the technical constraints of the experimental setting, the radioactive load, and the low temporal resolution, which is in the range of minutes.

Positron Emission Tomography

PET relies on the injection of a radioactive tracer that binds to specific molecules of the brain. It is not invasive but implies exposure to ionizing radiation. The gamma photon emission caused by the positrons emitted during the decay of the tracer is measured by the PET scanner. This allows imaging the local concentrations of the tracer, which depends on the concentration of molecules to which it is specifically binding. The particular appeal of the method for psychiatry is that specific radioligands can reflect the local energy consumption, with the glucose analogue fluorodeoxyglucose (FDG), and even local receptor densities of important neurotransmitters such as dopamine, serotonin, and opioids. In psychopharmacology, PET is used to see local receptor occupancy of new drugs that can be directly radiolabeled for animal studies or to investigate the competition of the studied drug with known tracers.

Magnetic Resonance Imaging

In the past two decades, MRI has contributed essentially to the understanding of cognitive processes. The first and still most applied technique is the BOLD method, which measures the regional changes in blood oxygenation. It has a very good spatial resolution in the millimeter range and a temporal resolution that is approximately real time for the observed phenomenon (i.e., the oxygenation change that occurs in the range of some seconds). fMRI is therefore very useful for the investigation of cognitive processes and of the related large-scale networks. The limitations depend on the measured parameter (local blood oxygenation), which is secondary to the electrical signal transduction; furthermore, the main effect is not directly related to the increase of oxygen consumption by neuronal activity but to the increase of oxygenated blood resulting from the local vessel reaction to hypoxia. Despite these theoretical limitations, fMRI has been proved to be extremely useful in normal and pathological cognition research and has yielded insights that appeared unreachable until one or two decades ago.

More recently, a new MRI technique, called DTI, has been developed that, strictly speaking, is not functional but structural. However, it is of particular interest in cognition research because it allows investigating the "hardwiring" (i.e., the fiber connections between distant brain regions). Major methodological limitations remain in understanding the physiological meaning of the signal changes in the white matter. However, increasing evidence indicates that the results can be used to study changes of white matter organization related to brain pathology and plasticity. Furthermore, methodological developments allow tracing fibers through the white matter with possible important insights about the pathways underlying the information exchange between distant brain regions. DTI measures the molecular movement that is restricted by cell membranes of the axons and therefore tends to be limited to their direction. The more the movement is directed in one dimension, the higher is the DTI signal (fractional anisotropy).

The limitation of fMRI to detect only relative blood oxygenation changes is important for the study of task-unrelated resting states and of absolute group differences. Arterial spin labeling is an MRI method that allows measuring the regional brain perfusion in absolute values and therefore the investigation of the basic metabolism in different pathological conditions without the need for an activating experimental paradigm. The spatial resolution is still lower than that of BOLD MRI, and the recording time is longer. However, for schizophrenia research, it has already been proved as a useful tool to investigate symptom- or syndrome-related metabolic changes and to compare them with those of other disorders.

Combination of Methods

The traditional approach of cognition research is to relate neuropsychological test results to diagnostic groups or clinically relevant features. With the increasing possibilities to study the underlying brain processes, neuropsychological tests have been combined with biological measurements such as neurophysiology or fMRI. Recent technical advances have allowed different biological measurements to be combined with new perspectives for the investigation of cognition. Of particular interest is the co-registering of fMRI and EEG or evoked potentials with their complementary spatial and temporal resolution (Jann et al. 2009; Muller et al. 2005).

Cognition and Schizophrenic Psychopathology

Consciousness, Cognition, and Psychotic Symptoms

In the field of schizophrenic psychopathology, disorders of cognition are described in terms of thought, perception, and self-consciousness. All of these terms explicitly refer to conscious, intrapsychic experiences. This is also the case for the domain of distorted perceptions, particularly for the typical auditory hallucinations and the ego disturbances. Especially in the case of thought disorders, the actual object of observation and its assessment are ambiguous. In fact, formal thought disorders do not refer to the subjective experience of thinking, as the term *thought* suggests, but primarily to structural abnormalities of spoken language.

Formal Thought Disorders

Formal thought disorders consist of syntactic, grammatical, associative, semantic, and logical errors, which are assessed by an examiner. Furthermore, the quantity of content and the speed of spoken language are considered. The implicit equation of these speech disorders to disorders of thought is, however, an unproven inference and should be handled with caution. At most, it appears legitimate to hypothesize that the formal disorders of spoken language may reflect similar dysfunctions in inner speech and silent verbal reasoning. As a matter of fact, patients do not necessarily feel their thoughts to be disordered.

Some refer to having too many ideas that they are not able to communicate or to feeling perplexed or confused. A further problem for cognitive psychology is that nothing is known about the relation between the classic psychopathological concept of formal thought disorder and other modalities of thinking such as operational planning, visual imagery, or mental arithmetic.

In recent years, increasing evidence for language-related dysfunctions in schizophrenia has been reported. In the wake of initial findings of associations between neuropsychological and neurophysiological abnormalities and impaired language-related performance in schizophrenia, several studies have shown that psychological dysfunctions and disorders in brain regions involved in the language system are most consistently related to the symptom complex of formal thought disorders. In particular, left hemispheric reductions in the event-related P300 potential were correlated with impaired performance on verbal memory tasks and with formal thought disorder (Heidrich and Strik 1997; Strik et al. 2008).

The pathophysiology of formal thought disorders appears to be related to a dynamic dysregulation of the left frontotemporal language system rather than to a local disorder of one single brain region or of an entire transmitter system. In functional activation studies, in fact, a reduced responsivity of left superior-posterior temporal regions has been described that was more pronounced in patients with more severe formal thought disorders (Kircher et al. 2001). In a recent combined perfusion and volumetric study (Horn et al. 2009), the gray matter in left temporal regions, corresponding to the Wernicke's area, was reduced in patients with severe formal thought disorders. Furthermore, the resting perfusion in both the left Broca's region and Wernicke's area correlated with the severity of formal thought disorders and reached values up to three times higher than normal (Horn et al. 2009). Such abnormally high perfusion values have been reported in neurological disorders such as migraine and epilepsy. At the current state of knowledge, this dysregulation pattern in formal thought disorder can be summarized as follows: A local reduction of gray matter in the sensory language area is related to a state of hyperexcitation of the left frontotemporal language system. The hyperactive system is less responsive to external activation, possibly because of a ceiling effect (i.e., there are no more perfusion reserves). At the behavioral level, this hyperactivity corresponds to a quantitatively sufficient or even increased language production along with the typical structural errors.

The combination of a local volume reduction and a hyperactivity of the entire system allows the hypothesis that a local dystrophy is the pathological trait at the basis of chronic or periodic states of language-related disorders in some schizophrenic patients. The trait may be responsible for both the negative symptoms such as alogia and perplexity and the positive symptoms such as logorrhea, incoherence, and derailments during states of functional excitation. It has not been clarified yet, however, whether the state of hyperactivity is triggered by a local disinhibition caused by the loss of γ-aminobutyric acid (GABA)ergic interneurons or by a compensatory hyperactivation driven by superordinate brain regions.

As described earlier, our current knowledge of the pathophysiology of formal thought disorders suggests that they are likely to refer to the specific domain of verbal communication (i.e., speech and language understanding) and verbal cognition (i.e., inner speech, logical reasoning, verbal associations, and meaning). This type of cognition can be understood as verbal imagery that follows the rules and contents of language. Consequently, formal thought disorders are central for social interactions as well as for verbal description and logical analysis of reality.

In a group of psychotic patients, the presence and severity of symptoms were rated on a psychopathological scale that also assigned each psychotic behavioral disorder to one of three system-specific domains: language, affectivity, or motor activity (Figure 5–3). These domains were defined on the basis of the relevance for interpersonal interactions and their reasonable affiliation to a brain system. The investigated domains and the respective candidate systems were language, affectivity, and motor activity. The principal components analysis of the data identified the three domains as major components from the symptom pool and showed that these domains had a certain degree of independence from one another (Strik et al. 2010). This means that in some patients, language-related symptoms—especially formal thought disorders—are predominant, whereas in others, motor or emotional symptoms prevail. This result indicates that subgroups of psychotic patients exist and that these subgroups are related to dysregulated brain systems that are important for interpersonal communication. In addition, this observation allows the individual symptomatology to be circumscribed in terms of defining the prevailing domain of psychotic communication.

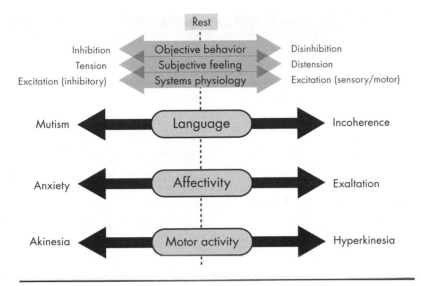

Figure 5–3. Bern Psychopathology Scale of systems-specific symptoms.
Upper part: deviations from resting state, referred to the level of observation. *Lower part:* deviations from normal communication behavior in three systems-specific domains, in terms of negative and positive symptom groups.
Source.   Strik et al. 2010.

Delusions

Another central symptom in schizophrenia is a delusion. Delusions are traditionally considered as disorders of thought content. Similar to formal thought disorders, however, delusions are assessed by an external observer who states that the patient has verbally communicated an erroneous conviction and that he or she is not able to consider alternative explanations. This criterion (i.e., that the erroneous subjective judgment defines the symptom) is, with the exception of neglect, probably unique in medicine; it excludes by definition that the patient can consider the symptom as an expression of a disorder. Nonverbal behavior, however, cannot be used by an observer as proof for delusional convictions. Although such inferences are sometimes used in clinical practice, they are highly speculative.

The presumptive intrapsychic disorder of thought is, in the case of delusions, an uncorrectable error of judgment. In classic psychopathology, this phenomenon cannot be explained by another psychic disorder. It is therefore considered a primary pathological phenomenon. This view states that delusions depend on a cognitive disorder (i.e., an error of logical reasoning) and contains the implicit assumption that eventual emotions are secondary or independent. This causal relation has never been proved, however, and indications are that some delusions may be intimately and consistently linked to pathological emotional states.

In fact, the delusion often consists of an existential threat or, on the contrary, outstanding personal abilities. Both types of content are of extraordinary affective relevance. Furthermore, logical reasoning is not only erroneous but also severely narrowed. Patients focus and overvalue the idiosyncratic content and exclude alternative interpretations. This pattern is typical for exceptional affective states. Finally, paranoid delusions are often associated with aggressive or sensitive avoidance behavior that can be easily interpreted as the human equivalent of fight or flight reactions, respectively. Thus. researchers have sound reasons to assume that some of the most typical schizophrenic delusions are in fact closely related to abnormal affective states and therefore also related to the activity of the limbic system. This has been confirmed by the earlier cited study, which reported that affectively relevant delusions actually covary with affective symptoms rather than with formal thought disorders (Strik et al. 2010).

An alternative interpretation therefore appears appealing: these affective states might be the primary disorder, in terms of a pathological limbic dysregulation. Consistently, recent studies indicate that dysfunctions in the striatal dopamine and the limbic system are a possible hub for paranoid symptoms such as delusional mood and threatening delusions (Heinz and Schlagenhauf 2010). Such dysfunctions could explain both the cognitive restriction as a physiological consequence of the state of affective hyperarousal and the logical distortion as a psychological reaction, adopting even absurd and inapprehensible explanations and false objectives for one's actions in a desperate attempt to control the unbearable affective state.

Hallucinations

Hallucinations are subjective sensory perceptions without the corresponding physical stimulation. They can occur in any sensory modality. In global organic damage of the brain, more or less structured hallucinations are most frequent in the visual, followed by the acoustic and tactile modality. It is re-markable, therefore, that in schizophrenia the most frequent and characteris-tic hallucinations occur in the auditory modality. Furthermore, the typical hallucinations contain speaking voices and only rarely less structured sounds or music. This pattern is similar to excitatory dysfunctional patterns involving brain regions that are part of function-specific brain systems rather than dys-functions of distributed transmitter systems or global brain noxae. In the case of the typical schizophrenic "speaking voices," it is intriguing to understand them as an excitatory dysfunction of the language system. This pathophysio-logical interpretation was formulated as early as in the 1900 edition of Carl Wernicke's textbook of psychiatry (Wernicke 1900).

Only a century later, the necessary methods were available to corroborate this hypothesis. First results from electrophysiological brain mapping in the late 1980s indicated a left temporal hyperactivity in terms of increased beta frequencies. However, the method was not sufficiently reliable to allow con-clusions about the localization of the corresponding brain regions. In 1999, a landmark fMRI study of hallucinating patients identified a characteristic brain activation pattern consistent with Wernicke's original idea (Dierks et al. 1999). The pattern consisted of an activation of left frontal regions corre-sponding to Broca's area. This is also observed during normal inner speech (verbal thoughts). In addition, however, a contemporary activation of the left primary auditory cortex (Heschl's gyrus) was seen. The activated auditory re-gion was congruent with the area activated by external acoustic stimulation. This result showed a pathological retrograde stimulation from motor to sen-sory areas in the language-related auditory system, resulting in coactivation of the primary cortex during verbal thoughts (Dierks et al. 1999). This abnormal activity may assign the physical quality of an external stimulus to an internally generated event, attributing a false origin to a verbal content of mind.

In subsequent studies, this result has been replicated, although it must be kept in mind that because of methodological restrictions, in principle, it ap-plies to patients with intermittent hallucinations who are able to indicate when they start and stop. The fact that different types of hallucinations have different activation patterns cannot be excluded. However, more recent studies have contributed consistent insights showing that the activation of Heschl's gyrus is not a general phenomenon of increased attention to external stimuli but a sign of increased internal demands during the hallucinatory phenomenon (Hubl et al. 2007b). A progressive volume loss of Heschl's gyrus may occur in schizophrenic patients (Salisbury et al. 2007). Although this result has not been specifically related to auditory hallucinations yet, it suggests a possible excitotoxic effect of a chronic local hyperactivity.

The pattern of contemporary activation of motor speech areas and sensory auditory regions during the presence of the hallucinatory perception of verbal contents of consciousness raises the question of the underlying pathways that represent the "hardwiring" between the active regions and physically allow the reciprocal stimulation and inhibition. The perception and production of language activate frontal and temporal regions in both hemispheres. However, most subjects have a pronounced asymmetry with higher activity in the dominant hemisphere. The left intrahemispheric fiber connections are therefore of particular interest in the study of the language system dynamics. The most important connection between the frontal and temporal language-related regions is the arcuate fasciculus, an intrahemispheric corticocortical fiber tract.

Modern MRI techniques such as DTI were developed to visualize the anisotropy of the white matter in the brain. This parameter indicates the "directedness" of fiber bundles, which is an indirect measure reflecting the quantity of parallel axons in a given location. In most studies, a general effect of reduced anisotropy occurs in almost all brain regions in schizophrenia, indicating a lower level of white matter organization. However, in a study of carefully selected groups of schizophrenic patients, an interesting specific alteration of the arcuate fasciculus was found. The authors compared white matter anisotropy among schizophrenic patients with frequent auditory verbal hallucinations, schizophrenic patients who had never heard voices, and a group of nonschizophrenic control subjects. Consistent with results of other studies, a general effect of the schizophrenia diagnosis was reduced white matter anisotropy. However, patients with frequent auditory verbal hallucinations showed increased local anisotropy in the left arcuate fasciculus compared with patients who never hallucinated and control subjects (Hubl et al. 2004). This finding indicates enhanced frontotemporal connections, which are an essential part of the language system.

It is reasonable to assume a relation between the pathological coactivation of the primary auditory cortex during verbal thoughts and the structural increase in white matter tracts connecting the motor speech area with the sensory parts of the language system. Functionally, this may be related to a neurophys-

Table 5–2. Phenomenology of auditory hallucinations and related conscious cognitive contents

	Self-generated	Alien
Silent	Normal thoughts	Thought insertion
Loud	Thoughts heard aloud	Hallucinations

iological facilitation of the retrograde stimulation of Heschl's gyrus. However, it is not known whether the increased anisotropy of the arcuate fasciculus is the result of neural plasticity caused by a state of hyperexcitation of the system or whether a primary constitutional feature causes the system dysfunction.

Evidence indicates that the content of auditory verbal hallucinations is generated within the language system rather than in superordinate concept areas. In a meticulous case study of a female patient with a hemorrhagic frontotemporal lesion with sensory/motor aphasia who developed auditory verbal hallucinations, it was shown that the hallucinated voices had the same aphasia as the patient herself, indicating the origin of the content to be in the injured motor speech area, whereas the excitatory stimulus driving the dysfunctional dynamic of the language system was localized in the region of the temporal lesions with electrophysiological measurements (Hubl et al. 2007a).

Several studies have confirmed positive effects of inhibitory repetitive transcranial magnetic stimulation (rTMS) on treatment-resistant auditory verbal hallucinations. The stimulation is applied in left temporal regions, and the success appears to be enhanced by neuronavigation (i.e., by adapting the locus of the rTMS application to the individual area of brain hyperactivity during hallucinations). Although interindividual variance in the clinical response is considerable, in some patients the hallucinations decrease consistently or even cease completely, with an effect lasting from some weeks to several months (Hoffman et al. 2007).

In the formal description of auditory verbal hallucinations, they have two distinctive features with respect to verbal thoughts (i.e., verbal imagery, verbal representations): the perception as "loud" (i.e., as coming from outside) and the sensation of being alien (i.e., not self-generated) (Table 5–2).

The described system dynamics involving hyperexcitation in the primary acoustic cortex can well account for the subjective phenomenon of verbal thoughts getting the physical quality of external voices. However, whether the second feature of hallucinations, the alien sensation, can be explained by the same mechanism is unclear. In other words, we do not know whether the fact of physically hearing one's own thoughts is sufficient to perceive them as alien. However, there might be two different mechanisms responsible; in particular, the fact that all four possible combinations—normal verbal thoughts (silent/ self-generated), thought insertion/intrusion (silent/alien), hallucinations (loud/alien), and audible thoughts (loud/self-generated)—are well known in psychopathology indicates two virtually independent mechanisms.

Therefore, besides the pathological activation of the primary auditory cortex, which may account for making thoughts be heard aloud, we postulate a failure of self-monitoring.

Ego Disturbances

Schizophrenic disturbances of self-perception, sometimes also called disorders of ego boundaries, are traditionally important in European psychiatry. They are considered as one of the major diagnostic criteria in ICD-10 (World Health Organization 1992), although they are exclusively subjective phenomena. Ego disturbances include the sensation that one's own thoughts or actions are alien-made or -controlled or that one's thoughts are read or even stolen by others. Auditory verbal hallucinations usually are not included in the category of ego disturbances. On the basis of the above considerations, they must be considered a misperception of one's own thoughts as made by someone else. At least this element corresponds to the definition of an ego disturbance.

The common denominator of this apparently very heterogeneous group of psychopathological symptoms can be identified in a putative mechanism of self-monitoring, which allows perceiving and recognizing one's own actions as self-generated. A disorder of this important function can account for some of the listed examples of ego disturbances—namely, for the sensation of intrusion and control of one's own thoughts and actions and for the aspect of alien-generated hallucinated voices. Less convincing is this function as a possible basis for alien-read or -stolen thoughts.

Self-monitoring has not yet been extensively studied in nonschizophrenic and schizophrenic psychology, and the relation to schizophrenic psychopathology remains to be elucidated. However, interesting hypotheses and first results have linked a known neurophysiological phenomenon to self-monitoring of vocalization and possibly to auditory hallucinations. The mechanism is the so-called efferent copy. It refers to the fact that brain motor areas generating the efferent stimulus also discharge a corollary corticocortical stimulus. This anticipates the sensory perception of self-generated actions, allowing one to recognize one's own actions and possibly also to modulate the perceptional filter. It appears reasonable to assume that this mechanism plays a role also in the corticocortical cross-talk between sensory and motor brain regions during mental imagery, including inner speech and verbal reasoning.

The efferent copy can be studied in humans with electrophysiological methods. The assumption is that the corollary discharge before motor actions can be detected by an electrical coupling between motor and sensory brain regions. Accordingly, shortly before a voluntary vocalization, synchronization between frontal and temporal brain regions is observed in the gamma frequency band (40 Hz) in healthy subjects. This synchronization is significantly reduced in schizophrenic patients with auditory verbal hallucinations (Ford et al. 2002; Mathalon and Ford 2008). Further studies will show whether this observation can be directly linked to the phenomenon of schizophrenic ego disturbances in general.

Cognition and Schizophrenia Outcome

Schizophrenia is a very heterogeneous disorder regarding cross-sectional psychopathology and the long-term course. Some patients recover completely after a single episode, even if the DSM-IV-TR (American Psychiatric Association 2000) criteria of 6-month duration are applied, whereas others will have a deleterious course with extensive emotional, intellectual, and social damage. The prediction of the course is of enormous importance for clinical handling of schizophrenia, especially at the beginning of the disorder when professionals are expected to advise their patients not only regarding the treatment of the acute psychotic episode but also regarding their professional career and the adequate social setting for the following years. The cross-sectional symptomatology and the traditional clinical subgroups can give some indications for the evaluation of outcome. However, the severity of the related impairments fluctuates interindividually with a wide range. Cognitive deficits, on the other hand, are present already at or even before the onset; they are not much influenced by antipsychotic medication and are usually stable over time. Therefore, it is reasonable to use these deficits as indicators of long-term performance in the various cognitive domains and to link them to clinical outcome.

Cognitive impairments have been shown to be more reliable than positive symptoms in predicting social functioning and integration, self-care, and employment for the current illness episode and for the future course of the schizophrenic disorder. In particular, the domains of attention and vigilance were found to be related to social functioning. Verbal learning and memory, on the other hand, were related to social and occupational integration. Executive functions were associated with independent living and processing speed with employment. However, the correlation between cognition and functional outcome is not yet sufficient for reliable predictions. The explained variance ranges from 20% to 60%, which leaves a consistent margin of uncertainty. To improve this relation and to increase the value of cognitive deficits for the prediction of outcome, additional factors have been postulated that may indirectly mediate or modulate the effect of cognition on important determinants of outcome, such as motivation, quality of life, self-esteem, satisfaction, hope, responsibility, or goals. As possible mediators between cognition and the subjective and social determinants of functional outcome, negative symptoms such as anhedonia, amotivation, and avolition have been considered. These motivational factors have been shown to be important for social integration and in particular for employment and have been found to mediate between symptoms and outcome. The relation between cognition and these factors is not yet conclusive, however.

Cognition and Schizophrenia Treatment

The investigation of cognition with neuropsychological methods has yielded important insights about possible basic mechanisms of schizophrenic pathology. In contrast to European schools of psychopathology, in American psychiatry the link between basic cognitive disorders and symptomatology is not the focus of interest. Rather, empirical measures of neuropsychological performance are related to objective and quantitative measures of behavioral performance rather than to the subjective and/or psychologically complex schizophrenic symptoms, especially in the positive symptoms domain. Consequently, important contributions link cognitive deficits to pervasive behavioral deficits, mostly found in the negative symptom domain, and to long-term social functioning.

Different approaches make the assessment of cognitive disorders useful for treatment. These approaches use the relation of cognitive symptoms with pervasive deficit symptoms to predict the course of the illness; the possibility of training cognitive performance with specific programs, thus addressing cognitive disorders as treatment targets; and the relation of specific cognitive disorders with interpersonal communication domains for individual clinical motivation and conflict management.

Treatment Programs Targeting Cognitive Deficits

Standardized recovery criteria go beyond symptom remission (Andreasen et al. 2005) and put special emphasis on an improved personal and social functioning in residence, work, and leisure (Bellack 2006; Brekke and Nakagami 2010; Leucht and Lasser 2006; Liberman and Kopelowicz 2005; Lieberman et al. 2008; Ralph and Corrigan 2005; Rosen and Garety 2005; Van Os et al. 2006). Functional impairments are an essential diagnostic feature of schizophrenia (American Psychiatric Association 2000), have a high prevalence (Bottlender et al. 2010), and are a huge burden for patients and their family members (Bellack et al. 2007). They are associated with high direct and indirect costs (König and Friemel 2006) and often endure after symptom remission and despite good response to pharmacological treatment (Penn et al. 2005b). Therefore, therapy and psychiatric rehabilitation efforts focus on restoring or gaining an adequate level of psychosocial functioning.

The psychological treatment best suited to reach this aim is cognitive-behavioral therapy that is based on an integrative model of functional outcome and recovery (see Figure 5–4).

A large body of cross-sectional and longitudinal studies provides empirical evidence for the postulated link between neurocognition and functional outcome in the model (e.g., Bowie et al. 2006; Cohen et al. 2006; Green et al. 2000, 2004; Milev et al. 2005). However, the amount of explained variance in functional outcome is 20%–40% (Couture et al. 2006). Consequently, 60%–80% of the variance in functional outcome is unaccounted for by traditional neurocognitive measures, prompting researchers to search for other contribut-

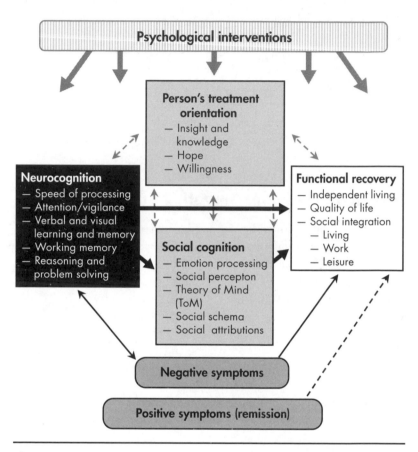

Figure 5–4.   Integrative model of treatment: possible mediators between neurocognition and functional outcome.

Source.   Adapted from Mueller and Roder 2010; Roder et al. 2010.

ing factors. More recently, social cognition and negative symptoms have been identified by structural equation modeling as mediating variables in the relation between basic neurocognition and various domains of functional outcome (e.g., Bell et al. 2008a; Bowie et al. 2010; Brekke and Nakagami 2010; Brekke et al. 2005; Gard et al. 2009; Roder and Schmidt 2009; Schmidt et al. 2010, 2011; Sergi et al. 2006; Vauth et al. 2004; Ventura et al. 2009). Moreover, the recovery concept highlights the importance of the patients' individual treat-

Table 5–3.   Cognitive-behavioral interventions

1.   Cognitive-behavioral therapy for persistent symptoms

2.   Cognitive remediation therapy

    2.1.   Neurocognitive remediation therapy

    2.2.   Social cognitive remediation therapy

3.   Integrated neurocognitive treatments

4.   Social competence approaches

5.   Psychoeducation and family therapy

ment orientation for a good intervention response. Variables such as insight into illness (Aleman et al. 2006), extrinsic and intrinsic motivation (Choi and Medalia 2010; Gard et al. 2009; Medalia and Lim 2004; Medalia and Richardson 2005; Velligan et al. 2006a), empowerment, hope, and knowledge (Corrigan 2006; Resnick et al. 2005) seem to be crucial for successful recovery.

Against this background, therapeutic interventions targeting cognitive and social deficits embedded in a multidimensional treatment concept are very promising. Five main approaches of cognitive-behavioral interventions (Table 5–3) can be distinguished, the first three of which are described in the following subsections. The remaining two approaches—social skills training and family psychoeducation programs—are beyond the scope of the current chapter; for a discussion of these interventions, see Chapters 10 ("Psychological Interventions for Schizophrenia," by Rossi et al.) and 11 ("Family Issues and Treatment in Schizophrenia," by Drapalski and Dixon) in this volume.

Cognitive-Behavioral Therapy for Persistent Symptoms

Over the past two decades, different working groups from England (e.g., Chadwick et al. 1996; Fowler et al. 1995; Kingdon and Turkington 2005; Tarrier 1992), North America (e.g., Beck and Rector 2000; Rector et al. 2003), Scandinavia (e.g., Perris 1989), and Australia (e.g., Jackson et al. 1998; Kingsep et al. 2003) have developed cognitive-behavioral therapy approaches. Although most of these approaches are administered in an individual setting, group settings also can be found in some studies, especially those conducted in the United States (overview in Wykes et al. 2008). In general, the primary goal of these interventions is to diminish positive symptoms. Some also aim to reduce negative symptoms and social anxiety and improve the level of functioning (Wykes et al. 2008). The cognitive treatment of irrational patterns of explanation building the basis of delusions and hallucinations is central to these therapeutic approaches. These irrational thinking patterns can be modified by cognitive therapy techniques of Beck (1970) and Ellis (1957) (e.g., Socratic dialogue, behavioral experiments for reality check, reattribution). Additionally, these approaches often contain psychoeducational elements, which impart the current state of knowledge about the causes of the disease, as well as a training of appropriate coping strategies.

Efficacy of Cognitive-Behavioral Therapy for Persistent Symptoms

Several meta-analyses have summarized the efficacy of such approaches. In contrast to earlier studies (e.g., Gould et al. 2001; Rector and Beck 2001), they report only moderate effect sizes (e.g., Lincoln et al. 2008; Pfammatter et al. 2006; Wykes et al. 2008; Zimmermann et al. 2005). In general, positive symptoms as well as the general psychopathology were significantly reduced at the posttreatment measurement (small to moderate effect sizes). The significant decrease in positive symptoms was maintained during a follow-up of 8.6 months (Lincoln et al. 2008). Significant moderate effects during the therapy phase also were found for negative symptoms, functioning, and mood (Wykes et al. 2008).

However, the methodological rigor of the ratings and the types of control conditions used seem to play an important role in relation to the outcome (Wykes et al. 2008; Zimmermann et al. 2005). Up to now, little evidence has shown that cognitive-behavioral therapy for (persistent) symptoms also influences the underlying cognitive functions, but these approaches seem to be the treatment of choice for reducing general psychopathology and positive symptoms in many schizophrenia patients.

Cognitive Remediation Therapy

Cognitive functions seem to be promising treatment targets, as a huge body of research suggests that they are consistent and reliable predictors of different domains of functional outcome and that they act as rate-limiting factors for the success of rehabilitative interventions (Bell et al. 2001; Couture et al. 2006; Green et al. 2000, 2004). This link implies that a reduction in cognitive deficits and/or an activation of cognitive resources may lead to an improvement in quality of life and social functioning in living, work, and leisure. These implications are the main reason for the increasing interest in cognitive deficits specific to schizophrenia and the most important premise of cognitive remediation therapy.

Depending on the therapeutic targets, cognitive remediation therapy can be categorized into neurocognitive remediation therapy and social cognitive remediation therapy. Each of these categories is discussed separately in the following subsections. (For an overview, see Roder and Medalia 2010.)

Neurocognitive Remediation Therapy

Neurocognitive remediation therapy has a long tradition, especially with war veterans and brain-injured patients (summary in Twamley et al. 2003). The first neurocognitive interventions for schizophrenia patients were developed 30 years ago. Most of these approaches aimed at improving a single neurocognitive function by means of laboratory tasks (Kurtz et al. 2001). However, over the past 20 years, broad-based and clinically oriented neurocognitive therapy approaches have been increasingly developed. The American Psychological Association Committee for the Advancement of Professional Practice (APA/CAPP) Task Force on Serious Mental Illness and Severe Emotional Disturbance (2007) included several of these neurocognitive approaches in their *Catalog of Clinical Training Opportunities: Best Practices for Recovery and Improved Outcomes for People With Serious Mental Illness* and denoted the state-of-the-art interventions.

Training for specific neurocognitive functions.

- Executive functions—Cognitive remediation therapy was originally developed in Australia (Delahunty and Morice 1993) and strongly influenced by Integrated Psychological Therapy (Roder et al. 2010). Later, it was adopted for use in the United Kingdom by Wykes and colleagues (Rose and Wykes 2008; Wykes and Reeder 2005; Wykes et al. 1999, 2003). Cognitive remediation therapy originally used paper-and-pencil exercises in an individual setting. It targets executive functioning and consists of three modules: cognitive flexibility, working memory, and planning. In recent years, the focus has been expanded to metacognitive functions that underlie certain symptoms. Cognitive remediation therapy places a strong emphasis on teaching methods and uses errorless learning principles adapted to each participant's own pace.
- Memory—Training procedures for memory are strongly based on the use of computer programs (e.g., Benedict et al. 1994; Medalia et al. 2000).

These interventions successfully improve the specifically targeted neurocognitive functions but generally fail to promote generalization effects and lack a theoretical foundation (Wykes and van der Gaag 2001).

*   **Attention**—Attention process training was originally designed to remediate attention deficits in individuals with brain injury (Sohlberg and Mateer 1987) and then adopted for cognitive rehabilitation of schizophrenia patients (Kurtz et al. 2001; Lopez-Luengo and Vasquez 2003; S.M. Silverstein et al. 2005). Attention process training provides an individualized, highly structured multilevel intervention for different components of attention and different modalities. Attention shaping is another attention training approach (S.M. Silverstein et al. 1999, 2001, 2005) designed for treatment-refractory schizophrenia. Shaping is an operant conditioning technique and involves the differential reinforcement of successive approximations toward an intended behavior. Attention shaping procedure also was combined with attention process training (S.M. Silverstein et al. 2005).

Broad-based neurocognitive remediation.   Various licensed computer programs, such as COGPACK (Olbrich 1996, 1998, 1999; www.markersoftware.com), Ben-Yishay's Orientation Remediation Module (Ben-Yishay et al. 1985), Captain's Log Software (Sandford and Brown 1988), and PSS-CogReHab (Bracy 1995), have been used in treatment evaluation studies with schizophrenia patients (e.g., Bellucci et al. 2002; Hogarty et al. 2004; Kurtz et al. 2007; Lindenmayer et al. 2008). In general, these remediation approaches contain repeated practice exercises based on errorless learning principles. Twamley and colleagues' (2008) cognitive training intervention also fits into this category but is a group-based, noncomputerized, and manualized approach with a focus on teaching and practicing compensatory and environmental strategies. The intervention includes tasks referred to prospective memory, attention and vigilance, learning and memory, and executive functions as well as to daily life. Cognitive training attempts to bridge the gap between traditional restorative approaches and compensatory approaches within neurocognitive remediation.

Compensatory approaches.   In contrast to the neurocognitive remediation approaches discussed earlier, compensatory approaches place their primary emphasis on bypassing neurocognitive impairments to improve broader aspects of functioning (Kern et al. 2009; Velligan et al. 2006b). An important compensatory approach is *errorless learning* (Kern et al. 2002, 2003, 2005), which is an integrated part of other cognitive remediation approaches. The key principle underlying this approach is the elimination of errors in the learning process and the automation of responses. Therefore, tasks are broken down to components with the simplest component trained first, followed by more complex components. Kern et al. (2009) have applied errorless learning procedure in laboratory-based studies but recently extended efforts to community settings. Another compensatory approach is represented by manual-based cognitive adaptation training (Maples and Velligan 2008; Velligan and Bow-Thomas 2000; Velligan et al. 2000, 2002, 2006b). *Cognitive adaptation training* uses at-home environmental support and structure (e.g., checklists, alarm signs for medication, reorganizing placement of belongings) to facilitate independent living by compensating especially for impaired executive functions.

Efficacy of neurocognitive remediation therapy. Meta-analyses by McGurk et al. (2007) and Pfammatter et al. (2006) quantitatively reviewed the results of randomized controlled trials ($N=26$ and 19, respectively) involving cognitive remediation as the experimental condition. Both meta-analyses found significant treatment effects in the neurocognitive domains of attention and executive functioning as well as in social functioning and symptom reduction (small to moderate effect sizes). Only in visual learning and memory were no effects found (McGurk et al. 2007). The effect sizes in neurocognition were maintained over an average follow-up period of 8 months (McGurk et al. 2007). Additionally, small to moderate generalization effects on functioning and symptoms were identified (McGurk et al. 2007; Pfammatter et al. 2006). In both meta-analyses, the highest effect sizes were found in social cognition. However, this may have been the result of a lack of studies addressing only social cognitive treatments. The combination of cognitive remediation and strategy learning methods led to significantly larger effects compared with the use of remediation techniques alone (McGurk et al. 2007).

Social Cognitive Remediation Therapy

A continuous increase of publications and interest in dealing with the construct of social cognition in schizophrenia patients was seen in the last 10 years (Green et al. 2005; Penn et al. 2008). As a result, the social cognitive dimensions have become an increasingly important intervention goal in cognitive remediation therapy approaches. Most of the existing treatments target one single social cognitive dimension defined as the primary target. Others include a broad-based focus on a combination of various social cognitive dimensions. Broad integrated therapy approaches combining intervention on social cognition with other treatment targets are discussed in the next section (see "Integrated Neurocognitive Treatments" below). Nonintegrated social cognitive remediation approaches are relatively new psychological interventions and can be categorized into 1) approaches targeting one single primary social cognitive dimension or 2) broad-based approaches addressing various social cognitive functions (Roder et al. 2010).

Training targeting specific social cognitive functions.

- **Emotion and social perception**—Training in social perception and perception of emotions (Van der Gaag et al. 2002) is an individually administered remediation program. Skills in social perception and perception of emotions are the primary treatment goal, and the included training to enhance basic skills, such as memory, attention, and executive functions, is necessary for perceptual social cognitive functions. Training of Affect Recognition (TAR; Wölwer et al. 2005) is administered to pairs of patients at a time with the goal of enhancing affect recognition by interpreting facial expressions, nonverbal behavior, and social context. Both treatments involve restoration and compensation strategies following errorless learning principles. Emotional Management Therapy (Hodel and Brenner 1996; Hodel et al. 2004) and Training of Emotional Intelligence (Vauth and Stieglitz 2008; Vauth et al. 2001) expand the treatment target by adding coping strategies and the concept of emotional intelligence.

- **Theory of mind**—The Instrumental Enrichment Program (Feuerstein 1980; Rancone et al. 2004) is based on mediated learning with a focus on the learning process and the patients' erroneous beliefs and thinking strategies. It includes exercises that aim to improve the perception of emotions, social intelligence, and finally role-played social situations, in which theory of mind issues are dealt with. Social Cognition Enhancement Training (Choi and Kwon 2006) aims to improve the theory of mind functions of context appraisal and perspective-taking abilities with cartoons.

Broad-based approaches addressing several social cognitive domains. Social Cognition and Interaction Training (SCIT), developed by Penn and colleagues (Combs et al. 2007a; Horan et al. 2009; Penn et al. 2005a, 2007; Roberts and Penn 2009; D. Roberts, D.L. Penn, D. Combs, "Social Cognition and Interaction Training," unpublished treatment manual, University of North Carolina, 2006), consists of three phases: 1) emotion perception linked to facial expression, 2) attribution bias and theory of mind in figured-out situations, and 3) integration and generalization of the learned social skills by applying them to realistic social situations. Metacognitive Skill Training for Patients With Schizophrenia (MCT; Moritz and Woodward 2007; Moritz et al. 2009) is a metacognitive remediation approach based on two components: knowledge translation and identification of the negative consequences of cognitive biases underlying positive symptoms (e.g., attributions, jumping to conclusions, theory of mind). The goal of MCT is to improve patients' thinking by minimizing cognitive errors. Horan et al. (2009) recently developed a social cognition intervention approach that includes tasks from SCIT and TAR. This social cognitive skills training primarily targets emotion and social perception and secondarily social attribution and theory of mind.

Efficacy of social cognitive remediation therapy. The preliminary results of a meta-analysis (Mueller et al. 2009), including almost 20 randomized controlled trials, to evaluate social cognitive remediation and combined treatment approaches are promising: over an average duration of 23 weeks, a significant global therapy effect could be seen, which was maintained during a follow-up period of 9.5 months on average. Superior effects of social cognitive remediation compared with control treatment were found in proximal and in distal outcome variables: the summarized social cognitive areas and the subareas of emotional processing, social perception, and theory of mind were significant. Additionally, the summarized neurocognitive area and the subareas of speed of information processing, planning/problem solving, verbal memory, and working memory provide evidence for an amelioration compared with the control groups. Significant effects were found in proximal outcome of reduced psychopathological symptoms and improved social functioning. Setting, control groups, and type of intervention were identified as moderators. This study provides strong evidence for social cognitive remediation and combined treatment (including social cognitive remediation).

Integrated Neurocognitive Treatments

Our definition of *integrated neurocognitive treatments* includes two aspects:

1. An intervention is integrated when the treatment of neurocognitive do-mains is combined with one or more of the following areas as an active therapeutic target: social cognition, knowledge of the disease or problems ("deficits," "resources"), social skills (e.g., residential, vocational, and rec-reational areas), and thinking styles (e.g., irrational beliefs).
2. The term *integrated* also points to the necessity that cognitive remediation therapy should always be embedded in a broad-based treatment concept tailored to the patients' rehabilitative goals and cognitive strengths and weaknesses.

Generally, these approaches are used in group-based settings, partially supplemented by individual sessions. The best-evaluated and most promising integrated cognitive therapy approaches are summarized below.

Integrated Psychological Therapy

Integrated Psychological Therapy (Brenner et al. 1997; Roder et al. 1988, 2006, 2010) was the first systematically structured, comprehensive, and manualized in-tegrated therapy program developed for schizophrenia patients. It combines neu-rocognitive and social cognitive interventions with a social and interpersonal problem-solving skills approach. Integrated Psychological Therapy is structured into five subprograms with increasing levels of complexity; these are taught se-quentially, as a building-block model is postulated (see Figure 5–5).

The first subprogram, "Cognitive Differentiation," aims at enhancing neurocognitive functioning (e.g., attention, verbal memory, cognitive flexibil-ity, concept formation). The second subprogram, "Social Perception," targets social cognitive deficits (e.g., social and emotional perception, emotional ex-pression). The third subprogram, "Verbal Communication," addresses verbal fluency and executive functioning—skills that affect interpersonal communi-cation directly. Moreover, it constitutes the link between the more cognitively oriented first two subprograms and the more behaviorally oriented last two subprograms. The fourth subprogram, "Social Skills," and the fifth, "Inter-personal Problem Solving," foster building social competence through the

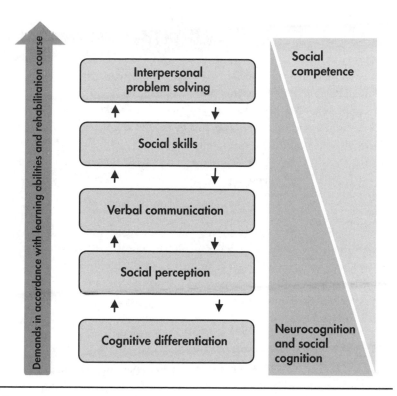

Figure 5–5. Integrated Psychological Therapy: content and conceptualization.

Source. Adapted from Roder et al. 2010.

development of interpersonal skills via role-plays and through group-based problem-solving exercises. Therapy is guided by a well-trained therapist and a cotherapist and takes place in small groups of five to eight participants in 60-minute sessions twice a week over at least a 3- to 4-month period. In addition, in vivo exercises and homework assignments as well as individualized sessions by request of patients or therapists are implemented.

Cognitive Enhancement Therapy

The conceptualization of cognitive enhancement therapy (CET) (Hogarty and Flesher 1999a, 1999b; Hogarty et al. 2004, 2006) was considerably influenced by Integrated Psychological Therapy. CET is a holistic, developmental approach aiming at the rehabilitation of social cognitive and neurocognitive deficits among patients with schizophrenia based on a neurodevelopmental model. CET attempts to facilitate the attainment of social cognitive milestones (e.g., cognitive flexibility, tolerance for ambiguity and uncertainty) to prepare patients to show appropriate behavior in social contexts and to create a personally relevant understanding of schizophrenia by psychoeducation. Neurocognitive deficits are addressed by administering computer-based training. In addition, patients receive social cognitive group exercises (e.g., categorization exercises, solving real-life social dilemmas).

Neurocognitive Enhancement Therapy

Neurocognitive enhancement therapy is a comprehensive approach to cognitive remediation developed by Bell et al. (2001, 2008b) with a particular focus on work rehabilitation and intense and repetitive practice to influence neurocognitive impairments. The program consists of three main components: computer-based cognitive training, a social information processing group, and a work feedback group.

Neuropsychological Educational Approach to Cognitive Remediation

The comprehensive, evidence-based, manualized Neuropsychological Educational Approach to Cognitive Remediation (NEAR) (Medalia and Freilich 2008; Medalia et al. 2002) constitutes a synthesis of knowledge derived from educational psychology, behavior and learning theories, and rehabilitation psychology. NEAR exercises are therefore designed to increase intrinsic motivation, independence, self-efficacy, and persistence on learning tasks. Tasks are taken from commercially available educational software.

Integrated Neurocognitive Therapy

Over the past 4 years, our research group has designed a cognitive-behavioral group therapy program, Integrated Neurocognitive Therapy (Mueller and Roder 2010), as a further development of the neurocognitive and social cognitive subprograms of Integrated Psychological Therapy. The treatment concept of Integrated Neurocognitive Therapy encompasses all 11 neurocognitive and social cognitive domains defined by the NIMH MATRICS Initiative (Green et

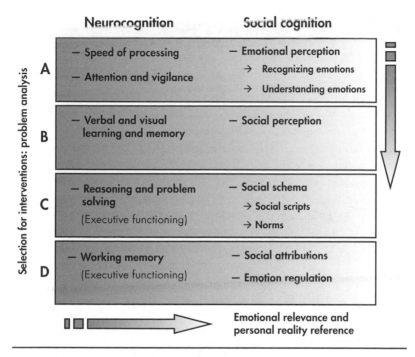

Figure 5–6. Integrated Neurocognitive Therapy: content and conceptualization.

Source. Adapted from Mueller and Roder 2010; Roder et al. 2010.

al. 2005; Nuechterlein et al. 2004). These domains are subsumed into four integrated neurocognitive treatment modules (see Figure 5–6).

The first modules are more structured, include more computer-based exercises, and are of less cognitive complexity and emotional strain than the last modules. This "bottom-up" and "top-down" approach puts a strong focus on the patients' daily life context to promote transfer and generalization. Enhancing insight into (illness-specific) cognitive resources and deficits, as well as possibilities of coping, represents a further aim of treatment. Integrated neurocognitive treatment also facilitates intrinsic motivation and resources. This new therapy approach was evaluated by an international randomized multicenter study in Switzerland, Germany, and Austria, which is supported by the Swiss National Foundation (Project no. 3200B0-108133/1).

Efficacy of Integrated Therapy Approaches

With the exception of the newly developed Integrated Neurocognitive Therapy program, integrated therapy approaches represent interventions with a broad empirical basis. Results are encouraging insofar as improvements have been found not only in proximal cognitive performance but also in the more distal areas of psychosocial functioning and psychopathology. Integrated Psychological Therapy, CET, neurocognitive enhancement therapy, and NEAR are all included in the *Catalog of Clinical Training Opportunities: Best Practices for Recovery and Improved Outcomes for People With Serious Mental Illness,* published by the APA/CAPP Task Force on Serious Mental Illness and Severe Emotional Disturbance (2007). Programs offering cognitive remediation with adjunctive rehabilitation interventions appear to have an advantage in comparison with programs providing cognitive remediation alone (McGurk et al. 2007). Moreover, research with Integrated Psychological Therapy has yielded strong empirical evidence for the efficacy of integrated therapy: a meta-analysis including 35 studies with 1,529 patients in 12 countries showed significant moderate effect sizes in neurocognition, social cognition, and functional outcome (Mueller and Roder 2010; Roder et al. 2010). Furthermore, an analysis of research examining a variety of different Integrated Psychological Therapy subprograms indicated that studies offering combined neurocognition/social perception subprograms had superior effects in terms of proximal and distal outcomes compared with studies providing neurocognition alone (Mueller and Roder 2008). Also, only Integrated Psychological Therapy treatment that included all subprograms was found to have long-lasting and still-increasing effects posttreatment. Treatments employing single subprograms did not show these effects (V. Roder, D. R. Mueller, "Integrated Neurocognitive Therapy (INT) for Schizophrenia Patients," unpublished manual, Bern, Switzerland, University Psychiatric Hospital, 2006).

Improved function is a key goal of recovery and is often defined as the ultimate goal of any therapeutic treatment (Mueller and Roder 2007; Spaulding and Nolting 2006), as well as of cognitive remediation. Integrated therapy seems to be a powerful and promising method to reach this goal within a multimodal rehabilitation process.

Conclusion

Cognitive dysfunction, encompassing both neurocognition and social cognition, is a hallmark of schizophrenia; deficits are present in the majority of patients, frequently precede the onset of other symptoms, persist even with successful pharmacological treatment, and account for a significant portion of enduring functional impairment. The importance of cognitive impairment in the course of schizophrenia suggests that interventions must address cognitive functioning if they are to positively influence long-term outcome. Against this background, therapeutic interventions that target cognitive and social deficits and are embedded in a multidimensional treatment concept show great promise:

- Cognitive-behavioral therapy for persistent symptoms is a good choice for reducing general psychopathology and positive symptoms in some patients.
- Cognitive remediation therapy seems to be effective in improving neurocognitive and social cognitive functioning.
- Integrated neurocognitive treatments in groups seem to be very promising approaches, especially for improving functional recovery.

Future research should aim at understanding the relationship between cognitive deficits in the residual state and clinical symptom domains. This will allow us to better define important behavioral dimensions of schizophrenic pathology, which can be mapped to higher brain functions such as language, emotions, and motor behaviour, and to the underlying brain circuits (Strik et al. 2010).

References

Addington J, Saeedi H, Addington D: The course of cognitive functioning in first episode psychosis: changes over time and impact on outcome. Schizophr Res 78:35–43, 2005

Aleman A, Hijman R, deHaan EHF, et al: Memory impairment in schizophrenia: a meta-analysis. Am J Psychiatry 156:1358–1366, 1999

Aleman A, Agrawal N, Morgan KD, et al: Insight in psychosis and neuropsychological function. Br J Psychiatry 189:204–212, 2006

Al-Uzri MM, Reveley MA, Owen L: Measuring memory impairment in community-based patients with schizophrenia. Br J Psychiatry 189:132–136, 2006

American Psychiatric Association: Diagnostic and Statistical Manual of Mental Disorders, 4th Edition, Text Revision. Washington, DC, American Psychiatric Association, 2000

Andreasen NC, Carpenter WT, Kane JM, et al: Remission in schizophrenia: proposed criteria and rationale for consensus. Am J Psychiatry 162:441–449, 2005

APA/CAPP Task Force on Serious Mental Illness and Severe Emotional Disturbance: Catalog of Clinical Training Opportunities: Best Practices for Recovery and Improved Outcomes for People with Serious Mental Illness. September 2007. Available at: http://www.apa.org/practice/resources/grid/catalog.pdf. Accessed April 6, 2011.

Beck A: Cognitive therapy: nature and relation to behavior therapy. Behav Ther 1:184–200, 1970

Beck AT, Rector NA: Cognitive therapy of schizophrenia: a new therapy for the new millennium. Am J Psychother 54:291–300, 2000

Bell M, Bryson G, Greig T, et al: Neurocognitive enhancement therapy with work therapy. Arch Gen Psychiatry 58:763–768, 2001

Bell M, Tsang HW, Greig TC, et al: Neurocognition, social cognition, perceived social discomfort, and vocational outcomes in schizophrenia. Schizophr Bull 35:738–747, 2008a

Bell M, Zito W, Greig T, et al: Neurocognitive enhancement therapy and competitive employment in schizophrenia: effects on clients with poor community functioning. Am J Psychiatr Rehabil 11:109–122, 2008b

Bellack AS: Scientific and consumer models of recovery in schizophrenia: concordance, contrasts, and implications. Schizophr Bull 32:432–442, 2006

Bellack AS, Green MF, Cook JA, et al: Assessment of community functioning in people with schizophrenia and other severe mental illnesses: a white paper based on an NIMH-sponsored workshop. Schizophr Bull 33:805–822, 2007

Bellucci DM, Glaberman K, Haslam N: Computer-assisted cognitive rehabilitation reduces negative symptoms in the severely mentally ill. Schizophr Res 59:225–232, 2002

Benedict RH, Harris H, Markow T, et al: Effects of attention training on information processing in schizophrenia. Schizophr Bull 20:537–546, 1994

Bentall RP, Corcoran R: Persecutory delusions: a review and theoretical integration. Clin Psychol Rev 21:1143–1192, 2001

Ben-Yishay Y, Piasetsky EB, Rattok J: A systematic method for ameliorating disorders in basic attention, in Neuropsychological Rehabilitation. Edited by Meir MJ, Benton AL, Diller L. New York, Guilford, 1985, pp 165–181

Birkett P, Sigmundsson T, Sharma T, et al: Reaction time and sustained attention in schizophrenia and its genetic predisposition. Schizophr Res 95:76–85, 2007

Bleuler E: Dementia Praecox or the Group of Schizophrenias (1911). Translated by Zinkin J. New York, International Universities Press, 1950

Bottlender R, Strauss A, Möller H-J: Social disability in schizophrenic, schizoaffective and affective disorders 15 years after admission. Schizophr Res 116:9–15, 2010

Bowie CR, Reichenberg A, Patterson TL, et al: Determinants of real-world functional performance in schizophrenia subjects: correlations with cognition, functional capacity, and symptoms. Am J Psychiatry 163:418–425, 2006

Bowie CR, Reichenberg A, McClure MM, et al: Age-associated differences in cognitive performance in older community dwelling schizophrenia patients: differential sensitivity of clinical neuropsychological and experimental information processing tests. Schizophr Res 106:50–58, 2008

Bowie CR, Depp C, McGrath JA, et al: Prediction of real-world functional disability in chronic mental disorders: a comparison of schizophrenia and bipolar disorder. Am J Psychiatry 167:1116–1124, 2010

Bracy O: CogRehab Software. Indianapolis, IN, Psychological Software Services, 1995

Brekke J, Nakagami E: The relevance of neurocognition and social cognition for outcome and recovery in schizophrenia, in Neurocognition and Social Cognition in Schizophrenia Patients: Basic Concepts and Treatment. Edited by Roder V, Medalia A. Basel, Switzerland, Karger, 2010, pp 23–26

Brekke J, Kay DD, Lee KS, et al: Biosocial pathways to functional outcome in schizophrenia. Schizophr Res 80:213–225, 2005

Brenner HD, Roder V, Hodel B, et al: Terapia Psicologica Integrata (IPT). Milan, Italy, McGraw-Hill, 1997

Brothers L: The social brain: a project for integrating primate behavior and neurophysiology in a new domain. Concepts Neurosci 1:27–51, 1990

Brüne M, Abdel-Hamid M, Lehmkämper C, et al: Mental state attribution, neurocognitive functioning, and psychopathology: what predicts poor social competence in schizophrenia best? Schizophr Res 92:151–159, 2007

Brunet-Gouet E, Decety J: Social brain dysfunctions in schizophrenia: a review of neuroimaging studies. Psychiatry Res 148:75–92, 2006

Buss A, Lang P: Psychological deficit in schizophrenia: affect reinforcement and concept attainment. J Abnorm Psychol 70:2–24, 1965

Chadwick P, Birchwood M, Trower P: Cognitive Therapy for Delusions, Voices and Paranoia. New York, Wiley, 1996

Chapman LJ, Chapman JP: Disordered thought in schizophrenia. Englewood Cliffs, NY, Prentice Hall, 1973

Chen EY, Hui CL, Dunn EL, et al: A prospective 3-year longitudinal study of cognitive predictors of relapse in first-episode schizophrenic patients. Schizophr Res 77:99–104, 2005

Chiaramonti R, Muscas GC, Paganini M, et al: Correlations of topographical EEG features with clinical severity in mild and moderate dementia of Alzheimer type. Neuropsychobiology 36:153–158, 1997

Choi J, Medalia A: Intrinsic motivation and learning in a schizophrenia spectrum sample. Schizophr Res 118:12–19, 2010

Choi KH, Kwon JH: Social cognition enhancement training for schizophrenia: a preliminary randomized controlled trial. Community Ment Health J 42:177–187, 2006

Cohen AS, Forbes CB, Mann MC, et al: Specific cognitive deficits and differential domains of social functioning in schizophrenia. Schizophr Res 81:227–238, 2006

Combs DR, Adams SD, Penn DL, et al: Social Cognition and Interaction Training (SCIT) for inpatients with schizophrenia spectrum disorders: preliminary findings. Schizophr Res 91:112–116, 2007a

Combs DR, Penn DL, Wicher M, et al: The Ambiguous Intentions Hostility Questionnaire (AIHQ): a new measure for evaluating hostile social-cognitive biases in paranoia. Cogn Neuropsychiatry 12:128–143, 2007b

Cornblatt B, Lenzenweger M, Dworkin R, et al: Childhood attentional dysfunctions predict social deficits in unaffected adults at risk for schizophrenia. Br J Psychiatry 161 (suppl 18):59–64, 1992

Corrigan PW: Recovery from schizophrenia and the role of evidence-based psychosocial interventions. Expert Rev Neurother 6:993–1004, 2006

Corrigan PW, Addis IB: The effects of cognitive complexity on a social sequencing task in schizophrenia. Schizophr Res 16:137–144, 1995

Corrigan PW, Penn DL (eds): Social Cognition in Schizophrenia. Washington, DC, American Psychological Association, 2001

Couture SM, Penn DL, Roberts DL: The functional significance of social cognition in schizophrenia: a review. Schizophr Bull 32:44–63, 2006

Cromwell RL, Spaulding W: How schizophrenics handle information, in The Phenomenology and Treatment of Schizophrenia. Edited by Fann WE, Karacan I, Pokorny AD, et al. New York, Spectrum, 1978, pp 127–162

Delahunty A, Morice R: A training program for the remediation of cognitive deficits in schizophrenia: preliminary results. Psychol Med 23:221–227, 1993

Dierks T, Linden DEJ, Jandl M, et al: Activation of Heschl's gyrus during auditory hallucinations. Neuron 22:615–621, 1999

Dollfus S, Lombardo C, Bénali K, et al: Executive/attentional cognitive functions in schizophrenic patients and their parents: a preliminary study. Schizophr Res 53:93–99, 2002

Duncan CC, Barry RJ, Connolly JF, et al: Event-related potentials in clinical research: guidelines for eliciting, recording, and quantifying mismatch negativity, P300, and N400. Clinical Neurophysiol 120:1883–1908, 2009

Edwards J, Jackson HJ, Pattison PE: Emotion recognition via facial expression and affective prosody in schizophrenia: a methodological review. Clin Psychol Rev 22:789–832, 2002

Ekman P, Friesen WV: Pictures of Facial Affect. Palo Alto, CA, Consulting Psychologists Press, 1976

Ellis A: Rational psychotherapy and individual psychology. J Individ Psychol 13:38–44, 1957

Engel AK, Fries P, Singer W: Dynamic predictions: oscillations and synchrony in top-down processing. Nat Rev Neurosci 2:704–716, 2001

Erlenmeyer-Kimling L, Rock D, Roberts SA, et al: Attention, memory, and motor skills as childhood predictors of schizophrenia-related psychoses: the New York High-Risk Project. Am J Psychiatry 157:1416–1422, 2000

Feuerstein R: Instrumental Enrichment. Baltimore, MD, University Park Press, 1980

Ford JM, Mathalon DH: Neural synchrony in schizophrenia. Schizophr Bull 34:904–906, 2008

Ford JM, Mathalon DH, Whitfield S, et al: Reduced communication between frontal and temporal lobes during talking in schizophrenia. Biol Psychiatry 51:485–492, 2002

Fowler D, Garety P, Kuipers E: Cognitive Behaviour Therapy for Psychosis: Theory and Practice. Chichester, UK, Wiley, 1995

Frith CD: Consciousness, information-processing and schizophrenia. Br J Psychiatry 134:225–235, 1979

Frith CD: The Cognitive Neuropsychology of Schizophrenia. Hillsdale, NJ, Lawrence Erlbaum, 1992

Gard DE, Fisher M, Garrett C, et al: Motivation and its relationship to neurocognition, social cognition, and functional outcome in schizophrenia. Schizophr Res 115:74–81, 2009

Gillis JS: Schizophrenic thinking in a probabilistic situation. Psychological Record 19:211–224, 1969

Gould RA, Mueser KT, Bolton E, et al: Cognitive therapy for psychosis in schizophrenia: an effect size analysis. Schizophr Res 48:335–342, 2001

Gray JA, Roth BL: Molecular targets for treating cognitive dysfunction in schizophrenia. Schizophr Bull 33:1100–1119, 2007

Green MF, Nuechterlein KH: The MATRICS initiative: developing a consensus cognitive battery for clinical trials. Schizophr Res 72:1–3, 2004

Green MF, Kern RS, Braff DL, et al: Neurocognitive deficits and functional outcome in schizophrenia: are we measuring the "right stuff"? Schizophr Bull 26:119–136, 2000

Green MF, Kern RS, Heaton RK: Longitudinal studies of cognition and functional outcome in schizophrenia: implications for MATRICS. Schizophr Res 72:41–51, 2004

Green MF, Olivier B, Crawley JN, et al: Social cognition in schizophrenia: recommendations from the Measurement and Treatment Research to Improve Cognition in Schizophrenia New Approaches Conference. Schizophr Res 31:882–887, 2005

Green MF, Nuechterlein KH, Kern RS, et al: Functional co-primary measures for clinical trials in schizophrenia: results from the MATRICS psychometric and standardization study. Am J Psychiatry 165:221–228, 2008a

Green MF, Penn DL, Bentall R, et al: Social cognition in schizophrenia: an NIMH workshop on definition, assessment, and research opportunities. Schizophr Bull 34:1211–1220, 2008b

Harris JG, Minassian A, Perry W: Stability of attention deficits in schizophrenia. Schizophr Res 91:107–111, 2007

Heaton RK, Chelune GJ, Talley JL, et al: Wisconsin Card Sorting Test Manual. Odessa, FL, Psychological Assessment Resources, 1993

Heidrich A, Strik WK: Auditory P300 topography and neuropsychological test performance: evidence for left hemispheric dysfunction in schizophrenia. Biol Psychiatry 41:327–335, 1997

Heinz A, Schlagenhauf F: Dopaminergic dysfunction in schizophrenia: salience attribution revisited. Schizophr Bull 36:472–485, 2010

Hemsley DR: What have cognitive deficits to do with schizophrenic symptoms? Br J Psychiatry 130:167–173, 1977

Hodel B, Brenner HD: Ein Trainingsprogramm zur Bewältigung von maladaptiven Emotionen bei schizophren Erkrankten. Erste Ergebnisse und Erfahrungen. Nervenarzt 67:564–571, 1996

Hodel B, Kern RS, Brenner HD: Emotion management training (EMT) in persons with treatment-resistant schizophrenia: first results. Psychiatry Res 68:107–108, 2004

Hoekert M, Kahn R, Pijnenborg M, et al: Impaired recognition and expression of emotional prosody in schizophrenia: review and meta-analysis. Schizophr Res 96:135–145, 2007

Hoffman RE, Hampson M, Wu K, et al: Probing the pathophysiology of auditory/verbal hallucinations by combining functional magnetic resonance imaging and transcranial magnetic stimulation. Cereb Cortex 17:2733–2743, 2007

Hogarty GE, Flesher S: Developmental theory for a Cognitive Enhancement Therapy of schizophrenia. Schizophr Bull 25:677–692, 1999a

Hogarty GE, Flesher S: Practice principles of cognitive enhancement therapy for schizophrenia. Schizophr Bull 25:693–708, 1999b

Hogarty GE, Flesher S, Ulrich R, et al: Cognitive enhancement therapy for schizophrenia: effects of a 2-year randomized trial on cognition and behavior. Arch Gen Psychiatry 61:866–876, 2004

Hogarty GE, Greenwald DP, Eack SM: Durability and mechanism of effects of cognitive enhancement therapy. Psychiatr Serv 57:1751–1757, 2006

Horan WP, Kern RS, Shokat-Fadai K, et al: Social cognitive skills training in schizophrenia: an initial efficacy study of stabilized outpatients. Schizophr Res 107:47–54, 2009

Horn H, Federspiel A, Wirth M, et al: Structural and metabolic changes in language areas linked to formal thought disorder. Br J Psychiatry 194:130–138, 2009

Hubl D, Koenig T, Strik W, et al: Pathways that make voices: white matter changes in auditory hallucinations. Arch Gen Psychiatry 61:658–668, 2004

Hubl D, Hauf M, van Swam C, et al: Hearing dysphasic voices. Lancet 370:538, 2007a

Hubl D, Koenig T, Strik WK, et al: Competition for neuronal resources: how hallucinations make themselves heard. Br J Psychiatry 190:57–62, 2007b

Huddy VC, Hodgson TL, Kapasi M, et al: Gaze strategies during planning in first-episode psychosis. J Abnorm Psychol 116:589–598, 2007

Jackson H, McGorry P, Edwards J, et al: Cognitively oriented psychotherapy for early psychosis (COPE). Br J Psychiatry 172:93–100, 1998

Jann K, Dierks T, Boesch C, et al: BOLD correlates of EEG alpha phase-locking and the fMRI default mode network. Neuroimage 45:903–916, 2009

Kern RS, Horan WP: Definition and measurement of neurocognition and social cognition, in Neurocognition and Social Cognition in Schizophrenia Patients: Basic Concepts and Treatment. Edited by Roder V, Medalia A. Basel, Switzerland, Karger, 2010, pp 1–22

Kern RS, Liberman RP, Kopelowicz A, et al: Applications of errorless learning for improving work performance in persons with schizophrenia. Am J Psychiatry 159:1921–1926, 2002

Kern RS, Green MF, Mintz J, et al: Does "errorless learning" compensate for neurocognitive impairments in the work rehabilitation of persons with schizophrenia? Psychol Med 33:433–442, 2003

Kern RS, Green MF, Mitchell S, et al: Extensions of errorless learning for social problem-solving deficits in schizophrenia. Am J Psychiatry 162:513–519, 2005

Kern RS, Liberman RP, Becker R, et al: Errorless learning for training individuals with schizophrenia at a community mental health setting providing work experience. Schizophr Bull 35:807–815, 2009

Kingdon A, Turkington D: Cognitive Therapy of Schizophrenia. New York, Guilford, 2005

Kingsep P, Nathan P, Castle D: Cognitive behavioural group treatment for social anxiety in schizophrenia. Schizophr Res 63:121–129, 2003

Kircher TT, Liddle PF, Brammer MJ, et al: Neural correlates of formal thought disorder in schizophrenia: preliminary findings from a functional magnetic resonance imaging study. Arch Gen Psychiatry 58:769–774, 2001

König HH, Friemel S: Gesundheitsökonomie psychischer Krankheiten. Bundesgesundheitsblatt 49:46–56, 2006

Kostova M, Passerieux C, Laurent JP, et al: N400 anomalies in schizophrenia are correlated with the severity of formal thought disorder. Schizophr Res 78:285–291, 2005

Kraepelin E: Psychiatrie: Ein Lehrbuch für Studierende und Ärzte [Psychiatry: a Textbook for Students and Practitioners], 8th Edition, Vol 3. Leipzig, Germany, Barth, 1913

Kurtz MM: Neurocognitive impairments across the lifespan in schizophrenia: an update. Schizophr Res 74:15–26, 2005

Kurtz MM, Moberg PJ, Mozley LH, et al: Effectiveness of an attention- and memory-training program on neuropsychological deficits in schizophrenia. Neurorehabil Neural Repair 15:23–28, 2001

Kurtz MM, Seltzer JC, Shagan DS, et al: Computer-assisted cognitive remediation in schizophrenia: what is the active ingredient? Schizophr Res 89:251–260, 2007

Lehmann D: Brain electrical mapping of cognitive functions for psychiatry—functional micro-states. Psychiatry Res 29:385–386, 1989

Lehmann D, Ozaki H, Pal I: EEG alpha map series: brain micro-states by space-oriented adaptive segmentation. Electroencephalogr Clin Neurophysiol 67:271–288, 1987

Lehmann D, Faber PL, Gianotti LR, et al: Coherence and phase locking in the scalp EEG and between LORETA model sources, and microstates as putative mechanisms of brain temporo-spatial functional organization. J Physiol Paris 99:29–36, 2006

Leonhard C, Corrigan PW: Social perception in schizophrenia, in Social Cognition in Schizophrenia. Edited by Corrigan PW, Penn DL. Washington, DC, American Psychological Association, 2001, pp 73–95

Leucht S, Lasser R: The concepts of remission and recovery in schizophrenia. Pharmacopsychiatry 39:161–170, 2006

Liberman RP, Kopelowicz A: Recovery from schizophrenia: a concept in search of research. Psychiatr Serv 56:735–742, 2005

Libet B, Gleason CA, Wright EW, et al: Time of conscious intention to act in relation to onset of cerebral-activity (readiness-potential)—the unconscious initiation of a freely voluntary act. Brain 106:623–642, 1983

Lieberman JA, Drake RE, Sederer LI, et al: Science and recovery in schizophrenia. Psychiatr Serv 59:487–496, 2008

Light GA, Braff DL: Sensory gating deficits in schizophrenia; can we parse the effects of medication, nicotine use, and changes in clinical status? Clin Neurosci Res 3:47–54, 2003

Light GA, Hsu JL, Hsieh MH, et al: Gamma band oscillations reveal neural network cortical coherence dysfunction in schizophrenia patients. Biol Psychiatry 60:1231–1240, 2006

Lincoln TM, Suttner C, Nestoriuc Y: Wirksamkeit kognitiver Interventionen für Schizophrenie. Eine Meta-Analyse. Psychologische Rundschau 59:217–232, 2008

Lindenmayer JP, McGurk SR, Mueser KT, et al: A randomized controlled trial of cognitive remediation among inpatients with persistent mental illness. Psychiatr Serv 59:241–247, 2008

Loong JWK: Wisconsin Card Sorting Test (WCST), Computerized Version. San Luis Obisbo, CA, Wang Neuropsychological Laboratory, 1989

Lopez-Luengo B, Vasquez C: Effects on Attention Process Training on cognitive functioning of schizophrenia patients. Psychiatry Res 119:41–53, 2003

Maples NJ, Velligan DI: Cognitive Adaptation Training: establishing environmental supports to bypass cognitive deficits and improve functional outcomes. Am J Psychiatr Rehabil 11:164–180, 2008

Martin JA, Penn DL: Attributional style in schizophrenia: an investigation in outpatients with and without persecutory delusions. Schizophr Bull 28:131–141, 2002

Mathalon DH, Ford JM: Corollary discharge dysfunction in schizophrenia: evidence for an elemental deficit. Clin EEG Neurosci 39:82–86, 2008

Mathalon DH, Faustman WO, Ford JM: N400 and automatic semantic processing abnormalities in patients with schizophrenia. Arch Gen Psychiatry 59:641–648, 2002

Matsui M, Sumiyoshi T, Yuuki H, et al: Impairment of event schema in patients with schizophrenia: examination of scripts for shopping at supermarket. Psychiatry Res 143:179ñ187, 2006

McGurk SR, Twamley EW, Sitzer DI, et al: A meta-analysis of cognitive remediation in schizophrenia. Am J Psychiatry 164:1791–1802, 2007

Medalia A, Freilich B: The Neuropsychological Educational Approach to Cognitive Remediation (NEAR) model: practice principles and outcome studies. Am J Psychiatr Rehabil 11:164–180, 2008

Medalia A, Lim RW: Self-awareness of cognitive functioning in schizophrenia. Schizophr Res 71:331–338, 2004

Medalia A, Richardson R: What predicts a good response to cognitive remediation interventions? Schizophr Bull 31:942–953, 2005

Medalia A, Revheim N, Casey M: Remediation of memory disorders in schizophrenia. Psychol Med 30:1451–1459, 2000

Medalia A, Revheim N, Herlands T: Remediation of Cognitive Deficits in Psychiatric Outpatients: A Clinician's Manual. New York, Montefiore Medical Center Press, 2002

Milev P, Ho BC, Arndt S, et al: Predictive values of neurocognition and negative symptoms on functional outcome in schizophrenia: a longitudinal first-episode study with 7-year follow-up. Am J Psychiatry 162:495–506, 2005

Moritz S, Woodward TS: Metacognitive Training for schizophrenia patients (MCT): a pilot study on feasibility, treatment adherence, and subjective efficacy. German Journal of Psychiatry 10:69–78, 2007

Moritz S, Woodward TS, Stevens C, et al: Metacognitive Training for Patients With Schizophrenia (MCT), British Version. Hamburg, Germany, VanHam Campus Verlag, 2009

Mueller DR, Roder V: Integrated psychological therapy for schizophrenia patients. Expert Rev Neurother 7:1–3, 2007

Mueller DR, Roder V: Empirical evidence for group therapy addressing social perception in schizophrenia, in Social Perception: 21st Century Issues and Challenges. Edited by Teiford JB. New York, Nova Science Publishers, 2008, pp 51–80

Mueller DR, Roder V: Integrated psychological therapy and integrated neurocognitive therapy, in Neurocognition and Social Cognition in Schizophrenia Patients: Basic Concepts and Treatment. Edited by Roder V, Medalia A. Basel, Switzerland, Karger, 2010, pp 118–144

Mueller DR, Roder V, Heuberger A: Efficacy of social cognitive remediation in schizophrenia patients: a meta-analysis. Schizophr Bull 35 (suppl 1):346–347, 2009

Muller TJ, Federspiel A, Horn H, et al: The neurophysiological time pattern of illusionary visual perceptual transitions: a simultaneous EEG and fMRI study. Int J Psychophysiol 55:299–312, 2005

Murray RM, O`Callaghan E, Castle DJ, et al: A neurodevelopmental approach to the classification of schizophrenia. Schizophr Bull 18:319–332, 1992

Naatanen R, Jacobsen T, Winkler I: Memory-based or afferent processes in mismatch negativity (MMN): a review of the evidence. Psychophysiology 42:25–32, 2005

Niendam TA, Bearden CE, Rosso IM, et al: A prospective study of childhood neurocognitive functioning in schizophrenic patients and their siblings. Am J Psychiatry 160:2060–2062, 2003

Norman RM, Malla AK, Cortese L, et al: Symptoms and cognition as predictors of community functioning: a prospective analysis. Am J Psychiatry 156:400–405, 1999

Nuechterlein KH: Signal detection in vigilance tasks and behavioral attributes among offspring of schizophrenic mothers and among hyperactive children. J Abnorm Psychol 92:4–28, 1983

Nuechterlein KH, Dawson ME: A heuristic vulnerability/stress model of schizophrenic episodes. Schizophr Bull 10:300–312, 1984

Nuechterlein KH, Dawson ME, Green MF: Information-processing abnormalities as neuropsychological vulnerability indicators for schizophrenia. Acta Psychiatr Scand Suppl 384:71–79, 1994

Nuechterlein KH, Barch DM, Gold JM, et al: Identification of separable cognitive factors in schizophrenia. Schizophr Res 72:29–39, 2004

Nuechterlein KH, Green MF, Kern RS, et al: The MATRICS Consensus Cognitive Battery, part 1: test selection, reliability, and validity. Am J Psychiatry 165:203–213, 2008

Olbrich R: Computer based psychiatric rehabilitation: current activities in Germany. European Psychiatry 11:60–65, 1996

Olbrich R: [Computer-assisted psychiatric rehabilitation]. Psychiatr Prax 25:103–104, 1998

Olbrich R: Psychologische Verfahren zur Reduktion kognitiver Defizite. Erfahrungen mit einem computergestutzten Trainingsprogramm. Fortschr Neurol Psychiatr 67 (suppl 2):74–76, 1999

Osler M, Lawlor DA, Nordentoft M: Cognitive function in childhood and early adulthood and hospital admission for schizophrenia and bipolar disorders in Danish men born in 1953. Schizophr Res 92:132–141, 2007

Pascual-Marqui RD, Esslen M, Kochi K, et al: Functional imaging with low-resolution brain electromagnetic tomography (LORETA): a review. Methods Find Exp Clin Pharmacol 24:91–95, 2002

Peer JE, Spaulding WD: Heterogeneity in recovery of psychosocial functioning during psychiatric rehabilitation: an exploratory study using latent growth mixture modeling. Schizophr Res 93:186–193, 2007

Penn DL, Corrigan PW, Bentall RP, et al: Social cognition in schizophrenia. Psychol Bull 121:114–132, 1997

Penn DL, Roberts D, Munt ED, et al: A pilot study of social cognition and interaction training (SCIT) for schizophrenia. Schizophr Res 80:357–359, 2005a

Penn DL, Waldheter MA, Perkins DO, et al: Psychosocial treatment for first-episode psychosis: a research update. Am J Psychiatry 162:2220–2232, 2005b

Penn DL, Addington J, Pinkham A: Social cognitive impairments, in The American Psychiatric Publishing Textbook of Schizophrenia. Edited by Lieberman JA, Stroup TS, Perkins DO. Washington, DC, American Psychiatric Publishing, 2006, pp 261–274

Penn DL, Roberts D, Combs D, et al: Best practices: the development of the Social Cognition and Interaction training program for schizophrenia spectrum disorder. Psychiatr Serv 58:449–451, 2007

Penn DL, Sanna LJ, Roberts DL: Social cognition in schizophrenia: an overview. Schizophr Bull 34:408–411, 2008

Perris C: Cognitive Therapy for Patients with Schizophrenia. New York, Cassel, 1989

Pfammatter M, Junghan UM, Brenner HD: Efficacy of psychological therapy in schizophrenia: conclusions from meta-analyses. Schizophr Bull 32 (suppl 1):S64–S80, 2006

Pfurtscheller G, Andrew C: Event-related changes of band power and coherence: methodology and interpretation. J Clin Neurophysiol 16:512–519, 1999

Pinker S: The Blank Slate: The Modern Denial of Human Nature. New York, Penguin, 2003

Pinkham AE, Penn DL: Neurocognitive and social cognitive predictors of interpersonal skill in schizophrenia. Psychiatry Res 143:167–178, 2006

Pinkham AE, Penn DL, Perkins DO, et al: Implications for the neural basis of social cognition for the study of schizophrenia. Am J Psychiatry 160:815–824, 2003

Pinkham AE, Hopfinger JB, Pelphrey KA, et al: Neural bases for impaired social cognition in schizophrenia and autism spectrum disorders. Schizophr Res 99:164–175, 2008

Piskulic D, Olver JS, Norman TR, et al: Behavioural studies of spatial working memory dysfunction in schizophrenia: a quantitative literature review. Psychiatry Res 150:111–121, 2007

Ralph RO, Corrigan PW: Recovery in Mental Illness: Broadening Our Understanding of Wellness. Washington, DC, American Psychological Association, 2005

Rancone R, Mazza M, Frangou I, et al: Rehabilitation of theory of mind deficits in schizophrenia: a pilot study of metacognitive strategies in group treatment. Neuropsychol Rehabil 14:421–435, 2004

Rappelsberger P, Pfurtscheller G, Filz O: Calculation of event-related coherence—a new method to study short-lasting coupling between brain areas. Brain Topogr 7:121–127, 1994

Rector N, Beck AT: Cognitive behavioral therapy for schizophrenia: an empirical review. J Nerv Ment Dis 189:278–287, 2001

Rector N, Seeman MV, Segal ZV: Cognitive therapy for schizophrenia: a preliminary randomised controlled trial. Schizophr Res 63:1–11, 2003

Reitan RM: Trail Making Test. Manual for Administration and Scoring. South Tucson, AZ, Reitan Neuropsychology Laboratory, 1992

Resnick S, Fontana A, Lehman AF, et al: An empirical conceptualization of the recovery orientation. Schizophr Res 75:119–128, 2005

Roberts D, Penn DL: Social Cognition and Interaction Training (SCIT) for outpatients with schizophrenia. Psychiatry Res 166:141–147, 2009

Roder V, Medalia A (eds): Neurocognition and Social Cognition in Schizophrenia Patients: Basic Concepts and Treatment. Basel, Switzerland, Karger, 2010

Roder V, Schmidt SJ: Social cognition as a possible mediator between neurocognition and social functioning. Eur Arch Psychiatry Clin Neurosci 259 (suppl 1):41, 2009

Roder V, Brenner HD, Kienzle N, et al: Integriertes Psychologisches Therapieprogramm (IPT) für schizophrene Patienten. Weinheim, Germany, Psychologie Verlags Union, 1988

Roder V, Mueller DR, Mueser KT, et al: Integrated psychological therapy (IPT) for schizophrenia: is it effective? Schizophr Bull 32:81–93, 2006

Roder V, Brenner HD, Kienzle N: Integriertes Psychologisches Therapieprogramm bei schizophren Erkrankten IPT. Weinheim, Germany, Beltz, 2008

Roder V, Müller D, Brenner HD, et al: Integrated Psychological Therapy (IPT) for the Treatment of Neurocognition, Social Cognition and Social Competency in Schizophrenia Patients. Göttingen, Germany, Hogrefe & Huber, 2010

Rose D, Wykes T: What do clients think of Cognitive Remediation Therapy? A consumer-led investigation of satisfaction and side effects. Am J Psychiatr Rehabil 11:181–204, 2008

Rosen K, Garety P: Predicting recovery from schizophrenia: a retrospective comparison of characteristics at onset of people with single and multiple episodes. Schizophr Bull 31:735–750, 2005

Rosvold HE, Mirsky AF, Sarason I, et al: A continuous performance test of brain damage. J Consult Clin Psychol 20:343, 1956

Ruckstuhl U: Schizophrenieforschung. Weinheim, Germany, Beltz, 1981

Rund BR, Melle I, Friis S, et al: The course of neurocognitive functioning in first-episode psychosis and its relation to premorbid adjustment, duration of untreated psychosis, and relapse. Schizophr Res 91:132–140, 2007

Salisbury DF, Kuroki N, Kasai K, et al: Progressive and interrelated functional and structural evidence of post-onset brain reduction in schizophrenia. Arch Gen Psychiatry 64:521–529, 2007

Salisbury DF, Taylor G, Hall MH: Early auditory gamma band response reduction in first hospitalized schizophrenia: a possible endophenotype for schizophrenia. Early Interv Psychiatry 2:A31–A31, 2008

Sandford JA, Browne RJ: Captain's Log Cognitive System. Richmond, VA, Brain Train, 1988

Schmidt SJ, Mueller DR, Roder V: Relevance of neurocognition, social cognition and negative symptoms for functional recovery and treatment in schizophrenia. Presentation at the World Congress of Behavioral and Cognitive Therapies, Boston, MA, June 2–5, 2010

Schmidt SJ, Mueller DR, Roder V: Social cognition as a mediator variable between neurocognition and functional outcome in schizophrenia: empirical review and new results by structural equation modeling. Schizophr Bull 37 (suppl 2):S41–S54, 2011

Sergi MJ, Rassovsky Y, Nuechterlein KH, et al: Social perception as a mediator of the influence of early visual processing on functional status in schizophrenia. Am J Psychiatry 163:448–454, 2006

Sergi MJ, Rassovsky Y, Widmark C, et al: Social cognition in schizophrenia: relationships with neurocognition and negative symptoms. Schizophr Res 90:316–324, 2007

Silver H, Goodman C: Impairment in error monitoring predicts poor executive function in schizophrenia patients. Schizophr Res 94:156–163, 2007

Silverstein ML, Harrow M, Bryson GJ: Neuropsychological prognosis and clinical recovery. Psychiatry Res 52:265–272, 1994

Silverstein ML, Mavrolefteros G, Close D: Premorbid adjustment and neuropsychological performance in schizophrenia. Schizophr Bull 28:157–165, 2002

Silverstein SM, Valone C, Jewell TC, et al: Integrating shaping and skills training techniques in the treatment of chronic treatment refractory individuals with schizophrenia. Psychiatric Rehabilitation Skills 3:41–58, 1999

Silverstein SM, Menditto AA, Stuve P: Shaping attention span: an operant conditioning procedure to improve neurocognition and functioning in schizophrenia. Schizophr Bull 27:247–257, 2001

Silverstein SM, Hatashita-Wong M, Solak BA, et al: Effectiveness of a two-phase cognitive rehabilitation intervention for severely impaired schizophrenia patients. Psychol Med 35:829–837, 2005

Singer W, Gray CM: Visual feature integration and the temporal correlation hypothesis. Annu Rev Neurosci 18:555–586, 1995

Sohlberg MM, Mateer CA: Effectiveness of an attention-training program. J Clin Exp Neuropsychol 9:117–130, 1987

Spaulding W, Nolting J: Psychotherapy for schizophrenia in the year 2030: prognosis and prognostication. Schizophr Bull 32 (suppl 1):94–105, 2006

Spring B, Weinstein L, Freeman R, et al: Selective attention in schizophrenia, in Handbook of Schizophrenia: Neuropsychology, Psychopathology, and Information Processing, Vol 5. Edited by Steinhauer SR, Gruzelier JH, Zubin J. Amsterdam, The Netherlands, Elsevier, 1991, pp 209–229

Sprong M, Schothorst P, Vos E, et al: Theory of mind in schizophrenia: meta-analysis. Br J Psychiatry 191:5–13, 2007

Straube E: The heterogeneous prognosis of schizophrenia: possible determinants of the short-term and five-year outcome, in Schizophrenia: Origins, Processes, Treatment, and Outcome. Edited by Cromwell RL, Snyder CR. New York, Oxford University Press, 1993, pp 258–274

Strauss E, Sherman E, Strauss O: A Compendium of Neuropsychological Tests: Administration, Norms, and Commentary, 3rd Edition. New York, Oxford University Press, 2006

Strik WK, Lehmann D: Data-determined window size and space-oriented segmentation of spontaneous EEG map series. Electroencephalogr Clin Neurophysiol 87:169–174, 1993

Strik WK, La Malfa G, Cabras P: A bidimensional model for diagnosis and classification of functional psychoses. Compr Psychiatry 30:313–319, 1989

Strik WK, Dierks T, Franzek E, et al: P300 asymmetries in schizophrenia revisited with reference-independent methods. Psychiatry Res 55:153–166, 1994

Strik WK, Fallgatter AJ, Stoeber G, et al: Specific P300 features in patients with cycloid psychosis. Acta Psychiatr Scand 95:67–72, 1997

Strik WK, Ruchsow M, Abele S, et al: Distinct neurophysiological mechanisms for manic and cycloid psychoses: evidence from a P300 study on manic patients. Acta Psychiatr Scand 98:459–466, 1998

Strik W, Dierks I, Hubl D, et al: Hallucinations, thought disorders, and the language domain in schizophrenia. Clin EEG Neurosci 39:91–94, 2008

Strik W, Wopfner A, Horn H, et al: The Bern psychopathology scale for the assessment of system-specific psychotic symptoms. Neuropsychobiology 61:197–209, 2010

Tarrier N: Management and modification of residual psychotic symptoms, in Innovation in the Psychological Management of Schizophrenia. Edited by Birchwood M, Tarrier N. Chichester, UK, Wiley, 1992, pp 147–170

Tecce JJ: Contingent negative variation and individual differences: a new approach in brain research. Arch Gen Psychiatry 24:1–16, 1971

Twamley EW, Jeste DV, Bellack AS: A review of cognitive training in schizophrenia. Schizophr Bull 29:359–382, 2003

Twamley EW, Savla GN, Zurhellen CH, et al: Development and pilot testing of a novel compensatory cognitive training intervention for people with psychosis. Am J Psychiatr Rehabil 11:144–163, 2008

Van der Gaag M, Kern RS, van den Bosch RJ, et al: A controlled trial of cognitive remediation in schizophrenia. Schizophr Bull 28:167–176, 2002

Van Os J, Burns T, Cavallaro R, et al: Standardized remission criteria in schizophrenia. Acta Psychiatr Scand 113:91–95, 2006

Vance A, Hall N, Casey M, et al: Visuospatial memory deficits in adolescent onset schizophrenia. Schizophr Res 93:345–349, 2007

Vauth R, Stieglitz RD: Training Emotionaler Intelligenz bei schizophrenen Störungen. Ein Therapiemanual. Göttingen, Germany, Hogrefe, 2008

Vauth R, Joe A, Seitz M, et al: Differenzielle Kurz und Langzeitwirkung eines "Trainings Emotionaler Intelligenz" und des "Integrierten Psychologischen Therapieprogramms" für schizophrene Patienten. Fortschr Neurol Psychiatr 69:518–525, 2001

Vauth R, Rüsch N, Wirtz M, et al: Does social cognition influence the relation between neurocognitive deficits and vocational functioning in schizophrenia? Psychiatry Res 128:155–165, 2004

Velligan DI, Bow-Thomas CC: Two case studies of cognitive adaptation training for outpatients with schizophrenia. Psychiatr Serv 51:25–29, 2000

Velligan DI, Bow-Thomas CC, Huntzinger C, et al: Randomized controlled trial of the use of compensatory strategies to enhance adaptive functioning in outpatients with schizophrenia. Am J Psychiatry 157:1317–1323, 2000

Velligan DI, Prihoda TJ, Ritch JL, et al: A randomized single-blind pilot study of compensatory strategies in schizophrenia outpatients. Schizophr Bull 28:283–292, 2002

Velligan DI, Kern RS, Gold JM: Cognitive rehabilitation for schizophrenia and the putative role of motivation and expectancies. Schizophr Bull 32:474–485, 2006a

Velligan DI, Mueller J, Wang M, et al: Use of environmental supports among people with schizophrenia. Psychiatr Serv 57:219–224, 2006b

Ventura J, Hellemann GS, Thames AD, et al: Symptoms as mediators of the relationship between neurocognition and functional outcome in schizophrenia. Schizophr Res 113:189–199, 2009

Wernicke C: Grundriss der Psychiatrie in klinischen Vorlesungen. Leipzig, Germany, Thieme, 1900

Whiteman M: The performance of schizophrenics on social concepts. J Abnorm Soc Psychol 49:266–271, 1954

Wölwer W, Streit M, Polzer U, et al: Facial affect recognition in the course of schizophrenia. Eur Arch Psychiatry Clin Neurosci 246:165–170, 1996

Wölwer W, Frommann N, Halfmann S, et al: Remediation of impairments in facial affect recognition in schizophrenia: efficacy and specificity of a new training program. Schizophr Res 80:295–303, 2005

World Health Organization: International Statistical Classification of Diseases and Related Health Problems, 10th Revision. Geneva, World Health Organization, 1992

Wykes T, Reeder C: Cognitive Remediation Therapy for Schizophrenia: Theory and Practice. New York, Routledge, 2005

Wykes T, van der Gaag M: Is it time to develop a new cognitive therapy for psychosis cognitive remediation therapy (CRT)? Clin Psychol Rev 21:1227–1256, 2001

Wykes T, Reeder C, Corner J, et al: The effects of neurocognitive remediation on executive processing in patients with schizophrenia. Schizophr Bull 25:291–307, 1999

Wykes T, Reeder C, Williams C, et al: Are the effects of cognitive remediation therapy (CRT) durable? Results from an exploratory trial in schizophrenia. Schizophr Res 61:163–174, 2003

Wykes T, Steel C, Everitt B, et al: Cognitive behavior therapy for schizophrenia: effect sizes, clinical models, and methodological rigor. Schizophr Bull 34:523–537, 2008

Zimmermann G, Favrod J, Trieu V, et al: The effect of cognitive behavioral treatment on the positive symptoms of schizophrenia spectrum disorders: a meta-analysis. Schizophr Res 77:1–9, 2005

6

Comorbidity in Schizophrenia

Stefano Pallanti, M.D.

Leonardo Quercioli, M.D.

The traditional approach to the diagnosis of schizophrenia led for many years to an underestimation of the problem of comorbidity. Until the publication of DSM-IV (American Psychiatric Association 1994), the diagnostic procedures were structured on a hierarchical basis, following a consolidated tradition in psychiatry to establish a hierarchy of diagnostic categories so that "psychiatric diagnoses are arranged in a hierarchy in which any given diagnosis *excludes* the symptoms of all higher members of the hierarchy and *embraces* the symptoms of the lower members" (Surtees and Kendell 1979, p. 438). For example, if a psychotic disorder were present, the possibly concomitant neurotic disorders would not be diagnosed because they would be regarded as part of the clinical picture of the psychotic condition. The diagnosis of "schizophrenia" in some way explained and included the presence of hierarchically lower syndromes, such as anxiety disorders. This assumption resulted in a diagnostic reductionism—namely, "the tendency to reduce all the symptoms and signs

213

presented by the person with schizophrenia only to schizophrenia" (Berman-zohn et al. 2001, p. 3). Considering the great difficulties of nosologists and cli-nicians to deal with complex sets of symptoms, undoubtedly the hierarchical approach contributed to the general orientation to treat schizophrenia as if it were a single and unitary disorder.

The concept of comorbidity in schizophrenia was recognized by DSM-IV; these diagnostic guidelines first permitted additional diagnoses on Axis I, such as anxiety disorder, in the presence of schizophrenia. At the same time, DSM-IV changed the formulation of the exclusion rules, stating that lower diag-noses would be excluded if they were "better accounted for" by a higher diag-nosis. Allowing more than one diagnosis on Axis I has been accompanied by numerous studies of "comorbidity," evidence of a broadened awareness of the co-occurrence of many syndromes with schizophrenia. However, the change in the wording of the exclusion rules from DSM-III (American Psychiatric As-sociation 1980) to DSM-IV has not solved the conceptual problem about the relation between schizophrenia and the "accounted for by schizophrenia" ex-cluded disorder.

Comorbid disorders must be considered a relevant cause of disability for patients with schizophrenia. Unfortunately, agreement has not been reached on setting guidelines for the treatment of disorders associated with schizo-phrenia, although the same disorders in the absence of schizophrenia are con-sidered treatable with effective and safe treatments.

Yet remnants of the old hierarchical diagnostic system remain, diverting attention from the pressing issue of managing what appear to be common— and treatable—disabling conditions, such as panic disorder and obsessive-compulsive disorder (OCD), that often occur with schizophrenia.

The issue of comorbid disorders in schizophrenia is receiving growing in-terest, widely supported by clinical and research data.

- Comorbid psychiatric conditions affect a large percentage of patients with schizophrenia. Data indicate percentages ranging from 48.6% to 76.7% (McMillan et al. 2009). These data suggest not only that these conditions have a large effect on schizophrenic psychopathology as a whole but also that these syndromes may be useful for classifying and subtyping a large percent-age of patients in the search for distinct phenotypes of schizophrenia.

- Comorbid conditions are persistent over time in schizophrenia and can occur across all phases of the course of the illness, including schizophrenia prodromes, first episode, and chronic schizophrenia (Buckley et al. 2009).
- Comorbid conditions in schizophrenia have a significant effect on the quality of life and are related to worse clinical outcomes (Buckley et al. 2009; McMillan et al. 2009).
- Comorbid conditions in schizophrenia have implications for treatment. Guidelines for treatment of such conditions in patients with schizophrenia remain to be defined; typically clinicians first follow the protocols used to treat the comorbid disorder when schizophrenia is not part of the clinical picture. This practice may in part explain the high rates of polypharmacy observed in the treatment regimens of schizophrenic patients. Unfortunately, the therapeutic implications of such clinical heterogeneity are still not well known, and treatment of comorbidity in schizophrenia is seen as a "trial and error" process, mostly based on personal clinical experience.
- Some comorbid conditions may provide clues about psychobiological hypotheses of schizophrenia itself (e.g., cannabis use and social phobia).
- Some comorbid conditions in schizophrenia may be related to treatments, specifically antipsychotics.

Mood Disorders in Schizophrenia

Depression

The measured rates of depressive phenomenology vary widely among literature data. Methodological problems make it difficult to compare these data, specifically because of varying definitions of schizophrenia (or psychotic illness), different clinical definitions of depression, different instruments used to assess depressive symptoms, nonhomogeneous study populations, and varying time intervals over which depressive symptom occurrence was considered (ranging from point prevalence to many years).

Estimates of the prevalence of depression in schizophrenia range from a point-prevalence rate of 7%–19.5% to a 5-year rate of 75% (Sands and Harrow 1999). The Epidemiologic Catchment Area Study (Fenton 2001) reported a 14-times-greater risk of having a depressive disorder for schizophrenic patients compared with the general population. The National Comorbidity Survey found an

81% lifetime risk of depression in patients with schizophrenia compared with a risk of 7%–25% in the general population (Gruenberg and Goldstein 1997). More recently, McMillan et al. (2009) studied the relation between self-reported schizophrenia and other mental disorders and found comorbid mood disorder in 73.9% of schizophrenic patients—specifically, major depressive disorder in 67.6%, dysthymia in 39.4%, and manic episodes in 39%. Data from the National Hospital Discharge Survey (Weber et al. 2009) on the prevalence of comorbid disorders among hospitalized patients indicated comorbid affective psychoses in 6.9% and depressive disorder not otherwise specified in 3.7% of the discharge records of patients with a primary diagnosis of schizophrenia.

Häfner et al. (2005) in their so-called ABC (Age, Beginning, Course) Schizophrenia Study and ABC Follow-Up Schizophrenia Study found an 83% lifetime prevalence rate for depressive mood at first admission for schizophrenia. Specifically, they observed that the onset of the prodromal stage in schizophrenia was marked by the appearance of depressive symptoms more than 4 years before first admission, whereas negative symptoms and cognitive and social impairment emerged thereafter (Figure 6–1). Depressive mood also was the most frequent symptom in 462 psychotic relapses in the controlled 12-year ABC follow-up study ($N=107$). As the psychosis remitted, the proportion of patients with depressive symptoms decreased and on average remained stable in the further course. The frequency of depressive symptoms in the prodromal stage and in relapse episodes of schizophrenia suggests that depression might at least to some degree be considered an early, milder stage of the same neurobiological process that eventually leads to psychosis.

More recently, Romm et al. (2010) found that almost 50% of the patients in their first year of treatment for a schizophrenia spectrum disorder had experienced one or more episodes of major depressive disorder at some point in their life. Of the patients who had such a lifetime history, 17% had experienced a major depressive episode more than a year before the onset of first-episode psychosis, whereas 30% experienced their first major depressive episode during or after onset of the initial psychotic episode.

Even though depressive symptoms often occur during schizophrenia, not all depressive symptoms are to be considered inevitably connected to the core symptomatology of schizophrenia. For example, their occurrence in many cases could constitute, from a purely psychodynamic point of view, a subjective reaction to the experience of psychotic decompensation.

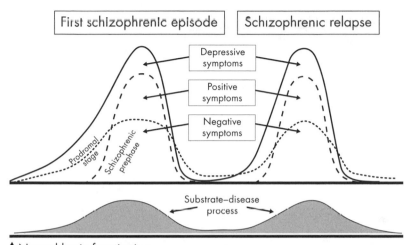

Figure 6–1. Model of sequence of depressive (negative) and psychotic syndromes in the prodromal stage and in psychotic episodes of schizophrenia. *Source.* Adapted from Häfner et al. 2005.

Differential Diagnosis for Depressive Symptoms in Schizophrenia

Medical/organic factors. The risk of developing depression linked to medical/organic factors is the same for patients with schizophrenia and for nonschizophrenic subjects. These possibilities include many common medical conditions (anemia, malignancies, neurological disorders, infectious diseases, metabolic or endocrine disorders), drugs taken for treatment of medical disorders (antihypertensives such as β-blockers, sedative-hypnotics, sulfonamides, and indomethacin), and the discontinuation of prescribed medications (steroids, psychostimulants). Alcohol, cocaine, cannabis, and other drugs may contribute to a depression on the basis of their acute or chronic use or their suspension. Even the suspension of caffeine or nicotine can generate states of withdrawal that may occur as depression.

Major depression. Close longitudinal follow-up is necessary for accurate diagnosis of depression in schizophrenia. In particular, it is important to ascertain that the person has met prior criteria for schizophrenia without prominent mood symptoms and that the diagnosis of depression in the course of schizophrenia is not mistakenly given to a person who had experienced a major depressive episode with psychotic features.

Negative symptoms of schizophrenia.   Whereas positive symptoms (hallucinations, delusions, grossly disorganized thought) represent the presence of a distinct abnormality in thought and perception, negative symptoms of schizophrenia (flattened affect, impoverished speech, apathy, avolition, anhedonia; Table 6–1) represent the absence or diminution of normal intellectual and emotional function and expression.

The main conditions to be distinguished from negative symptoms of schizophrenia are affective symptoms, cognitive symptoms, and psychomotor abnormalities; the clinician must also rule out the possibility that any of these symptoms represent drug-induced effects. In some patients, distinguishing negative symptoms from affective symptoms is relatively easy because several of the characteristic symptoms of depression (depressed mood, feelings of worthlessness, thoughts of death and suicide) do not correspond to negative symptoms. However, other depressive symptoms (anhedonia, apathy, avolition, psychomotor retardation) do resemble negative symptoms. Therefore, it may be difficult to distinguish among 1) schizophrenia with negative symptoms; 2) depressive-type schizoaffective disorder (documented major depressive episode concurrent with symptoms that satisfy Criterion A for schizophrenia [at least 1 month during which at least two of the following are significantly present: delusions, hallucinations, disorganized speech, grossly disorganized or catatonic behavior, or negative symptoms]; bizarre delusions or continual auditory hallucinations alone also fulfill the criteria); and 3) schizophrenia with comorbid depressive symptoms that do not fulfill the criteria for a major depressive episode (e.g., dysthymia or secondary depression related to the burden of schizophrenia or its drug treatment—a state almost identical to secondary negative symptoms).

Thus, the functional significance of depression in schizophrenia is obscured by its conceptual and operational overlap with the negative symptoms found in this disorder. Feelings of guilt and suicidal ideation may be suggestive of depression. However, features such as psychomotor retardation, impaired ability to concentrate, and decreased interest, pleasure, energy, or motivation could be part of negative and depressive symptomatology. Further evidence for the discriminant validity of negative symptoms and depression in schizo-

Table 6–1. Characteristic negative symptoms of schizophrenia

Symptom type	Clinical manifestation
Flattened affect	Unchanging facial expression, vocal tone, body position
Alogia	Lessening of speech fluency; reduced capacity to initiate or respond to speech; meager or impoverished content of speech
Avolition	Passivity; reduced capacity to initiate willful action
Apathy	Loss of interest; emotional disengagement; lack of spontaneity
Anhedonia	Lack of enjoyment in life; inability to experience pleasure or intimacy
Asociality	Social isolation due to active or passive social withdrawal
Psychomotor retardation	Slow or restricted physical movement
Impaired attention	Poor mental focus; poor persistence at tasks

Source. Adapted from Möller 2007.

phrenia was provided by reports of greater improvement in depressive as compared with negative symptoms after the use of antipsychotic medication (Mauri et al. 1999).

Negative symptoms, which can be confused with symptoms of depression, include low physical energy, reduction of interest, lack of pleasure in activities, less momentum, reduced motor activity, and reduced concentration. Other symptoms may be useful for differential diagnosis. The affect flattening is a strongly suggestive marker of negative symptoms, whereas sad mood, guilt, and suicidal ideation orient toward the depressive spectrum of psychopathology. Unfortunately, this distinction is not always easy for the clinician because patients with schizophrenia often have poor interpersonal skills and communication skills that are necessary to effectively present their own subjective states. A presumed diagnosis of negative symptoms is established by excluding other disorders associated with similar symptoms and by ascertaining that the suspected symptoms are in no way clinically dissimilar to negative symptoms. For that purpose, a clinical algorithm (Figure 6–2) can be helpful (Möller 2007).

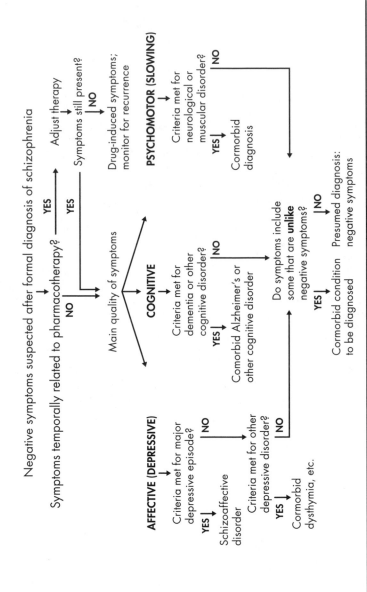

Figure 6–2.   Algorithm for the differential diagnosis of negative symptoms in schizophrenia.

Source.   Adapted from Möller 2007.

Clinicians should be mindful of the potential, in patients with schizophrenia, for negative symptoms to influence ratings of depression and should be aware that depressive symptoms in these patients might lead to functional limitations, particularly in the actual deployment of skills in the real world. Thus, for many patients with schizophrenia, depression may be an important treatment target for disability reduction.

Neuroleptic-induced dysphoria.   Unpleasant subjective effects induced by neuroleptics, leading to an instant dislike toward these drugs, were identified soon after the introduction of chlorpromazine in the 1950s. The term *dysphoria* was initially used in the context of studying the effects of neuroleptics, and the phrase has since remained as a convenient expression for describing the range of subtle and unpleasant subjective responses related to antipsychotic drug therapy. Dysphoric feelings have been described during antipsychotic therapy for a variety of clinical conditions (e.g., schizophrenia and other psychotic spectrum of disorders, Tourette's disorder, stuttering), and the prevalence rates varied considerably between 5% and 40% (Weiden et al. 1989). Dysphoric feelings have been reported to occur within a few hours of administering the first dose of antipsychotic medications and seem to persist over the following weeks and months, leading to several important clinical consequences. The immediate clinical manifestations include complaints of subjective intolerance, reluctance to take antipsychotic drugs, or even an outright refusal of treatment. Failure to address these problems may lead to long-term consequences such as nonadherence to treatment, clinical instability characterized by relapses and rehospitalizations, suicidal behavior, comorbid substance abuse, compromised quality of life, and increased health care costs. The emergence of early dysphoric responses also may have a predictive value in determining long-term clinical prognosis.

Neuroleptic-induced akinesia.   Akinesia is an extrapyramidal side effect (EPS) of antipsychotic drugs that resembles some aspects of the symptom profile seen in depression. Thus, apparent depression in some postacute schizophrenia patients may be closely linked to—or a part of—an extrapyramidal reaction such as akinesia. The classic symptom profile of neuroleptic-induced akinesia—which is particularly linked to the older-generation antipsychotics—involves stiffness of the large muscle groups leading to the typical parkinsonian posture with reduced accessory movements. More nuanced forms of akinesia are also possible, manifesting only as difficulty in initiating and sustaining spontaneous behavior, effort, or movement over time. These patients lack social initiative, and this state is accompanied by a decline in mood. On the subjective side, patients with this form of akinesia often report anhedonia, blame themselves, and complain of lack of energy. Medication-induced akinesia may benefit from reduction of the antipsychotic dosage, from addition of an antiparkinsonian drug, or from replacement of the current antipsychotic with a new-generation agent having a lower incidence of EPS.

Neuroleptic-induced akathisia.   Akathisia, an EPS mostly related to old-generation antipsychotics (e.g., phenothiazines, butyrophenones, sulpiride) can occur in more nuanced ways that are difficult to recognize when clinically expressed as a slight increase in motor behavior. The incidence of medication-induced akathisia has declined in the past decade as first-line therapy for schizophrenia has shifted from first- to second-generation antipsychotics, which have an overall lower rate of EPS. Unfortunately, akathisia may be overlooked as an adverse effect of second-generation antipsychotics. Untreated akathisia can have devastating effects, leading to severe agitation, aggression, medication nonadherence, and increased risk for suicide; therefore, early detection and effective treatment of akathisia are essential. A dosage reduction of the antipsychotic, or switching to a new-generation antipsychotic, may be indicated, but the addition of an antiparkinsonian agent appears to be less effective. More recently, mirtazapine has been suggested as a treatment option for antipsychotic-induced akathisia (Hieber et al. 2008).

Postpsychotic Depressive Disorder

According to DSM-IV-TR (American Psychiatric Association 2000), major depression and schizophrenia cannot be diagnosed concurrently. DSM-IV-TR Appendix B defines postpsychotic depressive disorder of schizophrenia (PPDD) as the presence of depressive symptoms that meet the criteria for major depressive episode during the residual phase of schizophrenia. Such depression may occur at any time during the residual phase but most commonly occurs following an acute psychotic episode.

For both DSM-IV-TR and ICD-10 (World Health Organization 1992) diagnostic criteria sets for PPDD are based on the respective criteria for depressive episodes, with some modifications and the addition of an item to avoid the diagnosis of a depressive episode during the acute psychotic episode. The DSM-IV-TR criteria have an item to exclude depressive symptoms that are better accounted for as medication side effects or negative symptoms. The main incompatibility between the two criteria sets is that the ICD-10 postschizophrenic depression criteria limit the diagnosis to the 12 months following the psychotic episode, whereas the DSM-IV-TR PPDD criteria do not have a time limitation.

In the ICD-10, postschizophrenic depression (F20.4) is defined as follows:

A depressive episode, which may be prolonged, arising in the aftermath of a schizophrenic illness. Some schizophrenic symptoms must still be present but no longer dominate the clinical picture. These persisting schizophrenic symptoms may be "positive" or "negative," although the latter are more common. It is uncertain, and immaterial to the diagnosis, to what extent the depressive symptoms merely have been uncovered by the resolution of earlier psychotic symptoms (rather than being a new development) or are an intrinsic part of schizophrenia rather than a psychological reaction to it. The depressive symptoms are rarely sufficiently severe or extensive to meet criteria for a severe depressive episode, and it is often difficult to determine which of the patient's symptoms result from depression and which result from antipsychotic medication or the impaired volition and affective flattening of schizophrenia itself. This depressive disorder is associated with an increased risk of suicide. (World Health Organization 1992)

Apparently, the concept of postschizophrenic depression tends to avoid a comorbidity in the stricter sense. This purpose becomes especially obvious in the last sentences of the ICD-10 diagnostic guidelines (see Table 6–2), which underline that in the case of mixed conditions, the diagnosis of either a depressive episode or a schizophrenic subtype should be given, depending on the prominent features (Möller 2005).

The bulk of the literature suggests that PPDD in the period following acute psychosis may represent the continuation of depression from the acute stage, whereas PPDD after a period of relative stability may herald the reemergence of psychosis. Perhaps the change in standard of care from typical to atypical antipsychotics as first-line medications in the treatment of acute schizophrenia is responsible for the reduced attention on PPDD. In fact, although efficacy of antidepressant drugs in association with antipsychotics has been observed, more recent observations have led to the conclusion that "at present, there is no

Table 6–2.   World Health Organization diagnostic guidelines for F20.4 postschizophrenic depression

The diagnosis should be made only if

a.   The patient has had a schizophrenic illness meeting the general criteria for schizophrenia (F20) within the past 12 months;

b.   Some schizophrenic symptoms are still present; and

c.   The depressive symptoms are prominent and distressing, fulfilling at least the criteria for a depressive episode, and have been present for at least 2 weeks.

If the patient no longer has any schizophrenic symptoms, a depressive episode should be diagnosed. If schizophrenic symptoms are still florid and prominent, the diagnosis should remain that of the appropriate schizophrenic subtype.

Source.   Reprinted from World Health Organization: *International Statistical Classification of Diseases and Related Health Problems,* 10th Revision. Geneva, World Health Organization, 1992. Used with permission.

convincing evidence to support or refute the use of antidepressants in treating depression in people with schizophrenia" (Whitehead et al. 2002, p. 10). In this context, atypical antipsychotics might be considered in the management of postpsychotic depression. In fact, olanzapine, risperidone, or ziprasidone may have antidepressant activity in patients with schizophrenia or schizoaffective disorders. Investigators supported that the therapeutic approach to be used in the management of depression in patients with schizophrenia first consisted of switching from a classic to an atypical antipsychotic before considering antidepressant drugs.

Schizoaffective Disorder

The schizoaffective psychoses represent a special type of the relevant modern conceptualization of a relation between schizophrenic and affective symptoms. The affective part occurs either simultaneously with the schizophrenic symptoms or sequentially (without concurrent schizophrenic symptoms), depending on the diagnostic system applied.

The concept of schizoaffective disorder was invoked in 1933 to describe "acute schizoaffective psychosis" (Kasanin 1933), in which patients presented with coterminous severe affective and psychotic symptoms. Clinically, schizoaffective disorder became a firmly established diagnostic category that gained further recognition on inclusion as a subtype of schizophrenia in DSM-I and DSM-II (American Psychiatric Association 1952, 1968).

Schizoaffective disorder is a prototypical boundary condition that had highlighted the disadvantages of a rigidly categorical classification system. The definition of schizoaffective disorder has changed during the last decades, and it is a highly "unstable" diagnosis, defined in different ways in Europe and in the United States (Table 6–3). In short, the DSM-IV-TR definition requires a co-occurrence of an affective episode and a schizophrenia active phase and at least 2 weeks without mood symptoms. At the same time, mood disorders with psychotic mood-incongruent symptoms could include schizophrenia symptoms. The ICD-10 classification defines only the co-occurrence of an affective syndrome and schizophrenia symptoms for 2 weeks of about the same extent and intensity as the affective symptoms. Schizophrenia symptoms are not allowed in psychotic affective disorders. However, despite the problems with the validity of the diagnosis, because of the large number of "in-between" patients, the diagnostic category of schizoaffective disorder is upheld.

In clinical practice, the use of schizoaffective disorder often solves diagnostic dilemmas associated with atypical presentation of mood symptoms within the context of schizophrenia but may not serve the patient well with respect to pharmacological or psychosocial management. Clinicians understandably find it difficult to discriminate between schizophrenia and bipolar disorder and, perhaps by virtue of personal bias, diagnose one or the other or compromise and use the term *schizoaffective disorder* to defer diagnostic exactness. These inconsistencies undermine the usefulness of diagnostic classification and highlight the need for careful deliberation of clinical and experimental data in future revisions of the nomenclature. In fact, studies on comorbidity indexes found a large overlap between the diagnostic categories of schizophrenia, schizoaffective disorder, and bipolar disorder, supporting the existence of an overlap between bipolar disorder and schizophrenia and thus challenging the categorical approach used in both DSM-IV-TR and ICD-10 classification systems. Growing evidence of an etiological overlap between schizophrenia, schizoaffective disorder, and bipolar disorder has become increasingly difficult to disregard (Laursen et al. 2009).

Table 6–3. Comparison of DSM-IV-TR and ICD-10 diagnostic criteria for schizoaffective disorder

	Mood criteria	Schizophrenic criteria	Duration criteria	Simultaneity criteria	Additional criteria
DSM-IV-TR	Major depressive, manic, or mixed episode	Meeting Criterion A for schizophrenia (two or more of delusions, hallucinations, disorganized speech, behavioral disturbances, or negative symptoms) One symptom if commenting on third-person voices or bizarre delusions	Major depressive episode: 2 weeks; mixed or manic episode: 1 week Psychotic symptoms: 1 month to meet Criterion A for schizophrenia	During the same period of the illness	Delusions or hallucinations for at least 2 weeks without prominent mood symptoms Mood symptoms as a substantial portion of the total duration of illness
ICD-10	Prominent manic, depressive, or mixed symptoms	One, preferably two of (a) to (d) symptoms for schizophrenia (does not include symptoms of speech)	Duration of the mood episode (manic: at least 1 week; major depressive: 2 weeks)	Preferably simultaneous, at least within a few days of each other	

Source.　Adapted from Malhi et al. 2008.

Assessment of Depressive Symptoms in Schizophrenia

The concern about what depression scales measure becomes of greater importance when the scales are used in populations for which they were not developed, such as a population with schizophrenia. This assessment has been hampered by the temporal variability of the depressive symptoms and by their overlap with both the negative symptoms of schizophrenia and the extrapyramidal effects of the antipsychotic treatment. So far, classic assessment instruments such as the Hamilton Rating Scale for Depression (Ham-D) and the Montgomery-Åsberg Depression Rating Scale have been used in those patients who have schizophrenia with depressive symptomatology, despite the important limitations concerning their use in subpopulations other than those they have been developed for. Earlier studies found that the rating of depression with the Ham-D is significantly influenced by negative symptoms in schizophrenia and by EPS (Collins et al. 1996; Yazaji et al. 2002).

The Beck Depression Inventory, a self-report instrument for depression, may be difficult to administer to inpatients with schizophrenia. The Depression subscale of the Positive and Negative Syndrome Scale (PANSS-D), which evaluates depression as a part of the comprehensive assessment of psychopathology in schizophrenia, is also widely used to assess depression in clinical trials (Siris et al. 2001). The PANSS-D, however, has been shown to have a significant correlation with the negative symptoms of schizophrenia (Collins et al. 1996).

To overcome some of the limitations, the Calgary Depression Scale for Schizophrenia (CDSS) was specifically developed to assess depression in schizophrenia (Addington et al. 1990). Derived from the Ham-D and the Present State Examination, the CDSS is a nine-item structured interview scale (Table 6–4) in which each item has a four-point anchored measure. The CDSS has been shown to be a reliable, valid, and specific measure of depression in patients with schizophrenia (Addington et al. 1993). Comparison studies (Kim et al. 2006; Yazaji et al. 2002) have reported that the CDSS is able to distinguish depression from negative psychotic symptoms and EPS. However, even though the CDSS appears to be less susceptible to confounding by positive symptoms, there have been inconsistent findings in the relationship between CDSS scores and positive symptoms in schizophrenia.

Table 6–4.   Items of the Calgary Depression Scale for Schizophrenia

1. Depressed mood

2. Hopelessness

3. Self-deprecation

4. Guilty ideas of reference

5. Pathological guilt

6. Morning depression

7. Early awakening

8. Suicide

9. Observed depression

Source.   Addington et al. 1990.

Strategies for Treatment of Depression in Schizophrenia

Treatment of depression in schizophrenia can be approached sequentially as outlined in Table 6–5.

Suicidality in Schizophrenia

In recent meta-analyses, the risk of suicide in schizophrenia was found to be 13 times greater than in the general population (Saha et al. 2007), and the lifetime risk of suicide in schizophrenia was estimated to be 4.9% (Palmer et al. 2005).

Approximately half of all patients with schizophrenia or schizoaffective disorder attempt suicide at some point in their patient careers, and from 4% to 13%, depending on the study, die of suicide, with the mortality risk higher in men than in women, although not markedly so. In the population at large, the risk of suicide is considered to be three times higher for men than for women. By contrast, in the population of individuals with schizophrenia, the odds ratio for suicide in men compared with women is approximately 1.57 (Hawton et al. 2005), meaning that whatever protects women from suicide in the general population (relative to men) does not appear to be operative in schizophrenia. Women with schizophrenia have been described as behaving

Table 6–5. Strategies for treatment of depression in schizophrenia

A. Is the current antipsychotic treatment contributing to depression?

   1) Reduce dosage.

   2) Change antipsychotic.

   3) Use atypical antipsychotics; avoid typical agents.

B. Use antidepressant agents.

   1) Selective serotonin reuptake inhibitor or serotonin-norepinephrine reuptake inhibitor (consider drug-drug interactions; avoid drugs that worsen weight gain)

   2) Tricyclic antidepressant

   3) Lithium

C. Add quetiapine, aripiprazole, or ziprasidone.

D. Use psychosocial intervention.

Table 6–6. Specific risk factors for suicide in schizophrenia

• Previous depressive disorder

• History of suicide attempt

• Hopelessness

• Poor adherence to treatment

• Higher educational attainment

• Age ≥30 years at onset of symptoms

like stereotypical men when it comes to suicide, acting impulsively and aggressively and choosing lethal means to end their lives.

A meta-analysis reported that the suicide risk in schizophrenia is strongly associated with previous depressive disorder, hopelessness, history of suicide attempt, and poor adherence to treatment (Hawton et al. 2005; Pompili et al. 2009; Table 6–6).

In a recent population-based case-control study, Reutfors et al. (2009) confirmed previous observations on higher educational attainment, age 30 years or older at onset of symptoms, and a history of a suicide attempt as associated with an increased risk of suicide within 5 years after a first clinical schizophrenia inpatient diagnosis. Tendencies for an increased risk of suicide being associated with having been married or cohabiting and with a longer total duration of hospitalization also were observed. Gender did not significantly affect the suicide risk, nor did a history of self-discharge, compulsory inpatient treatment, substance use disorder, or a family history of mental disorder or suicide.

Positive symptoms are generally less often included among risk factors for suicide in schizophrenia. However, several studies have found that the active and exacerbated phase of the illness and the presence of psychotic symptoms, as well as paranoid delusions and thought disorder, are associated with a high risk of suicide. Patients with the paranoid subtype of schizophrenia are also more likely to commit suicide. Suicides as a result of command hallucinations, although rare, have been reported in the literature. Kelly et al. (2004) reported that a large proportion of their patients with schizophrenia who committed suicide had poor control of thoughts or thought insertion, loose associations, and flight of ideas compared with those who died by other means.

Drug treatment of schizophrenia is generally associated with a reduced risk of suicide. In this regard, clozapine has been found to reduce suicide risk in schizophrenia (Pompili et al. 2009). However, because the administration of both clozapine and atypical antipsychotics may be accompanied by increased insight and illness awareness, and because sudden increases in insight may lead to increased suicidality in patients with schizophrenia, caution is needed, and patients should be followed up closely in an appropriate therapeutic relationship to monitor such abrupt increases in insight.

The SAD PERSONAS Scale (Patterson et al. 1983; Table 6–7) provides a mnemonic for assessing the most important risk factors for suicide. For each item on the SAD PERSONAS Scale that is present in an individual patient, 1 point is given. The total possible number of points is 11, which would represent very high risk for suicide.

The overrepresentation of violent suicide methods in schizophrenia as compared with those in the general population (Breier and Astrachan 1984) suggests that suicides among schizophrenia patients may be less preventable than suicides in the general population by restricting the availability of pharmacological means of suicide. Instead, other general preventive strategies, such as barriers at bridges and observation by cameras at railways, may be more valuable for decreasing suicides in this patient group.

Table 6–7. SAD PERSONAS Scale for assessment of suicide risk

S ex[a]

A ge[b]

D epression

P revious attempt

E thanol and drug abuse

R ational thought loss

S ocial supports lacking

O rganized plan

N o spouse

A ccess to lethal means

S ickness

[a]Men account for 75% of suicide deaths; women attempt suicide more often than men
[b]Elderly people and young adults are at greatest risk for suicide.

Source.   Adapted from Patterson et al. 1983.

Anxiety Disorders in Schizophrenia

The relation between anxiety and psychosis has been hypothesized in descriptive psychopathology at different moments of the schizophrenic process. At the onset, when delusional experiences begin, the phenomenological tradition has always reported the experiential dimension of anxiety as a dramatic and radically absolute uprooting from the interhuman dimension. Sullivan (1927) complained that psychiatrists too often see patients at only the end states of schizophrenia. If psychiatrists dealt professionally with more patients at a prepsychotic state, he argued, it would be easy to observe the gradations from the neurasthenic picture into schizophrenia. Fear states, ranging from phobia to terror, and from anxious feelings of apprehension to fully developed primitive panic, are important factors in many incipient conditions.

The recognition of co-occurrence of anxiety disorders in schizophrenia dates back to the early years of psychiatric nosology. However, the topic has long been neglected in both research and clinical settings; recently, such comorbidity has begun receiving growing attention. The first reason is related to the evolution of the diagnostic hierarchy rules in DSM with fewer current restrictions regarding diagnoses of anxiety disorder in patients with schizophrenia. In fact, DSM-IV-TR allows a diagnosis of anxiety disorder if the anxiety symptoms are "not better accounted for by" or "not restricted to" schizophrenic symptoms. Furthermore, there is an increasing awareness that positive outcomes can be achieved by a significant proportion of schizophrenic patients, and current treatment approaches favor individualized care and adopt a more holistic perspective. Recent evidence shows that comorbid anxiety disorder has a negative effect on patients' recovery and functioning (Karatzias et al. 2007; Pallanti et al. 2004); thus. recognizing and treating anxiety disorders, when present, in patients with schizophrenia spectrum disorders could contribute to more positive outcomes. Finally, pharmacological treatment of psychosis might precipitate an anxiety disorder, or pharmacological approaches to anxiety disorders might precipitate psychosis. Thus, the relationship between these two symptom clusters may be complex and multidetermined.

A recent meta-analysis from Achim et al. (2011) that combined data from 52 studies and a total of 4,032 patients confirmed that anxiety disorders are highly prevalent in schizophrenia spectrum psychotic disorders and that prevalence rates are higher than those reported for the general population, also highlighting the great variations in rates among studies (Table 6–8).

Panic Disorder

Estimation of the prevalence of panic disorder comorbidity in schizophrenia had been difficult prior to 1987, and some studies that used the stringent DSM-III exclusion criteria may have underestimated prevalence.

The lifetime prevalence of panic disorder in schizophrenia is about 30% in the general population and from 5% to nearly 40% in clinical samples (Buckley et al. 2009). The number of male patients with panic disorder is twofold higher than that of female patients (Ulas et al. 2007). Regarding the etiopathogenetic mechanisms underlying the co-occurrence of panic disorder in schizophrenia, the main hypotheses suggest that panic disorder may favor the onset of schizophrenia (Kahn and Meyers 2000) and that the comorbidity is the result of common underlying etiological factors. These factors, for instance, may run in families because panic disorder in relatives of schizophrenic patients might be the expression of attenuated familial susceptibility factors for schizophrenia.

Table 6–8. Co-occurrence of anxiety disorders in schizophrenia: overall prevalence rates

	OCD	PD	AGO	PTSD	SP	SPP	GAD	Any
No. of studies	34	23	12	20	16	11	14	16
No. of patients	3,007	1,393	862	1,388	1,259	925	939	958
Mean prevalence rate (%)[a]	12.1	9.8	5.4	12.4	14.9	7.9	10.9	38.3
95% CI	7.0%–17.1%	4.3%–15.4%	0.2%–10.6%	4.0%–20.8%	8.1%–21.8%	1.9%–13.8%	2.9%–18.8%	26.3%–50.4%
Range	0.6%–55.0%	0.0%–35.0%	0.0%–27.5%	0.0%–51.4%	3.6%–39.5%	0.0%–30.8%	0.0%–45.0%	10.4%–85.0%
Heterogeneity	317.98*	162.79*	83.52*	294.09*	127.37*	80.78*	142.52*	146.23*

Note. AGO = agoraphobia; Any = proportion of patients with at least one of the anxiety disorders assessed in the study; CI = confidence interval; GAD = generalized anxiety disorder; OCD = obsessive-compulsive disorder; PD = panic disorder; PTSD = posttraumatic stress disorder; SP = social phobia; SPP = simple phobia.

[a]Mean prevalence rates express main results.

*P < 0.001.

Source. Adapted from Achim et al. 2011.

This great variability of rates may be attributed to some methodological issues. First, different inclusion criteria have been used to select the samples. Indeed, most of the authors recruited in- or outpatients, but others recruited day hospital–treated subjects. Second, different diagnoses in the frame of psychosis have been considered. Some studies included acute schizophrenic patients, whereas other authors referred to chronic schizophrenia (Ulas et al. 2007). Third, time of assessment varied among the studies.

Finally, most of the authors did not precisely report the treatments received by the patients under study. Moreover, many studies did not consider drugs as a confounding variable in the statistical analyses, although it has been hypothesized that medication commonly used in the treatment of schizophrenia (i.e., antipsychotics, mood stabilizers, antidepressants, and benzodiazepines) may interfere with the level of anxiety (Buckley et al. 2009).

Hypotheses About Panic Disorder in Schizophrenia

Two main hypotheses have been proposed to explain the co-occurrence of panic disorder and schizophrenia. First, it was suggested that a "panic psychosis" does exist (Kahn and Meyers 2000). Panic may contribute to the development of a dopamine-mediated, panic-related psychosis. The Kahn hypothesis resembles a model in which chronic methamphetamine abuse may result in a lasting change in brain dopaminergic and nondopaminergic systems. The hypothesis of a panic psychosis has been strengthened by some clinical observations. In schizophrenic patients, panic attacks tend to precede the onset of hallucinations, auditory hallucinations and delusions might develop during severe anxiety attacks, and alprazolam or clonazepam may induce remission of both panic attacks and concomitant positive and negative symptoms.

Second, it was proposed that panic and schizophrenia may have common etiological factors. Assuming a multifactorial threshold model of liability for schizophrenia, panic disorder in relatives of schizophrenic patients might be seen as the expression of attenuated familial susceptibility factors for schizophrenia.

In patients with schizophrenia who also have panic symptoms, the two diatheses may interact in a dynamic way, creating a vicious cycle of symptoms.

Assessment of Panic Disorder in Schizophrenia

Clinicians may have had some difficulties in formulating a correct diagnosis of panic disorder in schizophrenic individuals because panic may have atypical (e.g., prolonged duration of episode) and uncommon clinical features (Savitz et al. 2011). Moreover, florid positive symptoms and debilitating negative symptoms may complicate the assessment of panic, and antipsychotic-treated patients may be difficult to evaluate for symptoms related to panic because of the confound of EPS (e.g., akathisia).

Furthermore, the formulation of the diagnosis of schizophrenia and panic disorder can be difficult because schizophrenic patients may tend to withhold descriptions of that experience when they feel a sense of shame or fear or are afraid to be hospitalized.

Panic symptoms may be more common in patients with paranoid schizophrenia, compared with other schizophrenia subtypes or schizoaffective disorder. Furthermore, panic attacks were frequently related to paranoid ideation in these studies. Bermanzohn et al. (1997) described the potential for a relation between panic attacks and paranoia. It has been suggested that the high association between panic disorder and the paranoid type of schizophrenia might be related to greater anxiety sensitivity or hyperarousal in these patients. Indeed, according to the cognitive-behavioral model, the likelihood of having a panic disorder increases with hypervigilance, hyperarousal, and the patient's tendency to attribute physical symptoms to the presence of an external threat. In patients with the paranoid subtype of schizophrenia, this perceived threat may parallel their delusional systems; hence they believe something bad is going to happen even before they start experiencing the symptoms of panic. The panic attack then reinforces this belief that something bad is going to happen and thus begins a vicious cycle.

Comorbid panic symptoms have been associated with a decrease in age at onset for schizophrenia, more severe psychopathology, and an increased risk of suicidal ideation and behavior and comorbid substance use (Buckley et al. 2009).

The assessment of panic disorder in schizophrenic patients is of relevant interest in research and in clinical settings, but unfortunately, specific standardized instruments aimed at evaluating panic in schizophrenia are still lacking. None of the available instruments should be considered a substitute for a skilled interview, especially in view of the confusing concurrence of panic symptoms with psychotic exacerbation. In fact, the assessment of panic disorder in schizophrenia requires specific interviewing skills (Table 6–9) and the motivation to investigate potential panic symptoms. Thus, for instance, in psychotic patients, the exploration may begin with questions about psychotic phenomena (i.e., auditory hallucinations, paranoid fear) potentially related to

Table 6–9.   Screening questions for possible panic symptoms in schizophrenia

Are you experiencing…

1. Sudden feelings of anxiety, fear, or panic? Feelings of anger or rage? Crying?

2. Sudden heart racing? Heart pounding?

3. Sudden chest pain? Chest pressure?

4. Sudden sweating?

5. Sudden trembling or shaking?

6. Suddenly feeling short of breath or like you can't catch your breath?

7. Sudden choking or a lump in your throat?

8. Suddenly nauseous or queasy?

9. Suddenly feeling dizzy, light-headed, or faint?

10. Suddenly feeling detached, sort of like you are in a glass box?

11. Suddenly afraid of losing control? Afraid of going crazy?

12. Suddenly afraid of dying? Afraid of having a heart attack?

13. Sudden numbness or tingling, especially in your hands or face?

14. Suddenly feeling hot or cold?

15. Sudden itching in your teeth?

16. Sudden fear that people want to hurt you?

17. Sudden voices?

Source.   Adapted from Savitz et al. 2011.

panic symptoms and then progress to focus on the sudden onset of paniclike symptoms. During nonpsychotic periods, panic attacks may continue without psychotic features. History of these episodes may be gathered through more conventional questions about abrupt onset of panic, chest pain, tachycardia, or shortness of breath. Because nonpsychotic panic attacks can seem milder to the patient, they may require careful inquiry for diagnosis. Also, the symptom chronology should be investigated. Indeed, patients often recall nonpsychotic panic attacks that preceded the onset of paroxysmal psychotic symptoms by months or years.

Table 6–10. Strategies for treatment of panic disorder in schizophrenia

A. Consider whether patient's current antipsychotic might be inducing panic symptoms.

B. Change antipsychotic medication.

C. Check thyroid function.

D. Reduce caffeine consumption.

E. Use of add-on treatment: only anecdotal reports are available that suggest imipramine, mirtazapine, or alprazolam as effective.

F. Treat panic as in patients without schizophrenia, taking into account drug-drug interactions and potential weight gain.

G. Use cognitive-behavioral therapy.

Strategies for Treatment of Panic Disorder in Schizophrenia

Treatment of panic disorder in schizophrenia can be approached as outlined in Table 6–10.

Social Anxiety Disorder (Social Phobia)

Social anxiety is itself a disabling disorder, and individuals who have comorbid conditions have a more severe level of disability (Wittchen and Fehm 2001). Subjects with social anxiety disorder have a higher risk of developing substance or alcohol abuse or dependence, and in patients with schizophrenia, as in the general population, substance abuse or dependence appears associated with higher impulsivity and suicidality.

Comorbid panic disorder and OCD have been widely investigated in schizophrenia patients, but, unfortunately, social anxiety in schizophrenia has received much less clinical attention. Frequently, schizophrenic patients express nervousness and anxiety during social interactions. Penn et al. (1994) suggested that social phobia is more frequent in schizophrenia patients than in nonpsychiatric control subjects.

According to a biodevelopmental shyness vulnerability model, Goldberg and Schmidt (2001) investigated the severity of shyness and early sociability troubles among adults who have a serious social dysfunction, such as schizophrenic patients. They reported that individuals with schizophrenia showed significantly more shyness, lower sociability, and more recollections of childhood social troubles compared with the control group. Within the schizophrenia group, both shyness traits and limited sociability were clearly associated with interpersonal dysfunction.

> Frank, a 24-year-old university student, received the diagnosis of paranoid schizophrenia 7 years ago. He had two hospitalizations at ages 18 and 20. He responded well to typical antipsychotics but stopped them because of EPS leading to relapse. Frank is currently taking clozapine, 250 mg/day, which resulted in remission of many of his symptoms (Brief Psychiatric Rating Scale score: 45% reduction after 6 weeks; 65% after 8 weeks).
>
> After 4 months of clozapine treatment, Frank began to complain of anxiety in various social situations. He reported difficulty speaking to others, particularly within his group of friends; feelings of shame; and extreme shyness toward women. Frank began to avoid certain situations and felt so anxious that he left the band in which he played guitar. In these anxious situations, he complained of tachycardia, tremor, and sweating. Clinical assessment showed stable remission of psychotic symptoms, no EPS, reduction of disturbing cognitive experience (67% reduction in Frankfurt Complaint Questionnaire score), and social phobic symptoms (Liebowitz Social Anxiety Scale [LSAS]—Fear or Anxiety score: 42 [percentage of subscale total score: 58%]; Avoidance score: 44 [61%]).
>
> Frank's anxiety symptoms were significantly reduced after 40 days of treatment with fluoxetine (up to 30 mg).

Epidemiological studies indicated that the rate of social anxiety disorder in schizophrenia ranges from 13% to 39% (Pallanti et al. 2004). Even if social anxiety disorder in schizophrenia appears as a stable phenomenon across assessments, it often remains unrecognized and therefore untreated because of its frequent confusion with negative symptoms in schizophrenia patients.

Social Anxiety and Negative and Positive Symptoms of Schizophrenia

In terms of symptomatology, social anxiety and schizophrenia have some superficial similarities: both involve social withdrawal, isolation, and feelings that others judge or perceive patients in a negative fashion that can veer into paranoia. This is the main reason that, within the schizophrenic population, social anxiety may be a greater problem in patients who predominantly express negative symptoms. This psychopathological debate was first discussed by Meehl (1962), who pointed out that anhedonia, a core negative symptom, could contribute to or be a consequence of what he described as "aversive drift" in schizophrenia (i.e., the tendency to take on a burdensome, threatening, gloomy, negative emotional valence). He suggested that this aversive drift is intense and pervasive in the interpersonal domain, manifesting itself as ambivalence and interpersonal fear.

Although patients with negative symptoms typically present with little emotional expression, flat affect does not necessarily correspond to blunted emotional experience. Thus, a patient may show flat affect but experience significant social anxiety.

Similar to individuals with severe social anxiety, patients with negative symptoms tend to be isolative. These individuals with predominantly negative symptoms have greater impairment in social relationships and quality of life relative to those expressing predominantly positive symptoms. Thus, the tendency of patients with negative symptoms to withdraw from social contact may represent attempts to cope with high levels of social anxiety.

A study by Pallanti et al. (2004) of outpatients with schizophrenia found higher levels of insight and avoidance-related behaviors in patients with comorbid social anxiety, supporting the hypothesis that the awareness of illness and its sequelae might lead to an increase in social phobia psychologically. On the other hand, this study also showed that an increase in negative symptoms correlated with a decrease in insight and avoidance-related behaviors. The authors believed that negative symptoms or primary psychosis led to more detachment-style behaviors, which could be confused with social phobia, than the actual interpersonal sensitivity and avoidant features that are associated with true social phobia in schizophrenic patients. However, the stress-induced anxiety also seemed to increase the levels of paranoia, suggesting that social anxiety may exacerbate positive symptoms.

Recently, Mazeh et al. (2009) suggested that the "fear" component of social anxiety may be associated with positive symptomatology of schizophrenia. It seems that patients in an acute phase of their disease have a higher degree of alertness, anxiety, and sensitivity to their surroundings, whereas the chronic stage of the disease is associated with avoidance. In the acute psychotic phase of schizophrenia, similar aspects of psychosis through the PANSS Positive scale and the Fear or Anxiety component of the LSAS could be indirectly rated.

Schizophrenia and Social Anxiety: Putative Neurobiological Links

A biological link between schizophrenia and social anxiety disorder has been postulated, suggesting abnormalities in dopaminergic transmission in social anxiety, apart from the presence of schizophrenia, that are not found in other anxiety disorders. Decreased basal ganglia volume, decreased dopamine re-uptake site densities, and decreased dopamine receptor binding sites in social phobia, especially low availability of striatal dopamine type 2 (D_2) receptors (Schneier et al. 2008), have been shown. Stein et al. (1990) noted increased rates of social anxiety in patients with Parkinson's disease, a disease character-ized by hypodopaminergic transmission in the basal ganglia. Social inhibition therefore could be related to the physiological substrata of the extrapyramidal pathway similar to those involved in Parkinson's disease.

Liebowitz et al. (1986) noted that monoamine oxidase inhibitors are more effective than tricyclic antidepressants in social anxiety. Increased social phobia has been seen in patients with Tourette's disorder during treatment with halo-peridol (Mikkelsen et al. 1981). The role of dopamine in the symptoms of so-cial phobia also was supported by the findings that novelty-seeking and exploratory behavior is correlated to the striatal uptake of dopamine (Clonin-ger 1987) and that long alleles of the D_4 receptor gene significantly character-ized novelty-seeking individuals more than did short D_4 receptor gene alleles (Benjamin et al. 1996).

A serotonergic central dysfunction may be involved in the pathogenesis of social phobia; the dopaminergic and the serotonergic neurotransmitter system have been found to modulate the amygdala-connected circuitries that are cru-cial in emotional modulation and response to fearful stimuli. The phenotype of social phobia may correspond to an etiological heterogeneity involving var-ious neurotransmitter systems.

Pallanti et al. (2000) reported a group of patients with paranoid schizo-phrenia, resistant or intolerant to typical antipsychotics, who developed symp-toms of social phobia 9–20 weeks after beginning clozapine treatment and required pharmacological augmentation. Fluoxetine, in addition to the cloza-pine treatment, was effective in ameliorating social anxiety disorder in most of the schizophrenic patients with social anxiety disorder according to the LSAS. The authors hypothesized that some vulnerable schizophrenic patients could develop social phobia as a combined effect of unbalanced dopaminergic and serotonergic systems produced by clozapine, as a kind of behavioral extrapyramidal disorder.

Assessment of Social Anxiety in Schizophrenia

A first step in investigating social anxiety in schizophrenia with specific measures of assessment was proposed by Penn et al. (1994) for inpatients with schizophrenia. The authors developed a six-item scale similar in format to the revised Fear Questionnaire (Marks and Mathews 1979). This scale, which the authors called the "Ward Fear Scale," assesses social anxiety in six situations the patient is likely to encounter while living on an inpatient psychiatric ward. The items on the scale were

1. Meeting a new patient for the first time
2. Having someone watch you learn a new task in a group, such as occupational therapy
3. Having to talk in a new therapy group in front of other people for the first time
4. Meeting a new psychiatrist or psychologist for the first time
5. Doing a role-play in front of other patients while in a group
6. Talking with the psychiatric technician on the way to the canteen or another part of the regional center

The range of possible scores on the Ward Fear Scale is 0 to 48, and the scale was highly correlated $(r=0.80)$ with the Social Phobia subscale on the Fear Questionnaire.

Useful screening questions for social anxiety in schizophrenia and findings suggestive of comorbid social anxiety in schizophrenia are presented in Tables 6–11 and 6–12, respectively.

Table 6–11. Screening questions for social anxiety

- Are you afraid of speaking in public?
- Do you avoid social events?
- Do you fear being watched closely while doing something?
- Are you afraid of embarrassment?
- Do you blush or sweat easily?

Table 6–12.   Findings suggestive of social anxiety in schizophrenia

• Low social adaptation with low subjective well-being and good family adaptation

• Comorbid substance abuse disorder

• Familiality for anxiety disorders

• Parental emotional overinvolvement—a construct that encompasses a variety of affective and behavioral features on the part of family members toward an ill relative: overconcern, unusually self-sacrificing and devoted behavior, extremely overprotective behavior, emotional displays, dramatization, lack of objectivity

• Suicidal ideation

• High Liebowitz Social Anxiety Scale score

To assess social phobia in schizophrenia outpatients and inpatients, the use of the LSAS has been established as adequate and reliable. Pallanti et al. (2004) found no differences on any single item score between schizophrenic patients with social anxiety disorder and patients with social anxiety disorder as a primary diagnosis. In other words, no differences were seen in social anxiety phenomenology when it appeared as a primary diagnosis or when comorbid with schizophrenia. Also, these groups could be reliably distinguished from schizophrenic patients without comorbid social anxiety disorder on the LSAS. However, in some preliminary assessments conducted with schizophrenic subjects before the beginning of the study, the authors found that in this group of patients the administration of the scale by a clinician makes the reliability higher than with the self-administration. Particularly, it was observed that the LSAS, the Scale for the Assessment of Negative Symptoms (SANS), and the Scale for the Assessment of Positive Symptoms (SAPS) should be administered by the same clinician to avoid possible ambiguity between social anxiety symptoms and positive and negative symptoms. A similar rate of positive and negative symptoms in both groups of schizophrenic patients, with and without comorbid social anxiety disorder, was observed. In the past few years, several other literature studies have adopted Liebowitz's scale to assess social anxiety among schizophrenic patients (Mazeh et al. 2009).

Table 6–13   Strategies for treatment of social anxiety in schizophrenia

A. Is the current antipsychotic treatment (especially clozapine) contributing to social anxiety?

   1) Reduce dosage.

   2) Change antipsychotic (aripiprazole is preferred).

B. Use add-on treatment.

   1) Selective serotonin reuptake inhibitor

   2) Venlafaxine

C. Use cognitive-behavioral therapy.

Strategies for Treatment of Social Anxiety in Schizophrenia

Treatment of social anxiety in schizophrenia can be approached sequentially as outlined in Table 6–13.

Obsessive-Compulsive Disorder

Obsessive-compulsive symptoms and OCD have been frequently studied in patients with schizophrenia, and their prevalence among patients with schizophrenia is higher than in the general population. A study from the Epidemiologic Catchment Area Program (Boyd 1986) found a 12.5-fold increased odds of having OCD given a diagnosis of schizophrenia.

By contrast, another study from the Epidemiologic Catchment Area Program found a 3.77-fold increased risk of schizophrenia among patients with OCD, suggesting that, for some patients, the presence of OCD may be part of the psychosis prodrome. Buckley et al. (2009) reported a total of 36 studies that investigated the epidemiology of obsessive-compulsive symptoms or OCD among patients with schizophrenia. The prevalence of obsessive-compulsive symptoms (10%–64%) and OCD (0%–31.7%) varies widely across the studies and may have been overestimated because of difficulties in evaluating obsessions in subjects with delusional symptoms. Determining whether the patient is experiencing an obsession or a delusion may not be easy, especially when obsessions are held with firm conviction. A weighted average of the available data from all the studies crudely estimates a 25% prevalence of obsessive-compulsive symptoms and a 23% prevalence of OCD in patients with schizophrenia.

Historical Perspective on Obsessive-Psychotic Comorbidity

Westphal (1878) first distinguished obsessive-compulsive symptoms ("Zwangsvorstellungen") from psychosis ("Verrücktheit," "Wahnideen"). He proposed a clear-cut distinction of both syndromes with respect to clinical presentation, treatment of choice, and prognostic outcome. The publication of Westphal might be considered as the starting point of antagonistic pathogenetic concepts and stimulated the hypothesis of protective effects of obsessive-compulsive symptoms against the development of psychosis.

In consequence, succeeding investigators integrated the concepts of psychoanalysis and assumed that obsessive-compulsive symptoms might indicate an internal defense strategy against psychosis, which could prevent the progression of schizophrenic illness. Stengel (1945) described 14 patients with both syndromes, concluding that there was a "special relationship between obsessional neurosis and paranoid states": he proposed that catatonic or hebephrenic syndromes did not occur while obsessive symptoms were present and that psychotic patients with obsessive comorbidity frequently recognized the irrationality of their psychotic cognitions. Moreover, a "tendency towards remission" was observed and led to the postulation of a "feature of comparative benignity." In agreement with Sigmund Freud and succeeding investigators, it was assumed that "psychosis often resulted in a release of primitive impulses which had previously been kept under control with the aid of obsessional symptoms" (Stengel 1945, p. 185). In 1957, Rosen, after studying a large sample of patients, hypothesized that obsessive-compulsive symptoms might delay psychosis-caused "personality disorganization" by preventing the development of "malignant schizophrenia." Of particular importance, Rosen further observed that none of his patients developed obsessive symptoms after the onset of schizophrenia.

These traditional psychopathological concepts merged into the view that obsessive-compulsive symptoms and psychosis should be categorized as antagonistic disorders, whereas obsessive-compulsive symptoms were considered as partially preventive and favorable regarding the prognosis of patients who developed second-line psychotic syndromes.

Table 6–14.   Strategies for identifying obsessive-compulsive symptoms in the presence of psychosis

Obsessions and compulsions in schizophrenia are phenomenologically similar to those present in pure obsessive-compulsive disorder (OCD), as described in DSM-IV-TR.

1. A repetitious act should be considered a compulsion only if it occurs in response to an obsession and not if it occurs in response to psychotic ideation (e.g., repetitive checking in response to paranoid fears does not constitute a compulsion).

2. A recurrent, intrusive, ego-dystonic thought should not be considered an obsession if it revolves exclusively around current delusional themes (e.g., violent images, which constitute a common type of obsession in OCD, may represent an entirely different phenomenological entity in the context of psychosis). In the acute psychotic phase, it may be necessary to exclude questionable "obsessions" and reassess for these after the psychotic symptoms have been treated.

3. Obsessive-compulsive symptoms may be difficult to distinguish in the presence of thought disorder; it may therefore be necessary to reassess for obsessive-compulsive symptoms once disordered thought has normalized.

4. Primary obsessional slowness may be mistaken for prodromal schizophrenia or thought disorder; such patients may be unable to articulate any obsessions and may show no compulsions.

5. In some cases, it may be difficult to discriminate real obsessive-compulsive symptoms in the presence of psychosis; in such cases, empirical cotreatment with an antipsychotic and a selective serotonin reuptake inhibitor may be necessary.

Source.   Adapted from Bottas et al. 2005.

Recent Evidence on Obsessive-Psychotic Comorbidity

Distinguishing between delusions, obsessions, ruminations, and preoccupations can be difficult in patients with thought disorder (Table 6–14). Classic teaching describes delusions as ego-syntonic and actively embraced by the patient, whereas obsessions are typically ego-dystonic and recognized as pathological intrusions. This distinction does not always hold true in clinical interviews of patients with psychosis. Obsessions and delusions seem to lie on a continuum of insight, and in patients with schizophrenia, delusions and obsessions may be overlapping.

Obsessive-compulsive symptoms may occur throughout the course of schizophrenia, and it has been suggested that obsessive-compulsive symptoms manifest as part of the psychosis prodrome. Three patterns of obsessive-compulsive symptoms can be identified in patients with schizophrenia: 1) patients with long-standing obsessive-compulsive symptoms preceding the onset of psychosis, 2) patients with new-onset obsessive-compulsive symptoms developing at or after the onset of schizophrenia, and 3) patients with transient obsessive-compulsive symptoms over the course of schizophrenic illness.

Obsessive-compulsive symptoms in patients with schizophrenia are important to identify because they seem to have prognostic significance, and they may be differentially responsive to conventional and specialized treatments.

Obsessive symptoms—as was the case with affective symptoms—were originally considered to be of favorable prognostic value, and some authors have considered obsessive-compulsive symptoms in these patients a defense against "personality disintegration" and a positive prognostic indicator (Rosen 1957). Several more recent studies suggest that obsessive-compulsive symptoms in schizophrenia are associated with greater psychopathology and worse outcome. Patients with obsessive-compulsive symptoms tend to be more socially isolated, have longer hospitalizations, and be less responsive to treatment than patients without this symptom complex.

Braga et al. (2005) found that patients with schizophrenia and comorbid OCD had greater disability as measured by the Sheehan Disability Scale global scale, Work subscale, and Social Life subscale scores. Berman et al. (1995) found that the presence of obsessive-compulsive symptoms among subjects with chronic schizophrenia was associated with earlier age at illness onset, increased rates of hospitalization in the previous 5 years, and a decreased likelihood of being employed or married. Sevincok et al. (2007) found that OCD was an independent risk factor for suicidal ideation and suicide attempts in patients with schizophrenia. OCD also was more prevalent among patients with (than those without) suicidal ideation. The authors also found that compulsions were a predictor of suicide attempts.

Dopamine and serotonin are key neurotransmitters involved in the pathophysiology of both schizophrenia and OCD. Although substantial overlap in neurobiology may well contribute to the association between these disorders, a potential confounding factor in epidemiological studies of this association is that second-generation antipsychotics with serotonergic 5-HT$_2$ receptor blockade may exacerbate or produce de novo obsessive-compulsive symptoms in patients with schizophrenia (Lykouras et al. 2003). By contrast, second-generation antipsychotics also have been effective as an adjunctive medication for treatment-refractory OCD. Additional studies are needed to investigate the neurobiology of this paradox, which has important treatment-related implications.

The Putative Entity of Schizo-Obsessive Disorder

Growing evidence indicates that patients with comorbid OCD and schizophrenia (termed *schizo-obsessive*) may represent a special category of the schizophrenia population. Contemporary investigators contend that this subgroup of patients may have a specific pattern of neurobiological dysfunction that accounts for symptom co-expression.

Several questions must be answered to determine whether this putative schizo-obsessive subtype represents a true diagnostic entity: Do obsessions and delusions lie on a continuum, or are these symptoms categorically distinct? Can investigators and clinicians accurately distinguish an obsession with poor insight from a delusion? Does the observed overrepresentation of OCD in schizophrenia represent a nonrandom association (i.e., true epidemiological comorbidity), or is this apparent relation merely a consequence of some confounding variable (i.e., artifactual comorbidity)? Do individuals with this symptom co-expression constitute a more severely ill patient population with a greater magnitude of brain involvement, or are distinct neuroanatomical substrates unique to this subgroup?

Also, a controversy centers on the fact that several clinically discrete groups were described as pertaining to the schizo-obsessive disorder: OCD patients who become psychotic; schizophrenic patients with comorbid OCD; schizophrenic patients with obsessive-compulsive symptoms; and patients with comorbid OCD and schizotypal personality disorder. Existence of these groups may explain the diversity in epidemiological data, clinical manifestations and course, outcomes of various treatments, and prognosis.

Nancy is a 22-year-old unmarried nurse whose father committed suicide 6 years ago; she has a family history of mood disorders and OCD.

Nancy had her first episode of psychosis a year ago, during her first serious romantic relationship. At that time, she developed an obsession of contamination, cleaning rituals, ideas of reference, and delusions of bodily transformation, and she believed that her thoughts were being removed and broadcast to others. Her treatment included chlorimipramine, 150 mg, plus haloperidol, 6 mg, for 4 weeks.

On diagnostic assessment, she had a Yale-Brown Obsessive Compulsive Scale (Y-BOCS) score of 32 and SANS and SAPS total scores of 14 and 12, respectively; the Structured Clinical Interview for DSM-IV (SCID) showed obsessive-compulsive personality disorder.

With treatment, Nancy's symptoms remitted, and she returned to work. However, when she spontaneously stopped her medication, she had an abrupt relapse. A retrial of her previous medications resulted in no improvement, so she was started on fluvoxamine, 300 mg, and risperidone, 4 mg, and after 8 weeks she was able to return to work. However, she still had residual symptoms, including ideas of reference and some magical thinking. She suspended autonomously the complete treatment and after 2 months had a relapse. Fluvoxamine, 300 mg, and risperidone, 4 mg, were again started, but Nancy did not improve and showed persisting experience of influencing. Because of these continued psychotic symptoms, risperidone was switched to olanzapine, 15 mg, and fluvoxamine was reduced from 300 to 200 mg/day. Nancy showed a complete remission of her symptoms after 6 weeks.

Schizo-obsessive patients are reported to have an earlier onset of schizophrenia and a poorer outcome (Berman et al. 1995), but one study reported better global functioning (Tibbo et al. 2003).

In terms of symptom profile, both higher and lower positive and negative symptoms have been reported in schizo-obsessive patients. Studies of first-episode patients with schizophrenia have reported less affective flattening in those with OCD than in those without (de Haan et al. 2005); it is even hypothesized that OCD may have a "protective" effect in first-episode schizophrenia. Higher levels of catatonic symptoms and drug-induced extrapyramidal symptoms have been reported in schizo-obsessive patients (Kruger et al. 2000).

Comorbidity with other disorders in schizo-obsessive patients has been explored, with studies finding higher rates of "obsessive-compulsive spectrum" disorders (Tibbo et al. 2003) and panic disorder (Bermanzohn et al. 2000) and that additional comorbidities contribute to disability (Bermanzohn et al. 2000). These findings suggest that patients with schizophrenia and OCD may represent a discrete group with a specific clinical profile, which needs to be delineated further given the inconsistent findings thus far.

Neuropsychological studies on schizo-obsessive patients have shown ambiguous results, either because of the neglect of comorbid conditions in schizophrenic patients or because of the lack of specificity in the tests used. Compared with schizo-obsessive patients, patients with pure schizophrenia reported decreased neuropsychological performance in frontal lobe tests, whereas OCD patients tended to have better performances. However, some studies could not confirm such differences. Lysaker et al. (2002) reported that impaired performance on frontal tasks was related to comorbid obsessive-compulsive symptoms. Finally, Poyurovsky et al. (2007) found a higher level of "neurological soft signs" in schizo-obsessive and schizophrenic patients compared with OCD patients but found no significant differences between them.

Recently, Pallanti et al. (2009) investigated the P300 event-related brain potential (ERP), an index of endogenous cognitive processes typically elicited by infrequent sensory stimuli that are either novel or task relevant, in schizo-obsessive subjects. In terms of ERP abnormalities, schizo-obsessive patients showed a distinct pattern compared with both OCD and schizophrenic patients: a lower nontarget P300 similar to that of schizophrenic patients as an expression of a response inhibition deficit but a higher amplitude compared with schizophrenic patients without OCD. These data may support the suggestion of a specific pattern of neurobiological deficits in the subgroup of patients that accounts for symptom co-expression and that schizo-obsessive disorder can be considered a specific disorder instead of a severe form of OCD or a complicated form of comorbidity with schizophrenia.

Assessment of Obsessive-Compulsive Symptoms in Schizophrenia

The types of obsessions and compulsions experienced by patients with schizophrenia are similar to those found in OCD in nonschizophrenic patients: contamination obsessions, washing rituals, and counting and checking compulsions are the most frequent subtypes. Several contemporary studies suggested that the Y-BOCS and Y-BOCS Symptom Checklists are appropriate for detecting obsessive-compulsive symptoms in schizophrenia.

Strategies for Treatment of Obsessive-Compulsive Disorder in Schizophrenia

Treatment of OCD in schizophrenia can be approached sequentially as outlined in Table 6–15.

Posttraumatic Stress Disorder

Trauma and posttraumatic stress disorder (PTSD) have high prevalence rates among individuals with severe mental illness, such as schizophrenia. Between

Table 6–15.   Strategies for treatment of obsessive-compulsive disorder (OCD) in schizophrenia

A. Is it reasonable to consider the current antipsychotic treatment (especially clozapine or quetiapine) as contributing to ex novo development or worsening of OCD?

  1) Add adjunctive selective serotonin reuptake inhibitor (SSRI).

  2) Change antipsychotic (risperidone or aripiprazole is preferred).

B. Use anti-OCD medication.

  1) SSRI (consider drug-drug interaction; avoid drugs that worsen weight gain)

  2) Clomipramine

C. Combine pharmacotherapy with cognitive-behavioral psychotherapy for optimal outcome.

69.5% and 98% of this population experienced a traumatic event in their life (Resnick et al. 2003), compared with 39%–56% in the general population.

Of the anxiety disorders, PTSD has received relatively little attention, and evidence is clear that trauma has been underreported and PTSD underdiagnosed in patients' charts, despite the presumed role of trauma and psychological stress in predicting onset and relapse in schizophrenia. Within the limited literature examining trauma and psychosis, individuals with schizophrenia and a comorbid PTSD diagnosis have been found to have more frequent violent thoughts, behaviors, and feelings; heightened paranoia; and greater severity of delusions and hallucinations (Resnick et al. 2003). Negative beliefs about the self and others may mediate the relation between trauma and paranoia, and reexperiencing symptoms may mediate the link between trauma and hallucinations (Gracie et al. 2007). Comorbid PTSD also has been associated with several poor outcomes, including lower quality of life, higher rates of suicidal ideation and behavior, and increased use of medical services. Thus, PTSD and trauma seem to have a clear link with functional disability and positive symptoms of schizophrenia.

Relations Among Trauma, PTSD, and Psychotic Disorders

Trauma histories are common in patients with schizophrenia, and childhood trauma is considered a risk factor for psychosis. Patients with schizophrenia may be at increased risk for exposure to trauma because of illness-related features, environmental influences, and/or comorbid substance use. Many factors complicate the diagnosis and investigation of co-occurring PTSD and schizophrenia, including the presence of psychotic symptoms within the context of PTSD or PTSD symptoms—such as reexperiencing the trauma—that may mimic psychotic symptoms. Furthermore, psychotic symptoms (e.g., hallucinations and delusions) or experiences (e.g., involuntary hospitalization, seclusion, restraint, and forced medications) may themselves be a traumatic event contributing to PTSD, although they have not been uniformly considered as potential precipitating stressors.

Although trauma and PTSD are more prevalent in people with psychosis compared with the general population, the precise relation between trauma, PTSD, and psychosis remains unclear. Three different kinds of possible relations seem most likely.

1. *Psychosis can cause PTSD.* According to the traditional view, a traumatic event must include actual or threatened death, serious injury, or a threat to one's physical integrity. However, this threat may be subjectively or objectively experienced: for example, psychosis can have the ability to threaten one's own or another's life. A study by Kilpatrick et al. (1989) supported the validity of subjective interpretations of threat, showing that the way assault was perceived by their victims was predictive of the development of PTSD, regardless of the objective threat, such as use of weapons. Moreover, people who have not had the direct experience of acute precipitating trauma may still have the full range of PTSD symptoms present in those who have experienced more catastrophic trauma (Morrison et al. 2003). A growing number of research studies suggest that the experience of a first psychosis and its treatment can be traumatic and lead to PTSD-like problems.

   Furthermore, a review by Morrison et al. (2003) showed that many studies that used different methodologies found consistently high rates of PTSD in response to psychosis. These findings make it reasonable to conclude that some people do develop PTSD as a response to psychotic experiences.

2. *Trauma can cause psychosis.* Because many people with psychotic symptoms may have endured experiences of trauma prior to the onset of their psychosis, especially childhood sexual and physical abuse, traumatic life events may contribute to the development of psychosis. A review on

childhood trauma and psychotic disorders showed that the prevalence of reported childhood traumas ranged between 28% and 73%, with childhood sexual abuse ranging from 13% to 61% and childhood physical abuse ranging from 10% to 61% (Bendall et al. 2008). Although the exact role of trauma is still unknown, childhood abuse seems to be implicated in the development of psychosis for a substantial portion of patients.

3. *Psychosis and PTSD can both be part of a spectrum of responses to a traumatic event.* Some evidence indicates a common developmental process because factors such as dissociation or attribution style may mediate the development of psychosis and PTSD following a traumatic event. Moreover, the symptom similarity of these two disorders suggests that they may be similar entities, which may be part of a spectrum of responses to a traumatic event.

Assessment of Posttraumatic Stress Disorder Symptoms in Schizophrenia

The assessment tools for trauma and PTSD developed for the general population are suggested as appropriate for use among people with schizophrenia (Resnick et al. 2003).

The Trauma History Questionnaire—Revised (THQ-R; Mueser et al. 1998) assesses experiences of traumatic events in childhood and over lifetime. This self-report questionnaire consists of 16 items, which are rated as 0 (no) or 1 (yes). All items met DSM-IV-TR Criterion A1 about the objective threat of the traumatic experience. This questionnaire was successfully used in previous studies of trauma and severe mental illness (Mueser et al. 2007; Resnick et al. 2003).

The severity of PTSD can be measured by the PTSD Symptom Scale–Self-Report Version (PSS-SR; Foa et al. 1999). The PSS-SR asks participants to rate how often they experienced each of the 17 PTSD symptoms specified in DSM-IV during the past month, ranging from 0 (not at all/only one time) to 3 (five or more times a week/almost always). The sum of these scores represents the severity of PTSD symptoms.

Strategies for Treatment of Posttraumatic Stress Disorder in Schizophrenia

Treatment of PTSD in schizophrenia can be approached sequentially as outlined in Table 6–16.

Table 6–16. Strategies for treatment of posttraumatic stress disorder (PTSD) in schizophrenia

A. No guidelines or reports exist on treatment of PTSD in schizophrenia.

B. Use trauma-focused cognitive-behavioral therapy.

C. Use pharmacological add-on treatment for core symptoms.

   1) Selective serotonin reuptake inhibitor

   2) Venlafaxine, mirtazapine, or trazodone

   3) Anticonvulsants (carbamazepine, valproate, topiramate, gabapentin)

Generalized Anxiety Disorder

Literature indicates that generalized anxiety disorder (GAD) is highly prevalent among subjects with schizophrenia (Table 6–17). Lifetime GAD comorbidity has been reported in 27% (McMillan et al. 2009) of schizophrenic subjects and has a point prevalence of 8.6%–12% (Seedat et al. 2007). Despite this frequency, clinicians and researchers rarely consider GAD as a comorbid condition in schizophrenia.

> Jane, a 46-year-old woman, has had a diagnosis of chronic paranoid schizophrenia for 19 years. She has taken antipsychotic depot therapy for many years, with stable remission of her paranoid symptoms and good social adaptation recovery.
>
> In the last 2 years, after having breast cancer, her treatment was changed to quetiapine, 900 mg/day, to avoid hyperprolactinemia, with good response. During her last clinic visit, Jane reported: "Most of the time, I feel on edge. I cannot relax and fall asleep easily. If I am expecting a visit from a relative, my anxiety grows, and I have to take a sublingual lorazepam. I feel tense even though there is no reason, I cannot watch movies or read about certain topics, such as health or death. Oddly, when I heard the voices, I didn't suffer from so much anxiety; indeed, the voices helped me to calm down. Even before my surgery for cancer, I didn't feel so tense. Now I don't hear voices, but I spend most days short of breath and feeling nauseated."
>
> After hearing Jane's history, her psychiatrist added venlafaxine, 75 mg/day, to her medication, with significant resolution of symptoms of anxiety after 20 days.

Seedat et al. (2007) found that the Hamilton Anxiety Scale and the DSM-IV Generalized Anxiety Disorder Severity Scale (Stein 2005), despite having

Table 6–17.   Key manifestations of generalized anxiety disorder in schizophrenia

Anxious mood/tension	A general, persistent feeling of fearfulness that the patient cannot specify because it relates to something indefinable. The patient feels physically tense and keyed up as well as feverish and agitated.
Worries over trivial matters	The patient feels apprehensive and is preoccupied with the little things in daily life. He or she worries over trifles—for example, how to get from one place to another, how to organize his or her day.
Hyperemotivity	The patient is hyperemotive, overwhelmed by his or her emotional reactions. He or she is hypersensitive to events and to other people's reactions.
Somatic complaints	*Muscular* (muscular tension and stiffness); *sensory* (buzzing in ears, blurry vision); *cardiovascular* (heart beating too hard or too fast); *respiratory* (sense of tightness or heaviness in chest and has trouble breathing); *gastrointestinal* (feeling nauseated, diarrhea); *autonomic* (feeling too hot or too cold and having swings from one condition to the other).

good internal consistency, were characterized by low kappa values and wide confidence intervals, indicating poor agreement and arguably existing cutoff scores on these measures that may not be appropriate for this population.

Treatment of GAD in schizophrenia can be approached sequentially as outlined in Table 6–18.

Conclusion

Comorbid psychiatric conditions in schizophrenia not only exist but also constitute a widespread phenomenon that is becoming a major focus of clinical attention. Causes of such a high rate of comorbidity need to be further investigated and clarified. Biological and environmental causes, effects of one disorder on the subsequent onset of another disorder, and uncertainty in defining diagnostic boundaries probably all play a role to some extent. Comorbidity varies along the course of the schizophrenic disease. Indeed, comorbid conditions can be identified as more specifically related to the acute phase of the illness, as

Table 6–18. Strategies for treatment of generalized anxiety disorder (GAD) in schizophrenia

A. No guidelines or reports exist on treatment of GAD in schizophrenia.

B. Check thyroid function.

C. Reduce caffeine consumption.

D. Use pharmacological add-on treatment for core symptoms.

  1) Selective serotonin reuptake inhibitor

  2) Venlafaxine or duloxetine

  3) Quetiapine (up to 150 mg)

  4) Pregabalin

more frequently detectable during the residual phase, or in the course of rehabilitation programs. We believe that a first, basic classification of the schizophrenic comorbidity should disaggregate the primary comorbid condition from the secondary comorbid condition, the latter including the treatment-derived and medical-derived form of psychiatric comorbidity.

It is widely assumed that the main objectives of investigating comorbidity are to help refine definitions and diagnoses and to improve treatment. In the case of schizophrenia, psychiatric comorbidity may be overshadowed by prominent psychotic disturbances or trivialized by clinicians when their intervention is mainly imposed on the identification and treatment of characteristic symptoms such as delusions, hallucinations, and behavioral abnormalities. Although specific guidelines are lacking, comorbid conditions should become one of the first therapeutic targets in schizophrenia in all the phases of the disease. Schizophrenia is a chronic and severe disease, during the course of which the diagnosis of a comorbid condition could help to improve quality of life and long-term prognosis.

References

Achim AM, Maziade M, Raymond E, et al: How prevalent are anxiety disorders in schizophrenia? A meta-analysis and critical review on a significant association. Schizophr Bull 37:811–821, 2011

Addington D, Addington J, Schissel B: A depression rating scale for schizophrenics. Schizophr Res 3:247–251, 1990

Addington D, Addington J, Maticka-Tyndale E: Assessing depression in schizophrenia: the Calgary Depression Scale. Br J Psychiatry Suppl (22):39–44, 1993

American Psychiatric Association: Diagnostic and Statistical Manual: Mental Disorders. Washington, DC, American Psychiatric Association, 1952

American Psychiatric Association: Diagnostic and Statistical Manual of Mental Disorders, 2nd Edition. Washington, DC, American Psychiatric Association, 1968

American Psychiatric Association: Diagnostic and Statistical Manual of Mental Disorders, 3rd Edition. Washington, DC, American Psychiatric Association, 1980

American Psychiatric Association: Diagnostic and Statistical Manual of Mental Disorders, 4th Edition. Washington, DC, American Psychiatric Association, 1994

American Psychiatric Association: Diagnostic and Statistical Manual of Mental Disorders, 4th Edition, Text Revision. Washington, DC, American Psychiatric Association, 2000

Bendall S, Jackson HJ, Hulbert CA, et al: Childhood trauma and psychotic disorders: a systematic, critical review of the evidence. Schizophr Bull 34:568–579, 2008

Benjamin J, Li L, Patterson C, et al: Population and familial association between the D4 dopamine receptor gene and measures of novelty seeking. Nat Genet 12:81–84, 1996

Berman I, Kalinowski A, Berman SM, et al: Obsessive and compulsive symptoms in chronic schizophrenia. Compr Psychiatry 36:6–10, 1995

Bermanzohn PC, Arlow PB, Pitch RJ, et al: Panic and paranoia. J Clin Psychiatry 58:325–326, 1997

Bermanzohn PC, Porto L, Arlow PB, et al: Hierarchical diagnosis in chronic schizophrenia: a clinical study of co-occurring syndromes. Schizophr Bull 26:517–525, 2000

Bermanzohn PC, Porto L, Siris SG, et al: Hierarchy, reductionism, and "comorbidity" in the diagnosis of schizophrenia, in Schizophrenia and Comorbid Conditions: Diagnosis and Treatment. Edited by Hwang MY, Bermanzohn PC. Washington, DC, American Psychiatric Press, 2001, pp 1–30

Bottas A, Cooke RG, Richter MA: Comorbidity and pathophysiology of obsessive-compulsive disorder in schizophrenia: is there evidence for a schizo-obsessive subtype of schizophrenia? J Psychiatry Neurosci 30:187–193, 2005

Boyd JH: Use of mental health services for the treatment of panic disorder. Am J Psychiatry 143:1569–1574, 1986

Braga RJ, Mendlowicz MV, Marrocos RP, et al: Anxiety disorders in outpatients with schizophrenia: prevalence and impact on the subjective quality of life. J Psychiatr Res 39:409–414, 2005

Breier A, Astrachan BM: Characterization of schizophrenic patients who commit suicide. Am J Psychiatry 141:206–209, 1984

Buckley PF, Miller BJ, Lehrer DS, et al: Psychiatric comorbidities and schizophrenia. Schizophr Bull 35:383–402, 2009

Cloninger CR: A systematic method for clinical description and classification of personality variants: a proposal. Arch Gen Psychiatry 44:573–588, 1987

Collins AA, Remington G, Coulter K, et al: Depression in schizophrenia: a comparison of three measures. Schizophr Res 20:205–209, 1996

de Haan L, Hoogenboom B, Beuk N, et al: Obsessive compulsive symptoms and positive, negative, and depressive symptoms in patients with recent-onset schizophrenic disorders. Can J Psychiatry 50:519–524, 2005

Fenton WS: Comorbid conditions in schizophrenia. Curr Opin Psychiatry 14:17–23, 2001

Foa EB, Ehlers A, Clark DM, et al: The posttraumatic cognitions inventory (PTCI): development and validation. Psychol Assess 11:303–314, 1999

Goldberg JO, Schmidt LA: Shyness, sociability, and social dysfunction in schizophrenia. Schizophr Res 48:343–349, 2001

Gracie A, Freeman D, Green S, et al: The association between traumatic experience, paranoia and hallucinations: a test of the predictions of psychological models. Acta Psychiatr Scand 116:280–289, 2007

Gruenberg AM, Goldstein RD: Depressive disorders, in Psychiatry, Vol 2. Edited by Tasman A, Kay J, Lieberman JA. Philadelphia, PA, WB Saunders, 1997, pp 990–1019

Häfner H, Maurer K, Trendler G, et al: The early course of schizophrenia and depression. Eur Arch Psychiatry Clin Neurosci 255:167–117, 2005

Hawton K, Sutton L, Haw C, et al: Schizophrenia and suicide: systematic review of risk factors. Br J Psychiatry 187:9–20, 2005

Hieber R, Dellenbaugh T, Nelson LA: Role of mirtazapine in the treatment of antipsychotic-induced akathisia. Ann Pharmacother 42:841–846, 2008

Kahn JP, Meyers JR: Treatment of comorbid panic disorder and schizophrenia: evidence for a panic psychosis. Psychiatr Ann 30:29–33, 2000

Karatzias T, Gumley A, Power K, et al: Illness appraisals and self-esteem as correlates of anxiety and affective comorbid disorders in schizophrenia. Compr Psychiatry 48:371–375, 2007

Kasanin K: The acute schizoaffective psychoses. Am J Psychiatry 90:97–126, 1933

Kelly DL, Shim JC, Feldman SM, et al: Lifetime psychiatric symptoms in persons with schizophrenia who died by suicide compared to other means of death. J Psychiatr Res 38:531–536, 2004

Kilpatrick DG, Saunders BE, Amick-McMullan A, et al: Victim and crime factors associated with the development of crime-related posttraumatic stress disorder. Behav Ther 20:199–214, 1989

Kim SW, Kim SJ, Yoon BH, et al: Diagnostic validity of assessment scales for depression in patients with schizophrenia. Psychiatry Res 144:57–63, 2006

Kruger S, Braunig P, Hoffler J, et al: Prevalence of obsessive-compulsive disorder in schizophrenia and significance of motor symptoms. J Neuropsychiatry Clin Neurosci 12:16–24, 2000

Laursen TM, Agerbo E, Pedersen CB: Bipolar disorder, schizoaffective disorder, and schizophrenia overlap: a new comorbidity index. J Clin Psychiatry 70:1432–1438, 2009

Liebowitz MR, Fyer AJ, Gorman JM, et al: Phenelzine in social phobia. J Clin Psychopharmacol 6:93–98, 1986

Lykouras L, Alevizos B, Michalopoulou P, et al: Obsessive-compulsive symptoms induced by atypical antipsychotics: a review of the reported cases. Prog Neuropsychopharmacol Biol Psychiatry 27:333–346, 2003

Lysaker PH, Bryson GJ, Marks KA, et al: Association of obsessions and compulsions in schizophrenia with neurocognition and negative symptoms. J Neuropsychiatry Clin Neurosci 14:449–453, 2002

Malhi GS, Green M, Fagiolini A, et al: Schizoaffective disorder: diagnostic issues and future recommendations. Bipolar Disord 10:215–230, 2008

Marks IM, Mathews AM: Brief standard self-rating for phobic patients. Behav Res Ther 17:263–267, 1979

Mauri MC, Bitetto A, Fabiano L, et al: Depressive symptoms and schizophrenic relapses: the effect of four neuroleptic drugs. Prog Neuropsychopharmacol Biol Psychiatry 23:43–54, 1999

Mazeh D, Bodner E, Weizman R, et al: Co-morbid social phobia in schizophrenia. Int J Soc Psychiatry 55:198–202, 2009

McMillan KA, Enns MW, Cox BJ, et al: Comorbidity of Axis I and II mental disorders with schizophrenia and psychotic disorders: findings from the National Epidemiologic Survey on Alcohol and Related Conditions. Can J Psychiatry 54:477–486, 2009

Meehl PE: Schizotaxia, schizotypy, schizophrenia. Am Psychol 17:827–838, 1962

Mikkelsen EJ, Detlor J, Cohen D: School avoidance and social phobia triggered by haloperidol in patients with Tourette's disorder. Am J Psychiatry 138:1572–1576, 1981

Möller HJ: Occurrence and treatment of depressive comorbidity/cosyndromality in schizophrenic psychoses: conceptual and treatment issues. World J Biol Psychiatry 6:247–263, 2005

Möller HJ: Clinical evaluation of negative symptoms in schizophrenia. Eur Psychiatry 22:380–386, 2007

Morrison AP, Frame L, Larkin W: Relationships between trauma and psychosis: a review and integration. Br J Clin Psychol 42(pt 4):331–353, 2003

Mueser KT, Goodman LB, Trumbetta SL, et al: Trauma and posttraumatic stress disorder in sever mental illness. J Consult Clin Psychol 66:493–499, 1998

Mueser KM, Bolton E, Carty PC, et al: The trauma recovery group: cognitive-behavioral program for post-traumatic stress disorder in persons with severe mental illness. Community Ment Health J 43:281–304, 2007

Pallanti S, Quercioli L, Pazzagli A: Social anxiety and premorbid personality in paranoid schizophrenic patients treated with clozapine. CNS Spectr 5:29–43, 2000

Pallanti S, Quercioli L, Hollander E: Social anxiety in outpatients with schizophrenia: a relevant cause of disability. Am J Psychiatry 161:53–58, 2004

Pallanti S, Castellini G, Chamberlain SR, et al: Cognitive event-related potentials differentiate schizophrenia with obsessive-compulsive disorder (schizo-OCD) from OCD and schizophrenia without OC symptoms. Psychiatry Res 170:52–60, 2009

Palmer BA, Pankratz VS, Bostwick JM: The lifetime risk of suicide in schizophrenia: a reexamination. Arch Gen Psychiatry 62:247–253, 2005

Patterson WM, Dohn HH, Bird J, et al: Evaluation of suicidal patients: the SAD PERSONS scale. Psychosomatics 24:343–349, 1983

Penn DL, Hope DA, Spaulding W, et al: Social anxiety in schizophrenia. Schizophr Res 11:277–284, 1994

Pompili M, Lester D, Grispini A, et al: Completed suicide in schizophrenia: evidence from a case-control study. Psychiatry Res 167:251–257, 2009

Poyurovsky, M, Faragian, S, Pashinian, A, et al: Neurological soft signs in schizophrenia patients with obsessive–compulsive disorder. J Neuropsychiatry Clin Neurosci 19:145–150, 2007

Resnick SG, Bond GR, Mueser KT: Trauma and posttraumatic stress disorder in people with schizophrenia. J Abnorm Psychol 112:415–423, 2003

Reutfors J, Brandt L, Jönsson EG, et al: Risk factors for suicide in schizophrenia: findings from a Swedish population-based case-control study. Schizophr Res 108:231–237, 2009

Romm KL, Rossberg JI, Berg AO, et al: Depression and depressive symptoms in first episode psychosis. J Nerv Ment Dis 198:67–71, 2010

Rosen I: The clinical significance of obsessions in schizophrenia. J Ment Sci 103:773–785, 1957

Saha S, Chant D, McGrath J: A systematic review of mortality in schizophrenia: is the differential mortality gap worsening over time? Arch Gen Psychiatry 64:1123–1131, 2007

Sands JR, Harrow M: Depression during the longitudinal course of schizophrenia. Schizophr Bull 25:157–171, 1999

Savitz AJ, Kahn TA, McGovern KE, et al: Carbon dioxide induction of panic anxiety in schizophrenia with auditory hallucinations. Psychiatry Res 189:38–42, 2011

Schneier FR, Martinez D, Abi-Dargham A, et al: Striatal dopamine D2 receptor availability in OCD with and without comorbid social anxiety disorder: preliminary findings. Depress Anxiety 25:1–7, 2008

Seedat S, Fritelli V, Oosthuizen P, et al: Measuring anxiety in patients with schizophrenia. J Nerv Ment Dis 195:320–324, 2007

Sevincok L, Akoglu A, Kokcu F: Suicidality in schizophrenia patients with and without obsessive-compulsive disorder. Schizophr Res 90:198–202, 2007

Siris SG, Addington D, Azorin JM, et al: Depression in schizophrenia: recognition and management in the USA. Schizophr Res 47:185–197, 2001

Stein DJ: Generalized anxiety disorder: rethinking diagnosis and rating. CNS Spectr 10:930–934, 2005

Stein MB, Heuser IJ, Juncos JL, et al: Anxiety disorders in patients with Parkinson's disease. Am J Psychiatry 147:217–220, 1990

Stengel E: A study on some clinical aspects of the relationship between obsessional neurosis and psychotic reaction types. J Ment Sci 91:166–187, 1945

Sullivan SH: The onset of schizophrenia. Am J Psychiatry 6:105–134, 1927

Surtees PG, Kendell RE: The hierarchy model of psychiatric symptomatology: an investigation based on Present State Examination ratings. Br J Psychiatry 135:438–443, 1979

Tibbo P, Swainson J, Chue P, et al: Prevalence and relationship to delusions and hallucinations of anxiety disorders in schizophrenia. Depress Anxiety 17:65–72, 2003

Ulas H, Alptekin K, Akdede B, et al: Panic symptoms in schizophrenia: comorbidity and clinical correlates. Psychiatry Clin Neurosci 61:678–680, 2007

Weber NS, Cowan DN, Millikan AM, et al: Psychiatric and general medical conditions comorbid with schizophrenia in the National Hospital Discharge Survey. Psychiatr Serv 60:1059–1067, 2009

Weiden PJ, Mann JJ, Dixon L, et al: Is neuroleptic dysphoria a healthy response? Compr Psychiatry 30:546–552, 1989

Westphal K: Über Zwangsvorstellungen. Arch Psychiatr Nervenkr 8:734–750, 1878

Whitehead C, Moss S, Cardno A, et al: Antidepressants for people with both schizophrenia and depression. Cochrane Database of Systematic Reviews 2002, Issue 2. Art. No.: CD002305. DOI: 10.1002/14651858.CD002305.

Wittchen HU, Fehm L: Epidemiology, patterns of comorbidity, and associated disabilities of social phobia. Psychiatr Clin North Am 24:617–641, 2001

World Health Organization: International Statistical Classification of Diseases and Related Health Problems, 10th Revision. Geneva, World Health Organization, 1992

Yazaji ME, Battas O, Agoub M, et al: Validity of the depressive dimension extracted from principal component analysis of the PANSS in drug-free patients with schizophrenia. Schizophr Res 56:121–127, 2002

7

Substance Use Disorders and Schizophrenia

Michael P. Bogenschutz, M.D.

Pamela B. Arenella, M.D.

Epidemiology and Clinical Overview of Schizophrenia and Substance Use Disorders

Substance use disorders in persons with schizophrenia are a highly prevalent and very serious problem. Although estimates vary, and exact numbers are difficult to obtain, the lifetime prevalence of co-occurring substance use disorders in those receiving treatment for serious mental illnesses is anywhere from 25.2% to 30.3% (U.S. Department of Health and Human Services 2009). Estimates of the lifetime prevalence of substance use disorder in schizophrenia are even higher and range from 47% to 70% (Green et al. 2002; Gupta et al. 1996; Regier et al. 1990) and as high as 80% when nicotine is included (Lasser et al. 2000). The most commonly abused substances in schizophrenic patients are nicotine, alcohol, cocaine, and cannabis (Selzer and Lieberman 1993).

Substance use disorders cause significant morbidity and mortality in those with schizophrenia. People with schizophrenia who have co-occurring substance use disorders have worse outcomes in terms of course of illness, compliance with treatment, violence, homelessness, legal problems, life functioning, and physical illnesses (Bennett and Gjonbalaj 2007). Additionally, patients with schizophrenia may experience greater severity of symptoms, more frequent and longer hospitalizations (Swofford et al. 2000), and increased suicidality (Potvin et al. 2003).

Differentiating substance-induced psychiatric disorders from primary mental illnesses is very difficult. Traditionally, it was thought that treatment of the substance use disorder had to be completed prior to treatment of the psychiatric illness. The theory was that after a period of abstinence, psychiatric symptoms would remit and perhaps obviate the need for psychotropic medications. However, the wisdom of this approach has recently been challenged and refuted. Many studies have shown that for patients with dual diagnoses of a serious mental disorder such as schizophrenia and a substance use disorder, treatment of the psychiatric disorder improves the outcome of the psychiatric illness and sometimes that of the substance use disorder as well. Also, treatment of the substance use disorder can decrease the severity of the comorbid psychiatric illness (Smelson et al. 2008). Because treatment of substance use disorders has such a profound effect on outcomes, accurate diagnosis and initiation of treatment are crucial in this population.

Understanding Substance Use Disorders

Neurobiology of Substance Use Disorders

Over the last 20 years, our understanding of the neurobiology of addiction has expanded significantly. The basic brain reward circuitry pathway has been described and continues to be identified and refined. This reward pathway presumably evolved to encourage the preservation of our species by stimulating positive emotional experiences in response to food intake, sex, social interactions, and so forth. Multiple substances of abuse can cause either direct or indirect stimulation of this pathway. Dopamine, serotonin, γ-aminobutyric acid (GABA), and opiates can stimulate dopaminergic neurons, particularly in the ventral tegmental area (VTA) of the brain. The VTA is located near the basal ganglia and sends projections to the nucleus accumbens. Stimulation of the VTA neurons causes release of dopamine in the nucleus accumbens, which is considered to be primarily responsible for the rewarding or pleasurable effects of most drugs of abuse. Because these reward structures overlap with the mesocorticolimbic circuits known to be abnormal in schizophrenia, it has been hypothesized that persons with schizophrenia may have an abnormal neural response to potentially rewarding stimuli (Green 2007).

More recently, brain circuitry involved in motivation and craving for drugs and decision making around drug use has been elucidated (Kalivas and Volkow 2005). These systems involve alteration in glutamatergic activity in cortical regions, including the cingulate gyrus and prefrontal cortex, as well as changes in other parts of the brain such as the amygdala. As our understanding of these systems evolves, we have begun to identify targets for pharmacological intervention and treatment of substance use disorders.

Diagnostic Criteria for Substance Use Disorders

Substance Abuse

Substance abuse can be diagnosed (American Psychiatric Association 2000) if the patient has evidence of a clinically significant maladaptive pattern of use, with one or more of the following occurring within a 12-month period: 1) work, school, or home obligation failures; 2) interpersonal or social consequences; 3) recurrent legal consequences; or 4) dangerousness (recurrent physically hazardous use). Additionally, criteria for substance dependence cannot have been met in the past. A useful mnemonic—WILD—is shown in Table 7–1 (Bogenschutz and Quinn 2001).

Table 7–1.   Substance abuse criteria: WILD mnemonic

W	Work, school, or home obligation failures
I	Interpersonal or social consequences
L	Legal consequences (recurrent)
D	Danger (recurrent physically hazardous use)

Source.   Bogenschutz and Quinn 2001.

Substance Dependence

Substance dependence can be diagnosed (American Psychiatric Association 2000) when three or more of the following criteria are present within a 12-month period, and significant impairment or distress is evident: 1) activities given up or reduced; 2) physical dependence as indicated by tolerance; 3) physical dependence as indicated by withdrawal symptoms; 4) intrapersonal (i.e., internal) consequences, either medical or psychiatric; 5) repeated attempts to cut down or control use over time; 6) excessive amounts of time obtaining, using, or recovering from the substance used; and 7) duration or amount often greater than intended (within episode). It is important to specify whether the person has physiological dependence in addition to meeting substance dependence criteria. When diagnosing psychological dependence, the following course specifiers should be included: active; or in remission, either early (>30 days and <1 year of abstinence) or sustained (≥1 year) and full (no criteria for dependence are met) or partial (presence of at least one but not three of the dependence criteria). It is also important to include whether remission has been achieved while on agonist therapy or in a controlled environment. A useful mnemonic for substance dependence—ADDICTD—is shown in Table 7–2 (Bogenschutz and Quinn 2001).

At the time this chapter was written, in the current draft of DSM-5, the revision for substance use disorder proposed to eliminate the distinction between substance abuse and dependence, subsuming them both under the general term *substance use disorder.*

Table 7–2.   Substance dependence criteria: ADDICTD mnemonic

A	Activities given up or reduced
D	Dependence, physical: tolerance
D	Dependence, physical: withdrawal
I	Intrapersonal (internal) consequences (medical or psychiatric)
C	Cannot cut down or control use (over time)
T	Time-consuming (obtaining, using, recovering)
D	Duration or amount often greater than intended (within episode)

Source.   Bogenschutz and Quinn 2001.

Etiology: Why Are Substance Use Disorders So Common in Schizophrenia?

Thinking About Comorbidity

Kraemer (1995) defined four distinct kinds of comorbidity: random, clinical, familial, and epidemiological. *Random comorbidity* refers to the chance co-occurrence of two disorders. The expected rate of co-occurrence of two disorders due to chance is just the product of the prevalence rates of the two disorders. *Clinical comorbidity* refers to the effects of one disorder on a second disorder in people who have both disorders. These effects could exist regardless of the nature of the association (random or nonrandom) between the disorders. *Familial comorbidity* exists when the presence of one disorder in relatives of an individual affects the probability of that individual having another disorder. It provides evidence of a common underlying diathesis. *Epidemiological comorbidity* is a nonrandom association (greater or less than that expected by chance) between two disorders in a defined population.

Clinical comorbidity is related to the effects of one disorder on the presentation, course, biological parameters, and treatment outcome of another disorder when they co-occur. Basically, two relations are possible: disorder A affects disorder B, and disorder B affects disorder A. These are not mutually exclusive and could be mediated by a third condition or disorder.

Epidemiological comorbidity can arise through one or all of the following processes. The first possibility is that the two disorders share common etiological factors (including other disorders) or a common diathesis (including genetic risk factors). For example, comorbidity of chronic renal failure and coronary artery disease could be increased by the association of both disorders with diabetes. The second and third possible causes of comorbidity (again, not mutually exclusive) are that disorder A causes (or increases the probability of) disorder B and that disorder B causes disorder A. The relation could be mediated by another condition or disorder (e.g., in the case of schizophrenia, elevated rates of lung cancer are mediated by elevated rates and intensity of smoking). Figure 7–1 illustrates these possible relations.

When we consider the relations between schizophrenia and substance use disorders, it is important to remember that these relations may be different for different substances and also could be different at each stage of illness. Sub-

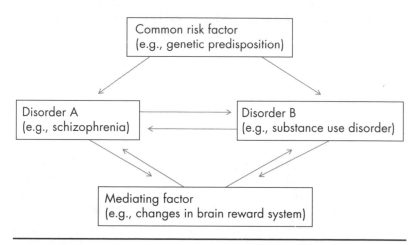

Figure 7–1.   Possible causal relations accounting for epidemiological co-morbidity.

stance use disorder is not a single disorder but a group of disorders describing multiple patterns of misuse of a variety of pharmacologically distinct compounds. Different subtypes of alcoholism have been identified, which have different patterns of inheritance, comorbidity, and response to pharmacotherapy. Although it is not clear that patients with schizophrenia are predisposed to misuse of any one class of drug over another, the observed comorbidity may be the result of an association between schizophrenia and particular types of substance use disorder and not others. Schizophrenia is also a heterogeneous construct, so different subtypes of schizophrenia (e.g., paranoid, undifferentiated, deficit syndrome) may have different relations to substance use disorders. In the following subsections, we review what is known about the causal relations between substance use and schizophrenia for each of the main classes of substance, considering both epidemiological and clinical comorbidity.

Is There a Common Diathesis Predisposing to Both Substance Use Disorder and Schizophrenia?

If schizophrenia and substance use disorder were different aspects of the same underlying process (disease, disorder), there would be a common etiology or pathophysiological mechanism. Considerable overlap is seen in the regions of the brain that have been shown to be involved in these disorders. Neurotransmitter systems, including dopamine, serotonin, and glutamate (N-methyl-D-aspartate [NMDA] receptors in particular), also have been implicated in both addictive disorders and schizophrenia. However, no clear link or common abnormality has been found. Furthermore, genetic studies have failed to establish any common genetic basis for schizophrenia and substance use disorders (Kendler 1985).

Ways in Which Substance Use May Cause or Exacerbate Schizophrenia

Cannabis

Cannabis use is now clearly implicated as a risk factor for the onset of schizophrenia (epidemiological comorbidity) and a cause of symptom exacerbation in patients who have schizophrenia. The risk of psychosis is approximately doubled in young people who use cannabis regularly (Moore et al. 2007). Cannabis-using schizophrenic patients may have fewer negative symptoms but more positive symptoms and more frequent hospitalizations than those who do not use cannabis. However, many schizophrenic patients who use marijuana regularly are quite stable with respect to psychosis. It is not clear why some individuals with schizophrenia appear to be more vulnerable to the effects of cannabis than others.

Stimulants

Stimulant use is very likely to exacerbate psychotic symptoms in schizophrenic patients (Curran et al. 2004). Stimulant intoxication can cause psychotic symptoms even in individuals with no predisposition to psychosis. These symptoms often persist for days or weeks after the use of stimulants has ceased. Although DSM-IV-TR (American Psychiatric Association 2000) defines substance-induced psychotic disorder as occurring within 1 month of the use of stimulants, it is thought that these symptoms can persist indefinitely (i.e., chronic, persistent psychosis caused by use of stimulants) through a process of sensitization or kindling (Yui et al. 2000). These psychoses are described as typically involving paranoid delusions, with or without auditory hallucinations, but can cause the full range of schizophrenic symptoms (Harris and Batki 2000). However, whether the disorder represents true schizophrenia (precipitated by stimulants) or a different disorder (chronic stimulant-induced psychosis) with similar symptomatology remains unclear.

> John had his first psychotic break when he was 20 years old and attending college. He had been abusing stimulants for 2 years prior to the onset of his illness. His stimulant use had gradually increased over the years to the point of using amphetamines daily for 1 month prior to his first psychiatric hospitalization. His psychotic symptoms did not remit in the hospital in the absence of stimulants, so he was started on antipsychotic medication.
>
> John was released from the hospital and stayed away from amphetamines for several months. Because his psychosis had remitted, he no longer felt it necessary to take his antipsychotic medications and discontinued them. The psychotic symptoms returned. John and his family reported that shortly thereafter, he resumed his stimulant abuse.
>
> John was rehospitalized and diagnosed with schizophrenia. He was restarted on antipsychotic medication and released. He then followed a downward course that included multiple hospitalizations, dropping out of college, and multiple failed attempts at employment. Despite treatment in a multidisciplinary co-occurring disorders specialty clinic, he was never able to maintain any significant periods of sobriety. He ended up living in a trailer on his parents' property so that they could monitor his adherence to treatment and his drug use.

Hallucinogens

Both the serotonergic hallucinogens and the NMDA receptor antagonist hallucinogens have been used as experimental models of schizophrenia. Hallucinogens can precipitate both brief psychotic episodes and chronic psychotic illness. The latter resembles first-break schizophrenia in presentation and clinical course and is thought to be more common in people with a family history of schizophrenia. Hallucinogens also can exacerbate psychotic symptoms in patients with schizophrenia. Several distinct classes of drugs are included in the general category of hallucinogens, and their effects are quite different.

The classic serotonergic hallucinogens include lysergic acid diethylamide (LSD), psilocybin (contained in certain species of mushrooms), mescaline (found in cactus species, including *Lophophora williamsii,* peyote), and dimethyltryptamine. Methylenedioxymethamphetamine (MDMA; Ecstasy) is a drug that has weak serotonergic hallucinogenic effects combined with stimulant effects. The typical effects of intoxication with these drugs include unusual sensory experiences, intense and labile emotions, and altered sense of self in relation to external reality. True hallucinations or paranoia are unusual but can occur. These symptoms generally resolve when the drug intoxication wears off (less than 12 hours for most of these substances), but occasionally a true persistent psychosis can occur.

NMDA receptor antagonist hallucinogens include phencyclidine (PCP), ketamine, and dextromethorphan (found in over-the-counter cough medicines). Acutely, these drugs produce not only altered perceptions and subjective sense of self and reality but also cognitive impairment and formal thought disorder. Because glutamate appears to play a significant role in the pathophysiology of schizophrenia, the effects of these drugs may have more in common with schizophrenia than those of the serotonergic hallucinogens. Psychotic episodes persisting for days are relatively common in people who use these drugs.

Opioids

Cases of psychosis have been reported in association with both opioid intoxication and opioid withdrawal. However, evidence from older studies indicates that opioids have a moderate but significant antipsychotic effect in patients with schizophrenia (Gold et al. 1977). No evidence shows that opioid abuse or dependence can cause a persistent psychosis or exacerbate psychotic symptoms in patients with schizophrenia.

Alcohol

Other than nicotine, alcohol is the most commonly used and abused substance among people with schizophrenia. Psychosis can occur as a consequence of heavy alcohol use, most commonly in patients with severe chronic alcohol dependence. This psychosis can resemble paranoid schizophrenia, but average age at onset is older, and alcohol-induced cognitive deficits (e.g., dementia) also may be present. Schizophrenic patients with alcohol and other substance use disorders have significantly more positive and fewer negative symptoms than do patients without substance use disorders (Talamo et al. 2006).

Inhalants

Inhalants include a wide range of volatile solvents, as well as nitrous oxide and vasodilators such as amyl nitrate. Many of the volatile solvents (such as gasoline, toluene, and difluoroethane) are neurotoxic and are known to cause brain damage, particularly white matter changes, leading to cognitive impairment. This brain damage also can cause symptoms of psychosis. Because inhalants are most commonly used by adolescents, it can be difficult to determine whether the onset of psychosis in a teenager who uses inhalants represents a first break of a primary psychotic disorder or a consequence of inhalant use. Neuroimaging abnormalities suggest but do not prove that inhalant use is the cause of the psychosis.

Nicotine

Tobacco dependence is found in more than half of patients with schizophrenia. Acutely, nicotine appears to improve cognitive function and to normalize sensory gating in schizophrenia and possibly to offset some of the side effects of antipsychotic medications. Thus, it has been proposed that schizophrenic patients use nicotine in an effort to self-medicate their negative symptoms and possibly even positive symptoms (Conway 2009). However, whether long-term use of nicotine has positive or negative effects on cognitive or other symptoms of schizophrenia is unclear. Any benefits are more than offset by the severe health consequences of smoking, which are one of the principal reasons that life expectancy in people with schizophrenia is about 20 years less than in the general population. Nicotine also lowers blood levels of antipsychotics, including haloperidol, chlorpromazine, olanzapine, and clozapine, by inducing hepatic enzymes such as cytochrome P450 (CYP) 1A2 and uridine 5′-diphospho (UDP)-glucuronosyltransferase.

Ways in Which Schizophrenia May Cause or Exacerbate Substance Use Disorders

Self-Medication

Self-medication is an attractive and frequently invoked theory stating that individuals with psychiatric disorders use substances in an effort (successful or unsuccessful) to control their psychiatric symptoms (Khantzian 1997). It follows that there should be specificity in the relation between the psychiatric symptoms and the particular substance that is used. In general, research has not been able to confirm such specific relationships, but it remains possible that self-medication is driving drug use in certain psychiatric diagnoses or subpopulations within diagnoses.

Schizophrenic patients have much higher rates of substance use disorders than do people without psychiatric diagnoses; however, the substances commonly misused by patients with schizophrenia appear to be the same as those commonly misused by others. There have been reports of a selective elevation in the rate of stimulant use disorders among schizophrenic patients. Whereas it may seem counterintuitive that people with psychosis would preferentially use psychotogenic drugs, the theory was proposed that stimulants help schizophrenic patients by ameliorating negative symptoms such as anhedonia and anergia. Although this may happen in some cases, more recent studies have not replicated the finding of preferential use of stimulants. The case for self-medication with nicotine is more persuasive. People diagnosed with schizophrenia have strikingly high rates of nicotine dependence relative to both the general population and patients with other psychiatric disorders, and nicotine appears to ameliorate cognitive and sensory gating deficits, as noted earlier. However, it is difficult to prove that this is actually why schizophrenic patients smoke.

Use of Drugs Because of Abnormal Functioning of Brain Reward Systems

Because of the lack of specificity of substances used by schizophrenic patients, more general hypotheses have been developed to attempt to explain why schizophrenic patients use drugs. One of the most persuasive explanations invokes abnormalities in neural reward circuitry to explain the propensity of schizophrenic patients to misuse substances. Because of abnormalities in the reward system, schizophrenic patients are hypothesized to experience less reward in response to naturally occurring reinforcers. The rewarding effects of drugs are more salient to schizophrenic patients because of what has been termed *reward deficiency syndrome* (Green et al. 1999). However, the same abnormalities in reward circuitry may make schizophrenic patients more sensitive to the rewarding effects of substances and less able to control impulses to use drugs (Chambers et al. 2001). All common drugs of abuse reliably cause the release of dopamine in the nucleus accumbens, which is thought to be responsible for at least some of the rewarding and pleasurable effects of drugs of abuse. Because antipsychotic drugs block dopamine receptors to varying degrees, taking these drugs also could cause reward deficit and heighten the risk of addiction. If this were true, one would expect lower rates of substance use in patients taking atypical antipsychotics than in patients taking typical dopamine type 2 (D_2) receptor blockers. Indeed, naturalistic studies of patients taking clozapine have shown a dramatic decrease in substance use over time with this medication (Zimmet et al. 2000). Also, atypical antipsychotics, including olanzapine and quetiapine, have been shown to have antiaddictive effects in preclinical and clinical studies in nonschizophrenic alcohol-dependent subjects. However, no large randomized trials have been designed to compare changes in drug or alcohol use among substance-abusing schizophrenic patients taking different antipsychotic medications. *No evidence indicates that schizophrenic patients are more likely to have problems with drugs or alcohol if they are given antipsychotics than if they are not.*

Assessment of Substance Use Disorders

Substance use disorders are very common but are often overlooked and underdiagnosed in patients with schizophrenia. Therefore, all patients in treatment for schizophrenia should be screened for co-occurring substance use disorders. A positive screening must be followed by a more thorough assessment of the severity of the substance use problem. Screening tools can be an effective first step in determining whether a patient is abusing substances. Multiple tools exist to screen for substance use disorders, but none has been extensively tested in the schizophrenic population. A recent analysis of the literature has shown that the CAGE questionnaire, the Michigan Alcoholism Screening Test (MAST), and the alcohol consumption questions of the Alcohol Use Disorders Identification Test (AUDIT-C) all have fairly good sensitivity and reliability when used in this population (Bennett 2009). The Alcohol, Smoking, and Substance Involvement Screening Test (ASSIST) screens for all substances of abuse and also has been shown to be reliable and valid in patients with first-episode psychosis (Hides et al. 2009). An example of one of these scales, the AUDIT-C, is shown in Table 7–3 (Bush et al. 1998). An AUDIT total score of greater than 4 will identify 86% of men who report heavy drinking or who meet criteria for alcohol use disorders, and a total score of greater than 2 will identify 84% of women who report heavy drinking or alcohol use disorders. This scale can be easily modified for other substances of abuse as a useful screening instrument.

Table 7–3. Alcohol consumption questions of the Alcohol Use Disorders Identification Test (AUDIT-C)

How often do you have a drink containing alcohol?

| Never (0) | Monthly or less (1) | 2–4 times a month (2) | 2–3 times a week (3) | 4 or more times a week (4) | Score: ___ |

How many drinks containing alcohol do you have on a typical day when you drink?

| 1 or 2 (0) | 3 or 4 (1) | 5 or 6 (2) | 7–9 (3) | 10 or more (4) | Score: ___ |

How often do you have six or more drinks on one occasion?

| Never (0) | Less than monthly (1) | Monthly (2) | 2–4 times a week (3) | 4 or more times a week (4) | Score: ___ |

Note. Add the numbers for each question to get total score. A total score >4 indicates a problem in males; a total score >2 indicates a problem in females.
Source. World Health Organization 1990.

Once a problem with alcohol or drugs is identified, a more thorough assessment of the extent of the problem is indicated. A good substance abuse history includes the following elements: substance used, route of administration, age at first use, period of heaviest use, frequency of use and amount used at heaviest use, frequency of use and amount used at present, date of last use, and any periods of abstinence. A thorough assessment will obtain these parameters for each substance used.

Because patients often minimize and deny substance use, clinicians must ask about use of alcohol and illicit substances in a matter-of-fact, nonjudgmental way. For example, rather than asking, "Do you drink?" one might ask, "How much do you drink?" If the patient denies drinking or is vague, the clinician should continue to ask progressively more specific questions. For example, "I'm not here to judge you, but in order for me to understand what your life is like for you, it's important for me to have an accurate understanding about your use of substances." "Do you drink/use every day?" If the answer is no, ask "How many days in a week?" Once the frequency of use is established, the clinician must inquire about the amount used in each episode. Again, if the answers are vague, the clinician should offer some choices, such as "Do you drink hard liquor or beer? Beer? How much? A six pack?"

In addition to using a nonjudgmental approach to interviewing, the assessment of substance use in this population requires information from multiple sources. Family members, therapists, and case managers often have a better knowledge of the day-to-day activities of the patient. They are often more concerned about the use of alcohol and drugs than the patients are. Random urine drug and alcohol screens are also important to obtain additional information. Patients must be informed and willing to allow the clinician to obtain information from these alternative sources, unless it is volunteered, unsolicited, because of concern.

Treatment of Substance Use Disorders in Schizophrenia

Models of Treatment

Traditionally, separate systems have existed in the United States for treatment of mental illnesses and treatment of addictions. This has greatly complicated the treatment of co-occurring disorders. Mentally ill patients with substance use disorders were often excluded from mental health programs, and those seeking drug and alcohol treatment were frequently not allowed in addiction treatment programs if they had serious mental illness. Beginning in the 1980s, there has been a great increase in awareness of the frequency of co-occurring disorders ("dual diagnosis") and a corresponding increase in efforts to modify the treatment systems to better accommodate those with dual disorders.

At the most general level, conceptually three models of treatment of co-occurring disorders are possible. In the *sequential* model, the disorders are treated one at a time in separate programs. This is typically how treatment was provided in the past. This model was supported by beliefs such as "The patient can't deal with his psychiatric issues until he is clean and sober." It was frequently reinforced by a lack of training and experience on the part of program staff regarding treatment of the "other" disorder. For those with a chronic, serious mental illness such as schizophrenia, this model is highly problematic. Because schizophrenia is usually a chronic condition, treating the schizophrenia first would result in the addiction never being treated. Treating the addiction first would result in frequent exacerbations and relapses as a result of untreated schizophrenia.

The *parallel* model recognizes that both disorders should be treated simultaneously but keeps treatment of the mental disorder and the substance use disorder separate. Although this is a major improvement over the sequential model, splitting the treatment can result in a lack of coordination and consistency in the treatment. Participation in two separate programs is more complicated for the patient, particularly if the programs are at separate locations. Because of ideological differences or simple lack of coordination, patients can be given conflicting messages and inconsistent treatment plans. However, with careful coordination, parallel treatment can be effective.

Integrated treatment models were developed in the 1980s and 1990s and continue to be elaborated today. In integrated treatment, psychiatric and substance use disorders are treated in a single program by a team of clinicians with expertise in both sets of disorders. Integrated team models typically have emphasized outreach into the community through services such as case management. Addiction treatments include both pharmacotherapies and psychosocial treatments, which typically use evidence-based addiction treatment models but may be modified for use with dual diagnoses (see section "Psychosocial Treatments for Addictions and Their Application With Schizophrenic Patients" later in this chapter). Although the research to date has significant methodological limitations, favorable outcomes have been reported for many such integrated treatment programs and high-quality parallel treatments (Horsfall et al. 2009).

Effects of Psychiatric Medications on Substance Use

Antipsychotics

The possible effects of antipsychotic medications on substance reward have been discussed earlier. This provides a theoretical argument for preferentially using weak D_2 blockers in substance-abusing patients, but this idea does not yet have convincing empirical support. More important, because adherence to medications is an even greater problem in patients with co-occurring substance use disorders than in those with schizophrenia alone, consideration should be given to using long-acting injectable formulations if adherence to oral medications is in question.

Antimanic Agents

Lithium and most of the anticonvulsants used as mood stabilizers (including carbamazepine and valproate) have been studied as potential treatments for alcohol dependence and cocaine dependence but have not been shown to be effective. Carbamazepine and valproate are effective in the treatment of alcohol withdrawal. Topiramate, an anticonvulsant that is not known to have antimanic properties, has produced consistent decreases in alcohol consumption in two randomized alcohol dependence trials.

Benzodiazepines

Benzodiazepines are frequently used as adjunctive medications in schizophrenia and appear to be useful to decrease anxiety, although they have no effect on psychosis. The abuse potential of benzodiazepines is fairly low in the general population but is somewhat higher among patients with substance use disorders. It is not known how the diagnosis of schizophrenia affects the abuse potential of benzodiazepines. Caution is always indicated when prescribing benzodiazepines to patients with substance use disorders. Benzodiazepines should be used rarely in patients who are actively misusing alcohol or opioids because of the potential for synergistic effects leading to respiratory depression. When benzodiazepines are prescribed in the context of a substance use disorder, it is good practice to use a "benzodiazepine contract" that spells out the expectations for safe use of the medication, including taking only as prescribed, not obtaining additional prescriptions from other doctors, not attempting early refills, and requiring discontinuation of the medication if the participant misuses it or relapses to alcohol or opioid use.

Antiparkinsonian Medications

Although antiparkinsonian medications are not usually thought of as addictive, they can be misused by the patients to whom they are prescribed. Rarely, they can become a primary substance of abuse. Clinicians should be vigilant for signs of abuse in all patients prescribed these medications. When it occurs, misuse of these medications can be managed by use of a contract such as that described in the previous subsection for benzodiazepines, by use of frequent prescriptions (e.g., weekly refills), by changing to another medication, by using a lower effective dose of the antipsychotic, or by changing to another antipsychotic medication with less potential for extrapyramidal side effects.

Antidepressants

For the most part, antidepressants have not been shown to have significant effects on substance use disorders. However, bupropion and desipramine are both effective in promoting smoking cessation. Selective serotonin reuptake inhibitor (SSRI) antidepressants may have effects on alcohol use that vary in different subgroups of alcoholic patients. In several trials involving sertraline or fluoxetine, Type I alcoholic patients (less severe, later onset) have had a more favorable response, in some cases reducing their drinking, and Type II alcoholic patients (more severe, earlier onset) have had a less favorable response, in one case actually drinking more when receiving fluoxetine. It is not clear how these findings would extrapolate to schizophrenic populations or whether the I versus II typology is valid among alcohol-dependent schizophrenic patients.

Use of Antiaddictive Medications in Schizophrenia

Four medications have been approved by the U.S. Food and Drug Administration (FDA) for the treatment of alcohol dependence: disulfiram, oral naltrexone, depot naltrexone, and acamprosate. The use of these medications has not been extensively studied in schizophrenia. However, some preliminary evidence indicates that naltrexone and disulfiram may be beneficial in this population (Smelson et al. 2008). Methadone and buprenorphine have been approved for the treatment of opiate dependence. These medications are considered safe and effective in schizophrenic patients, and they are commonly used, although data are lacking in this area. Several medications have been FDA approved for nicotine dependence, including nicotine replacement (patches, gum, nasal sprays), bupropion, and varenicline. Current data are insufficient to determine the effectiveness of any of these medications in schizophrenic patients, but added caution may be necessary in these patients taking varenicline and disulfiram (see subsections later in this chapter). No FDA-approved medications exist for the treatment of cocaine, stimulant, or marijuana dependence. Some medications, however, have shown promise in the treatment of cocaine dependence, including topiramate, modafinil, disulfiram, vigabatrin (Brodie et al. 2009), and a cocaine vaccine (Martell et al. 2009).

These medications are reviewed in the following subsections and summarized in Table 7–4.

Disulfiram

Disulfiram is an irreversible inhibitor of aldehyde dehydrogenase, which is one of the enzymes responsible for metabolizing ethyl alcohol. When a person taking a therapeutic dose of disulfiram drinks alcohol, acetaldehyde accumulates and causes the characteristic alcohol-disulfiram reaction. Acetaldehyde causes nausea, vomiting, facial flushing, tachycardia, hypotension, and physical discomfort. Disulfiram has not been found to be consistently effective in placebo-controlled studies, primarily because of issues related to compliance and a large placebo effect. Dosing ranges from 250 mg three times weekly to 500 mg/day. Treatment is recommended from 3 months to a year. Disulfiram should be used carefully and with close monitoring in this population because it can cause psychosis resulting from inhibition of dopamine β-hydroxylase. In practice, this does not appear to be a major concern for schizophrenic patients who are taking antipsychotic medication. Disulfiram requires extensive dietary and hygiene product restrictions, and patients can have severe adverse reactions when alcohol is ingested or absorbed through the skin. In addition, disulfiram has multiple drug interactions. Patients must be provided with extensive information about the alcohol-disulfiram reaction, products containing alcohol, and potential drug interactions. Therefore, patients must be reliable and able to follow instructions. Disulfiram should not be given to people who are highly impulsive. Common side effects (in the absence of alcohol) include headache and sedation. Potential serious adverse events include hepatotoxicity and peripheral neuropathy. Liver function test (LFT) results must be monitored prior to initiation and at intervals (2 weeks, 1 month, then every 6 months).

Naltrexone

Naltrexone is a μ-opioid antagonist. The proposed mechanism is attenuation of the rewarding effects of alcohol, thereby decreasing quantity of alcohol consumed. Naltrexone has also decreased craving for alcohol in some studies. Naltrexone has been shown to have a consistent moderate effect on drinking outcomes over multiple studies. There may be genetic variations in response to naltrexone. Naltrexone is available as an oral preparation and a long-acting injection. Compliance may be enhanced with the long-acting injectable formulation. Dosing of the oral formulation is 50 mg/day or 100 mg Monday and Wednesday and 150 mg on Friday. Compliance with the oral formulation may be enhanced by monitoring of administration. The long-acting formulation (Vivitrol) is given in 380-mg intramuscular injections each month. Potential serious adverse effects include hepatocellular injury, suicidal ideation or behavior, and severe injection site reactions such as cellulitis, abscess, and necrosis. More common side effects include gastrointestinal distress, nausea, and headache. Baseline LFTs should be obtained prior to initiation of naltrexone. LFT results should be rechecked after initiation. Naltrexone is contraindicated in patients who are physically dependent on opioids or in need of opioid analgesia. Naltrexone may precipitate withdrawal in those who have used opiates within the past 7–10 days.

> Sara had a long history of schizophrenia and comorbid alcohol dependence. Despite multiple attempts to treat her alcohol use disorder, she repeatedly relapsed to very severe heavy drinking. Treatments had included disulfiram, oral naltrexone, 12-step facilitation therapy, motivational interviewing techniques, and intensive case management. Sara's life was in shambles. She was involved in a relationship with a physically abusive man who beat her to the point of requiring hospitalization on several occasions, she had legal problems as a result of destructive behaviors when intoxicated, and she was beginning to develop liver disease.
>
> Sara's case was quite discouraging because she had repeatedly refused long-acting injectable treatment with naltrexone. Then, one day, she spontaneously asked for a trial of the long-acting formulation of naltrexone. Remarkably, her

Table 7–4.   U.S. Food and Drug Administration–approved antiaddictive medications

Medication	Indication/use	Usual dosing[a]	Common side effects	Serious side effects	Monitoring
Disulfiram	Alcohol dependence	250 mg/day or 500 mg M, W, F	Nausea, headache, sedation	Hepatotoxicity, psychosis, neuropathy, optic neuritis	LFTs at baseline, 2 weeks, 1 month, and every 6 months
Naltrexone	Alcohol dependence	50 mg/day orally or 380 mg/month intramuscularly	Nausea, vomiting, headache, injection site reactions	Acute opiate withdrawal, hepatocellular injury, increased suicidality; injection site cellulitis and necrosis	LFTs at baseline, 1 month, and every 6 months; suicidal thoughts and behaviors
Acamprosate	Alcohol dependence	666 mg three times a day	Diarrhea, nervousness, insomnia. fatigue	Increased suicidality	Suicidal thoughts and behaviors
Methadone	Opiate dependence	80–120 mg/day	Sedation, constipation, sweating	Severe cardiovascular problems, including arrhythmias, cardiac arrest, QTc prolongation; hypotension; CNS and respiratory depression	ECG, urine toxicology
Buprenorphine	Opiate dependence	4–24 mg/day sublingually (initial target dosage is 16 mg/day)	Headache, pain, nausea, constipation, sweating	Acute opiate withdrawal; CNS and respiratory depression (particularly in combination with other CNS depressants, such as intravenous benzodiazepines)	Urine toxicology with buprenorphine metabolites

Table 7–4. U.S. Food and Drug Administration–approved antiaddictive medications (*continued*)

Medication	Indication/use	Usual dosing[a]	Common side effects	Serious side effects	Monitoring
Nicotine replacement	Nicotine dependence	Gum 2–4 mg every hour as needed; lozenges 2–4 mg every 1–2 hours as needed; patch 21 mg/day; inhaler 6–16 cartridges/ day; nasal spray 1–2 sprays/hour	Headache, insomnia, oropharyngeal irritation, gastro- intestinal distress	Nicotine toxicity, including severe headache, arrhythmias, dizziness, vomiting, cold sweats, confusion	Heart rate, blood pressure, concomitant nicotine use
Bupropion	Nicotine dependence	150 mg twice a day	Nausea, headache, anxiety, insomnia, anorexia, tremor	Seizures, hypertension, tachycardia; increased suicidality, agitation, hostility	Heart rate, blood pressure, weight, suicidal thoughts and behaviors, agitation, and aggression
Varenicline	Nicotine dependence	1 mg twice a day	Nausea, constipation, insomnia, headache	Increased suicidality, agitation, hostility	Suicidal thoughts and behaviors, agitation, and aggression

Note. CNS = central nervous system; ECG = electrocardiogram; LFTs = liver function tests.
[a]Individual dosing may vary; please refer to text.

drinking decreased and eventually stopped. She was able to maintain 6 months of total abstinence. She also reengaged in a 12-step support group and psychosocial rehabilitation and even left her abusive partner.

Acamprosate

Acamprosate is an NMDA glutamate receptor antagonist. Its exact mechanism of action is unknown, but it is thought to balance excitatory (glutamate) and inhibitory (GABA) neurotransmission. It may be more effective for relapse prevention than for initiation of abstinence. Dosing is 666 mg three times a day, which makes compliance more difficult. In addition, some patients with religious delusions have been unwilling to take the medication because of the connotations of the number "666." The only major severe adverse effect is a possible increase in suicidal ideation and behavior. More common side effects include diarrhea, nervousness, insomnia, and fatigue. Clearance is decreased in renal insufficiency, so the dosage must be adjusted in patients with kidney disease.

Topiramate

Topiramate is not FDA approved for use in alcohol dependence. However, it has been shown in controlled studies to have a moderate but consistent benefit for decreasing quantity of alcohol consumption (Johnson et al. 2007) and may have some benefit in cocaine dependence as well (Kampman et al. 2004). Topiramate is an antiepileptic medication with multiple mechanisms of action. Dosages up to 300 mg/day have been used in some studies. Topiramate dosage must be increased gradually over 6 weeks to reduce the risk of intolerable common side effects such as nausea, memory or concentration impairment, anorexia, and paresthesias. More serious adverse effects include metabolic acidosis, kidney stones, hyperthermia, glaucoma, and significant cognitive impairment. Additionally, all antiepileptic medications now have a black box warning of increased suicidal ideation and behaviors. Monitoring of serum bicarbonate, electrolytes, serum urea nitrogen, and creatinine is required. Topiramate is metabolized in the liver, but it is excreted 70%–80% unchanged in the kidneys. Dosages may need to be adjusted in patients with liver or kidney disease.

Methadone

Methadone, a long-acting opiate agonist, has been used for detoxification and for maintenance in those with opiate dependence. Methadone has been in use for decades and has been found to be efficacious and safe. Side effects are moderate and may include constipation and sedation at high dosages. Methadone is metabolized by the CYP 3A4 isoenzyme, and blood levels may be increased when combined with medications that are competing for this isoenzyme such as SSRIs. Carbamazepine, on the contrary, is an inducer of this enzyme and may actually decrease blood levels of methadone. Maintenance treatment consistently improves functioning and health in patients who have failed attempts at abstinence. Patients must have documented evidence of physiological dependence prior to being started on methadone. If they are younger than 18, they must have two previous failed attempts at detoxification or abstinence. Typical dosages for maintenance range from 80 to 120 mg/day, while lower, tapering dosages are generally used for detoxification. Methadone for this indication must be dispensed at programs that are licensed and accredited for this purpose. Methadone may cause multiple cardiovascular problems, including arrhythmias, cardiac arrest, and increased QTc intervals. Patients should be screened for risk of arrhythmias, and electrocardiograms should be monitored at baseline and at least annually while receiving treatment. Other serious side effects include respiratory depression, central nervous system depression, and hypotension.

Buprenorphine

Buprenorphine is FDA approved for use in opiate dependence. It is a partial agonist of μ-opioid receptors with a high affinity for these receptors and a weak κ antagonist. Buprenorphine is available in several different formulations, including sublingual tablets (as either buprenorphine alone or buprenorphine plus naloxone). Buprenorphine may be prescribed in a physician's office, and induction must be monitored. A special Drug Enforcement Administration license is required to prescribe buprenorphine. Induction dosages range from 12 to 16 mg/day, and maintenance dosages can range from 4 to 24 mg/day. Naloxone, an opiate antagonist, is added to the sublingual form to decrease diversion and injection. Naloxone is poorly absorbed through the oral mucosa, so it is not active unless it is injected. Common side effects include headache, pain, nausea, constipation, and diaphoresis. Caution must be used with patients who are taking benzodiazepines because concomitant intravenous benzodiazepine use has caused respiratory depression and death.

Tom lived in a rural area and had a diagnosis of schizoaffective disorder when he developed opiate dependence. Despite multiple attempts to quit injecting heroin, he was unable to remain abstinent. He requested a trial of methadone but was unable to comply with the daily dosing schedule at the methadone clinic because of the extensive travel required each day. Instead, Tom was started on office-based buprenorphine, which initially required weekly but now only monthly trips into town. He has not used opiates for more than 3 years and has resumed working on his family farm.

Nicotine Replacement

Nicotine replacement comes in multiple forms, including gum, lozenges, inhalers, and patches. Most are used for a period of 12 weeks and then gradually tapered and discontinued. All may cause symptoms of nicotine toxicity if overused or used in conjunction with nicotine. Patients must be able to follow instructions and be reliable to not use concurrently with nicotine. Symptoms of nicotine toxicity include severe headache, dizziness, irregular heart rate, vomiting, cold sweats, and confusion. More common side effects are headache, insomnia, oropharyngeal irritation, and gastrointestinal distress. All forms of nicotine replacement are available over the counter and come with dosing instructions.

Bupropion

Bupropion, which was initially FDA approved for the treatment of depression, has subsequently been FDA approved for use in nicotine dependence. The mechanism of action is largely unknown, although it is a weak inhibitor of the neuronal uptake of norepinephrine and dopamine. The target dosage for nicotine dependence is 150 mg twice a day. Bupropion should be started at 150 mg/day and increased to twice-daily dosing as tolerated. Serious adverse events include seizures, hypertension, tachycardia, and neuropsychiatric symptoms including increased suicidal thoughts and behaviors, hostility, and agitation. More common and less severe side effects include headache, nausea, anxiety, insomnia, anorexia, and tremor.

Varenicline

Varenicline, a partial nicotine agonist, works by decreasing cravings and urges to use tobacco. It also has been shown to cause an increase in neuropsychiatric symptoms in some patients, including increased agitation, aggressive behavior, and suicidal ideation and behaviors. Schizophrenic patients receiving this medication should be closely monitored for worsening psychiatric symptoms. Varenicline also causes gastrointestinal symptoms, including nausea (which can be severe) and constipation; insomnia; and headache. Varenicline is started 1 week prior to the quit date and the dosage gradually raised as follows: 0.5 mg at bedtime for the first 3 days, 0.5 mg twice a day for the next 4 days, and 1 mg twice a day thereafter. Varenicline may be continued for 3–6 months, depending on success and tolerability.

Psychosocial Treatments for Addictions and Their Application With Schizophrenic Patients

Three important general points must be kept in mind before discussing specific psychosocial treatment. First, the evidence base for these treatments in dually diagnosed populations is much thinner than in standard addiction treatment populations. Second, very few studies of psychosocial treatments have limited their samples to patients with schizophrenia—much more often, the sample is a mixed group of patients with serious mental illness. Third, the modalities discussed in this subsection are in practice often used in combination rather than as stand-alone treatments. As an example, one of the most successful recent psychosocial treatment trials in a seriously mentally ill population used an intervention combining three of the modalities described later in this chapter: motivational interviewing, contingency management, and skills training (Bellack et al. 2006).

Cognitive-Behavioral Therapy

Cognitive-behavioral therapy for substance use disorders has multiple components. Patients work with therapists either one-to-one or in groups to identify the proximate causes and consequences of substance use (functional analysis) and work on changing behaviors and learning the skills necessary to avoid relapse (Carroll and Onken 2005). Psychoeducation about effects of drug use is often provided. Some time is generally focused on identifying triggers and behaviors that lead to relapse. Social skills training is incorporated into practicing behaviors that will reinforce sobriety, such as using drink refusal skills, asking for help, going to meetings, and calling a sober friend or sponsor. Obviously, considerable overlap exists between these methods and the social skills training methods used for treatment of social deficits in schizophrenia (Bellack 2004).

Motivational Interviewing and Motivational Enhancement Therapy

Motivational interviewing techniques, which focus on enhancing motivation to change rather than teaching specific skills, are effective in the treatment of substance use disorders in the general population (Hettema et al. 2005). Motivational enhancement therapy (MET; Miller et al. 1995) is a brief structured intervention that incorporates motivational interviewing techniques with feedback and goal setting. Motivational interviewing approaches are widely recommended and used in populations with serious mental illness including schizophrenia, although relatively few studies have been done in such populations. Adjustment of the interviewing techniques in the schizophrenic population appears to be helpful. Some of these adjustments include using more structured activities, prompts, examples, lists of options, frequent review and reminders, active reflection, and summarizing to promote cognitive organization and processing (Carey et al. 2007). Focus on concrete issues such as negative consequences of substance use disorders appears to be more beneficial than asking about motivating factors that continue use. These techniques have not been rigorously studied in well-designed studies but appear to be more effective than traditional motivational interviewing strategies.

Contingency Management

Contingency management is an effective drug abuse treatment approach that uses operant conditioning principles to increase the probability of target behaviors during treatment (Stitzer and Petry 2006). Typically, participants in drug abuse treatment receive rewards (cash, vouchers, or prizes) for producing drug-free urine samples, participating in treatment, or both. Contingency management is usually used as an adjunct to other treatments rather than as a stand-alone treatment. The effects of contingency management on these behaviors during treatment are quite strong, but they often become attenuated fairly rapidly when the contingencies are removed. This approach has not been widely used in populations with serious mental illness but has shown some promise (see, e.g., Tracy et al. 2007). Contingency management can be applied to a variety of target behaviors. including medication adherence.

Residential Treatment

Residential treatment with a dual-diagnosis focus is associated with improved outcomes across several studies (Drake et al. 2008). Although both substance use disorders and schizophrenia are typically long-term illnesses, it appears that an acute episode of intensive treatment can affect the course of both disorders. A period of stabilization in a drug-free and medication-adherent state may bring about benefits that cannot always be realized in an outpatient setting.

Twelve-Step Groups and 12-Step Facilitation

The 12-step approach has been less influential in the treatment of serious mental illness than in general addiction treatment. Schizophrenic patients are less likely to become involved with 12-step programs than are other people with addictions. Many patients with schizophrenia and comorbid substance use disorder avoid traditional self-help groups because of fears of stigmatization, paranoia, and negative reactions of others to disclosing use of psychiatric medications. However, those who do attend appear to benefit from 12-step participation about as much as anyone else. As a result, several specialized groups such as Double Trouble in Recovery (DTR) and Dual Recovery Anonymous (DRA) have been created. These groups focus on the 12-step model approach to recovery of both substance use disorder and psychiatric illness. As such, participants are encouraged to discuss the problems they face in relation to both problems and to take an active role in their recovery.

Conclusion

Substance use disorders are a prevalent co-occurring problem in those with schizophrenia. Substance use disorders have a significant adverse effect on morbidity and mortality in this population. The etiology is multifactorial, involving neurobiological, genetic, and environmental factors. Multiple substances of abuse are common, especially nicotine, alcohol, marijuana, and cocaine. Screening, diagnosis, and treatment of substance use disorders are important and can have profound effects on an individual's outcome. Treatments include psychopharmacological, psychotherapeutic, and multidisciplinary interventions. Several medications have been FDA approved for the treatment of substance use disorders and also appear to be helpful in treating schizophrenic patients with substance use disorders, although few controlled trials have been done in this population. Psychosocial and psychological interventions have been adapted for use in patients with schizophrenia as well. Treatment of both the psychotic illness and the substance use disorder will improve overall functioning and outcomes in these patients.

References

American Psychiatric Association: Diagnostic and Statistical Manual of Mental Disorders, 4th Edition, Text Revision. Washington, DC, American Psychiatric Association, 2000

Bellack AS: Skills training for people with severe mental illness. Psychiatr Rehabil J 27:375–391, 2004

Bellack AS, Bennett ME, Gearon JS, et al: A randomized clinical trial of a new behavioral treatment for drug abuse in people with severe and persistent mental illness. Arch Gen Psychiatry 63:426–432, 2006

Bennett ME: Assessment of substance use and substance-use disorders in schizophrenia. Clin Schizophr Relat Psychoses 3:50–63, 2009

Bennett ME, Gjonbalaj S: The problem of dual diagnosis, in Adult Psychopathology and Diagnosis, 5th Edition. Edited by Hersen M, Turner S, Beidel D. New York, Wiley, 2007, pp 34–77

Bogenschutz MP, Quinn DK: Acronyms for substance use disorders. J Clin Psychiatry 62:474–475, 2001

Brodie JD, Case BG, Figueroa E, et al: Randomized, double-blind, placebo-controlled trial of vigabatrin for the treatment of cocaine dependence in Mexican parolees. Am J Psychiatry 166:1269–1277, 2009

Bush K, Kivlahan DR, McDonell MB, et al: The AUDIT alcohol consumption questions (AUDIT-C): an effective brief screening test for problem drinking. Ambulatory Care Quality Improvement Project (ACQUIP). Alcohol Use Disorders Identification Test. Arch Intern Med 158:1789–1795, 1998

Carey KB, Leontieva L, Dimmock J, et al: Adapting motivational interventions for comorbid schizophrenia and alcohol use disorders. Clin Psychol (New York) 14:39–57, 2007

Carroll KM, Onken LS: Behavioral therapies for drug abuse. Am J Psychiatry 162:1452–1460, 2005

Chambers RA, Krystal JH, Self DW: A neurobiological basis for substance abuse comorbidity in schizophrenia. Biol Psychiatry 50:71–83, 2001

Conway JL: Exogenous nicotine normalises sensory gating in schizophrenia; therapeutic implications. Med Hypotheses 73:259–262, 2009

Curran C, Byrappa N, McBride A: Stimulant psychosis: systematic review. Br J Psychiatry 185:196–204, 2004

Drake RE, O'Neal EL, Wallach MA: A systematic review of psychosocial research on psychosocial interventions for people with co-occurring severe mental and substance use disorders. J Subst Abuse Treat 34:123–138, 2008

Gold MS, Donabedian RK, Dillard M Jr, et al: Antipsychotic effect of opiate agonists. Lancet 2:398–399, 1977

Green AI: Pharmacotherapy for schizophrenia and co-occurring substance use disorders. Neurotox Res 11:33–40, 2007

Green AI, Zimmet SV, Strous RD, et al: Clozapine for comorbid substance use disorder and schizophrenia: do patients with schizophrenia have a reward-deficiency syndrome that can be ameliorated by clozapine? Harv Rev Psychiatry 6:287–296, 1999

Green AI, Salomon MS, Brenner MJ, et al: Treatment of schizophrenia and comorbid substance use disorder. Curr Drug Targets CNS Neurol Disord 1:129–139, 2002

Gupta S, Hendricks S, Kenkel AM, et al: Relapse in schizophrenia: is there a relationship to substance abuse? Schizophr Res 20:153–156, 1996

Harris D, Batki SL: Stimulant psychosis: symptom profile and acute clinical course. Am J Addict 9:28–37, 2000

Hettema J, Steele J, Miller RW: Motivational interviewing. Annu Rev Clin Psychol 1:91–111, 2005

Hides L, Cotton SM, Berger S, et al: The reliability and validity of the Alcohol, Smoking and Substance Involvement Screening Test (ASSIST) in first-episode psychosis. Addict Behav 34:821–825, 2009

Horsfall J, Cleary M, Hunt GE, et al: Psychosocial treatments for people with co-occurring severe mental illnesses and substance use disorders (dual diagnosis): a review of empirical evidence. Harv Rev Psychiatry 17:24–34, 2009

Johnson BA, Rosenthal N, Capece JA, et al: Topiramate for treating alcohol dependence: a randomized controlled trial. JAMA 298:1641–1651, 2007

Kalivas PW, Volkow ND: The neural basis of addiction: a pathology of motivation and choice. Am J Psychiatry 162:1403–1413, 2005

Kampman KM, Pettinati H, Lynch KG, et al: A pilot trial of topiramate for the treatment of cocaine dependence. Drug Alcohol Depend 75:233–240, 2004

Kendler KS: A twin study of individuals with both schizophrenia and alcoholism. Br J Psychiatry 147:48–53, 1985

Khantzian EJ: The self-medication hypothesis of substance use disorders: a reconsideration and recent applications. Harv Rev Psychiatry 4:231–244, 1997

Kraemer HC: Statistical issues in assessing comorbidity. Stat Med 14:721–733, 1995

Lasser K, Boyd JW, Woolhandler S, et al: Smoking and mental illness: a population-based prevalence study. JAMA 284:2606–2610, 2000

Martell BA, Orson FM, Poling J, et al: Cocaine vaccine for the treatment of cocaine dependence in methadone-maintained patients: a randomized, double-blind, placebo-controlled efficacy trial. Arch Gen Psychiatry 66:1116–1123, 2009

Miller WR, Zweben A, DiClemente CC, et al: Motivational Enhancement Therapy Manual: A Clinical Research Guide for Therapists Treating Individuals With Alcohol Abuse and Dependence (Project MATCH Monograph Series, Vol 2; NIH Publ No 94-3723). Rockville, MD, National Institute on Alcohol Abuse and Alcoholism, 1995

Moore TH, Zammit S, Langford-Hughes A, et al: Cannabis use and risk of psychotic or affective mental health outcomes: a systematic review. Lancet 370:319–328, 2007

Potvin S, Stip E, Roy JY: Clozapine, quetiapine and olanzapine among addicted schizophrenic patients: towards testable hypotheses. Int Clin Psychopharmacol 18:121–132, 2003

Regier DA, Farmer ME, Rae DS, et al: Comorbidity of mental disorders with alcohol and other drug abuse: results from the Epidemiologic Catchment Area (ECA) Study. JAMA 264:2511–2518, 1990

Selzer JA, Lieberman JA: Schizophrenia and substance abuse. Psychiatr Clin North Am 16:401–412, 1993

Smelson DA, Dixon L, Craig T, et al: Pharmacological treatment of schizophrenia and co-occurring substance use disorders. CNS Drugs 22:903–916, 2008

Stitzer M, Petry N: Contingency management for treatment of substance abuse. Annu Rev Clin Psychol 2:411–434, 2006

Swofford CD, Scheller-Gilkey G, Miller AH, et al: Double jeopardy: schizophrenia and substance use. Am J Drug Alcohol Abuse 26:343–353, 2000

Talamo A, Centorrino F, Tondo L, et al: Comorbid substance-use in schizophrenia: relation to positive and negative symptoms. Schizophr Res 86:251–255, 2006

Tracy K, Babuscio T, Nich C, et al: Contingency management to reduce substance use in individuals who are homeless with co-occurring psychiatric disorders. Am J Drug Alcohol Abuse 33:253–258, 2007

U.S. Department of Health and Human Services, Substance Abuse and Mental Health Services Administration, Office of Applied Studies: National Survey on Drug Use and Health, 2008. Ann Arbor, MI, Inter-University Consortium for Political and Social Research, 2009

Yui K, Ikemoto S, Ishiguro T, et al: Studies of amphetamine or methamphetamine psychosis in Japan: relation of methamphetamine psychosis to schizophrenia. Ann N Y Acad Sci 914:1–12, 2000

Zimmet SV, Strous RD, Burgess ES, et al: Effects of clozapine on substance use in patients with schizophrenia and schizoaffective disorder: a retrospective survey. J Clin Psychopharmacol 20:94–98, 2000

8

Pharmacological Treatment of Schizophrenia

Seiya Miyamoto, M.D., Ph.D.

W. Wolfgang Fleischhacker, M.D.

The goals and strategies of treatment of schizophrenia vary according to the phase and severity of the illness. Clinicians are faced with several considerations and decisions about them. Pharmacological treatment is the most important element of the management, and antipsychotic drugs represent the mainstay of pharmacological treatment of schizophrenia. However, currently available antipsychotic drugs are less than optimal because a substantial proportion of schizophrenia symptoms fail to respond to these drugs and because they cause undesirable acute and chronic side effects. Consequently, there has been an intensive search for more effective and safer antipsychotic agents (Biedermann and Fleischhacker 2009; Miyamoto et al. 2008). In this chapter, we provide an updated overview of pharmacological treatment of schizophrenia and offer information with respect to the adjunctive treatments and safety and tolerability of antipsychotic drugs on the basis of currently available evidence.

Treatment During the Acute Phase

Therapeutic Goals

During the acute phase, patients usually have active symptoms of schizophrenia, which can occur during a first episode or as a relapse in a patient with multiepisode schizophrenia. The primary therapeutic goal is to alleviate or reduce the most severe symptoms of the illness, particularly pathological excitement or agitation, hostility, and exacerbated psychotic symptoms (Miyamoto et al. 2003b). Patients also have a substantial risk of self-injury or suicide and other unpredictable, dangerous behaviors to themselves, others, or property. Among patients with schizophrenia, 40% report suicidal thoughts, 20%–40% attempt suicide, and 9%–13% die by suicide (Meltzer 1998). Thus, rapid treatment of these acute symptoms and behavioral disturbances is essential to reduce these risks.

The second goal is to formulate short-term treatment plans and to lay the foundation for long-term maintenance treatment (Lehman et al. 2004; Miyamoto et al. 2003b). Nearly all acute episodes of schizophrenia should be treated with antipsychotic medications to reduce psychotic symptoms (Lehman et al. 2004). In this chapter, the term *antipsychotic* refers to several classes of medications, including first-generation antipsychotics (FGAs) and second-generation antipsychotics (SGAs) (see Table 8–1). Given that aripiprazole has a distinctly different mechanism of action from FGAs and SGAs, it is considered a third-generation antipsychotic (TGA) by most psychopharmacologists.

After initial assessment of the patient's diagnosis and clinical and psychosocial circumstances, including determination of the etiology of the psychotic exacerbation (e.g., nonadherence), pharmacotherapy should be applied as early in this phase as possible (Falkai et al. 2005). Patients should be provided with information on the nature and treatment of the disease, including the potential risks and benefits of the medication, in a manner that is appropriate to the patient's ability to understand (Falkai et al. 2005; Lehman et al. 2004). If patients experience clinical improvement from pharmacological treatment with minimal adverse effects, they will be more likely to continue medications after they recover from the acute episode. Therefore, the initial selection of an appropriate antipsychotic drug at a reasonable dose is critical. Decisions should be made collaboratively with the patient and the family to further strengthen the therapeutic effort. Patients' preferences appear to be a particularly important factor in determining the course of treatment.

Table 8–1. Dosing parameters of first-, second-, and third-generation antipsychotics

	Half-life (hours) (Mean)	Starting dosage (total mg/day)	Target dosage range (mg/day)		Average maintenance dosage range (mg/day)	Route of administration
			First episode	Recurrent episodes		
First-generation antipsychotics						
Chlorpromazine	16–30	50–150	300–500	300–1,000	300–1,000	Oral Short-acting IM
Haloperidol	14–20	1–4	2–8	3–15	5–20	Oral Short- and long-acting IM
Perphenazine	8–12 (10)	4–24	6–36	12–42	16–64	Oral Short- and long-acting IM
Second-generation antipsychotics						
Amisulpride	12–20 (12)	50–100	50–300	400–800	400–800	Oral
Asenapine	24	10	10	10	10–20	Sublingual
Blonanserin	68	4–8	4–12	8–16	8–16	Oral

Table 8–1.   Dosing parameters of first-, second-, and third-generation antipsychotics (*continued*)

	Half-life (hours) (Mean)	Starting dosage (total mg/day)	Target dosage range (mg/day) First episode	Target dosage range (mg/day) Recurrent episodes	Average maintenance dosage range (mg/day)	Route of administration
Second-generation antipsychotics (*continued*)						
Clozapine	10–105 (16)	25–50	150–300	400–600	400	Oral
Iloperidone	18–33	2	12	12–24	12–24	Oral
Olanzapine	20–70 (30)	5–10	10–20	15–30	10–20	Oral Short- and long-acting IM
Paliperidone	23	6	3–12	6–12	3–12	Oral Long-acting IM
Perospirone	2–3	4–8	8–16	12–48	12–48	Oral
Quetiapine	4–10 (7)	50–100	300–400	500–800	400–500	Oral
Risperidone	3–24 (15)	1–2	2–4	3–6	2–6	Oral Long-acting IM
Sertindole	72	4	4–12	8–24	12–20	Oral

Table 8–1. Dosing parameters of first-, second-, and third-generation antipsychotics (continued)

		Target dosage range (mg/day)			
	Half-life (hours) (Mean)	Starting dosage (total mg/day)	First episode	Recurrent episodes	Average maintenance dosage range (mg/day)	Route of administration

	Half-life (hours) (Mean)	Starting dosage (total mg/day)	First episode	Recurrent episodes	Average maintenance dosage range (mg/day)	Route of administration
Second-generation antipsychotics *(continued)*						
Ziprasidone	4–10 (7)	40–80	80–120	120–200	120–160	Oral Short-acting IM
Zotepine	12–30 (15)	50–100	75–150	150–450	75–300	Oral
Third-generation antipsychotic						
Aripiprazole	75–146 (94)	5–15	10–30	15–30	15–30	Oral Short-acting IM

Note. IM = intramuscular.

Source. Adapted from Falkai et al. 2005; Lehman et al. 2004; Miyamoto et al. 2008.

The third therapeutic goal is to attain a rapid return to the best level of functioning or to achieve full remission of the episode (Lehman et al. 2004). At present, schizophrenia has a chronic and progressive course in most patients (J.A. Lieberman 1999). It has been suggested that antipsychotic drug treatment can interrupt and ameliorate the pathophysiological process that causes psychotic symptoms and leads to clinical deterioration (J.A. Lieberman 1999). Studies of maintenance antipsychotic treatment also have shown its prophylactic effect in preventing relapse (Miyamoto et al. 2008). Thus, adequate acute pharmacological treatment not only treats the symptoms of schizophrenia but also mitigates the following course of the illness and produces more favorable outcomes (Miyamoto et al. 2003b). To develop a therapeutic alliance between clinicians, institutions, the patient, and the family, a relationship based on cooperation and trust is essential to achieving successful remission of the episode (R.P. Liberman and Kopelowicz 1995). Also, the quality of life (QOL) during the first years of illness likely will be better when full remission of an episode is achieved (Miyamoto et al. 2003b). Figure 8–1 provides a graphic overview of the considerations for the pharmacological management of schizophrenia.

Selection of an Antipsychotic Agent

When choosing the optimal antipsychotic drug for each individual patient, clinicians need to assess which medication is likely to provide the most suitable combination of efficacy and safety or tolerability and is able to improve the patient's QOL and social functioning (Miyamoto et al., in press). Primary considerations include the patient's prior response to antipsychotic medications and side-effect experience, adherence history, stated preference, and presence of comorbid medical conditions; and the drug's pharmacology and safety profiles, available formulations, and potential for drug interactions (Buchanan et al. 2010; Falkai et al. 2005). The patient and, if available, significant others should be included in a discussion of these considerations, and informed consent should precede medication administration. When selecting antipsychotics, the risk of both acute and chronic adverse effects should be weighed against the profound disability that can accompany severe mental illness and the potential for antipsychotic medication to greatly improve the

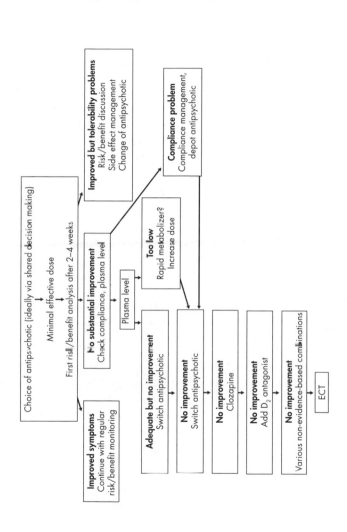

Figure 8–1.   Overview of pharmacological management of schizophrenia. D_2 = dopamine type 2 receptor; ECT = electroconvulsive therapy.

lives of patients and their families. It is prudent for clinicians to document their reasoning when selecting an antipsychotic medication.

At present, SGAs (excluding clozapine) are recommended in several authoritative guidelines as first-line agents for acute therapy for schizophrenia (Falkai et al. 2005, 2006; Lehman et al. 2004; Moore et al. 2007). The high costs of SGAs, however, have led to a continuing debate about their benefits compared with FGAs, although this discussion is currently becoming increasingly irrelevant given the advent of several generic SGAs. Moreover, there has been increased concern over the safety profile of SGAs, such as weight gain and metabolic abnormalities, in the last 10–15 years. These side effects are associated with potential long-term health risks in an already at-risk population as well as decreased adherence to treatment regimens. In addition, recent meta-analyses and government-funded large-scale, practical clinical trials have provided conflicting information about the relative advantages of FGAs and SGAs (Davis et al. 2003; Geddes et al. 2000; Jones et al. 2006; Kahn et al. 2008; Leucht et al. 2002b, 2009; Lewis et al. 2006; J.A. Lieberman et al. 2005; McEvoy et al. 2006; Rosenheck et al. 2006; Stroup et al. 2006).

In the most recent meta-analysis comparing SGAs with FGAs, four SGAs (clozapine, amisulpride, risperidone, and olanzapine) were more efficacious than FGAs for overall improvement in symptoms and for positive and negative symptoms (Leucht et al. 2009). However, the other SGAs (sertindole, quetiapine, ziprasidone, and zotepine) and the TGA aripiprazole were not superior to FGAs in efficacy, even for negative symptoms. In addition, only amisulpride, clozapine, and sertindole were superior to FGAs in terms of QOL. Thus, there may be a modest advantage for some but not all SGAs compared with FGAs.

Several studies of first-episode psychosis suggest that no clinically meaningful differences in short-term efficacy are seen between and among FGAs and SGAs (Buchanan et al. 2010), whereas most longer-term clinical trials have found at least some efficacy advantages for SGAs (A.I. Green et al. 2006; Kahn et al. 2008; Schooler et al. 2005). In contrast, significant differences in adverse effects have been found between and among FGAs and SGAs, especially with regard to extrapyramidal symptoms (EPS) (Table 8–2). Considering the effect of EPS on attitude toward treatment and compliance behavior, it would appear prudent to favor the SGAs with their lower EPS risk in this population, although the recently updated Schizophrenia Patient Outcomes

Research Team (PORT) recommendations exclude clozapine and olanzapine as first-line medications because of their metabolic risks (Buchanan et al. 2010). On the other hand, clozapine has the best-documented evidence for treatment-resistant schizophrenia (Tandon et al. 2008).

Antipsychotic Dosage

The goal of pharmacological treatment is to maximize efficacy and minimize adverse effects with the lowest effective dose (Davis and Chen 2004). Data from recent effectiveness trials, naturalistic studies, and various guidelines provide evidence of specific dosage levels and titration schedules for antipsychotics that may be appropriate in clinical practice (Buchanan et al. 2010; Buckley and Correll 2008; Falkai et al. 2005) (see Table 8–1). Dosages recommended in these guidelines, however, often differ considerably, sometimes by threefold or more (Davis and Chen 2004).

Determination of optimum antipsychotic dosage is complicated by the fact that response as well as susceptibility to side effects may differ from patient to patient and across phases of the illness (Buckley and Correll 2008). For example, first-episode patients generally respond to lower antipsychotic dosages than do patients with recurrent episodes (Robinson et al. 2005). Poor or partial responders may benefit from somewhat higher dosages than consistent responders (Davis and Chen 2005). The physiology of this variability is not well known, but it seems likely that individual variation in pharmacokinetic factors and in brain receptor density and sensitivity plays a role.

After more than 50 years of clinical use, the optimum dose of FGAs is still debated. To establish a therapeutic response, low-potency FGAs require higher dosages, but high-potency FGAs require much lower dosages. Most experts would agree that therapeutic effects do not continue to increase with very high FGA dosages, but considerable controversy persists regarding whether the efficacy of FGAs actually diminishes at higher dosages. Few good dose-finding studies exist for both older and newer antipsychotics. They usually provide better information about the lower level of the effective dosage range than about upper levels of efficacy and safety (Kinon et al. 2008; Peuskens 1995; Van Putten et al. 1992; Volavka et al. 1992). Geddes et al. (2000) argued, on the basis of a meta-analysis, that dosages greater than 12 mg/day in haloperidol equivalents are less efficacious than lower dosages because of the negative effects of EPS and perhaps other side effects such as sedation. In contrast, a meta-analysis of 42 randomized

Table 8–2. Side-effect profiles of antipsychotic drugs

Side effect	FGAs		SGAs				
	Haloperidol	Perphenazine	Amisulpride	Asenapine	Blonanserin	Clozapine	Iloperidone
Extrapyramidal symptoms	+++	++	0 to ++	0 to ++	+	0	0
Tardive dyskinesia	+++	++	+	?	?	0	?
Prolactin elevation	+++	++	+++	0 to +	++	0	0
Weight gain	+	+	+	0	0	+++	++
Glucose abnormalities	0	+?	+	0	++	+++	+
Lipid abnormalities	0	+?	+	0	++	+++	0
QTc prolongation	+	0	+	0 to +	0?	0	++
Sedation	++	+	0 to +	+	+?	+++	+
Hypotension	0	+	0	+	0	+++	+
Anticholinergic side effects	0	+	0	0	0	+++	0

Table 8–2. Side-effect profiles of antipsychotic drugs *(continued)*

Side effect	SGAs *(continued)*							TGA
	Olanzapine	Paliperidone	Perospirone	Quetiapine	Risperidone	Sertindole	Ziprasidone	Aripiprazole
Extrapyramidal symptoms	0 to +	0 to ++	0 to +	0	0 to ++	0	0 to +	+
Tardive dyskinesia	+	+	0 to +	0 to +	+	0 to +	+	+
Prolactin elevation	+	+++	+	0	+++	0 to +	+	0
Weight gain	+++	+	0	++	+	+	0	0
Glucose abnormalities	+++	0 to +	+	++	++	?	0	0
Lipid abnormalities	+++	0	0?	++	++	?	0	0
QTc prolongation	0 to +	0 to +	0?	+	+	+++	++	0
Sedation	+	+	+	++	+	0 to +	0 to +	0 to +
Hypotension	+	0 to +	0	++	+	+	+	0
Anticholinergic side effects	++	0	0	+	0	0	0	0

Note. This table is not based on direct quantitative comparative data of all the drugs listed. Data from many studies with varying methodology were reviewed to produce this one view. In addition, it is well known that interindividual variability is considerable with regard to drug safety and that most antipsychotic-induced adverse effects are dose-dependent. FGAs=first-generation antipsychotic drugs; SGAs=second-generation antipsychotic drugs; TGA=third-generation antipsychotic drug; 0=minimal to no risk; +=low risk; ++=moderate risk; +++=high risk; ?=unknown risk.

Source. *Adapted from* Falkai et al. 2005; Lehman et al. 2004; Miyamoto et al. 2008.

controlled trials (RCTs) comparing various dosages of FGAs found that dosages lower than 3.3 mg/day, expressed in haloperidol equivalents, were clearly less effective than higher dosages but that all dosages above this threshold were fully efficacious (Davis and Chen 2005). Brain imaging studies further support the use of low to moderate dosages of FGAs in acute schizophrenia (Janicak and Davis 1996). For example, positron emission tomography research has found that a haloperidol dosage of 2–5 mg/day induces 53%–74% striatal dopamine type 2 (D$_2$) receptor occupancy, with substantial clinical improvement (Kapur et al. 1996, 2000). These studies do not preclude the requirement of some patients for a higher-than-normal antipsychotic dose, but they do suggest that when groups of patients are assigned to very high dosages, such as more than 2,000 mg/day of chlorpromazine or 40 mg/day of haloperidol, the average rate and amount of improvement are likely to be no greater than for those assigned to more moderate dosages and may in fact be lower (Marder 1996).

The dosage recommendations for SGAs are summarized in Table 8–1. As with FGAs, optimal dosing of SGAs is a controversial issue. In general, doses tend to be lower in clinical trials than doses typically used in clinical practice (Buckley and Correll 2008).

Among SGAs, high dosing is used rarely with clozapine or risperidone, likely because of the disproportionate rise in the risk of seizures, sedation, and anticholinergic side effects for clozapine at dosages greater than 900 mg/day and the risk of EPS and hyperprolactinemia for risperidone at dosages greater than 8 mg/day, without evidence of substantial gains in efficacy (Buckley and Correll 2008). Controversies in dosing recommendations are exemplified by olanzapine, for which studies regarding dosages beyond 20 mg/day (the highest dosage recommended in the package insert) have produced inconsistent results (Kinon et al. 2008; Meltzer et al. 2008), and by clozapine, for which dosing practice differs widely between the United States and Europe (Pollack et al. 1995). Quetiapine and ziprasidone seem to have a linear dose-response curve within the therapeutic range, such that higher dosages will move a patient toward higher levels of response.

Route of Administration of Antipsychotics

Antipsychotic medications may be available as tablets, liquid concentrates, orally dissolving formulations, sublingual preparations, short-acting intramuscular (IM) preparations, or long-acting preparations (Miyamoto et al., in press). Except for emergency situations in which involuntary IM administration may be needed, the choice of route of application should be adjusted to the preferences of patients. One disadvantage of oral administration is that it may be less dependable than parenteral administration (Marder 1997). For example, patients sometimes will appear to accept oral medication but will actually "cheek" or spit the drug. Liquid concentrates, orally disintegrating tablets, or sublingual preparations are available for some antipsychotics and may be used to avoid such problems. Another disadvantage of oral administration is that pharmacokinetic factors such as hepatic disease or slow gastrointestinal absorption may increase the half-life of the drug and the time required to attain steady-state concentration (Marder 1997). Oral extended-release formulations such as paliperidone extended-release tablets and quetiapine fumarate extended-release tablets with generally more consistent peak-to-trough plasma levels have been suggested to provide more sustained plasma drug concentrations (Pani 2009).

Short-acting IM formulations are particularly useful in the treatment of severely disturbed patients who cannot be verbally redirected, who may be violent, and who may require medication over objection (Pereira et al. 2006). In these situations, many clinicians favor a combination of an antipsychotic and a rapid-acting parenteral benzodiazepine (e.g., lorazepam). Among the FGAs, a single IM injection of high-potency drugs such as haloperidol can result in rapid calming, and this effect is thought to be the result of sedation. True antipsychotic effect was formerly believed to develop after only several days or weeks (Lehman et al. 2004), but Kapur et al. (2005) presented evidence that the onset of antipsychotic action of IM haloperidol may occur within 24 hours of the first injection. A disadvantage of IM administration is the risk of injury to the patient (or the treatment team), usually by needle stick or accompanying physical restraint. In addition, high dosages of high-potency drugs can lead to acute dystonia or akathisia, which may increase the patient's agitation. Coadministration of an anticholinergic medication may reduce this risk.

Among the newer-generation antipsychotics, short-acting IM formulations of the SGAs olanzapine and ziprasidone and the TGA aripiprazole are available in some countries (see Table 8–1). The IM formulations of these drugs have been consistently shown to be well tolerated and have superior efficacy compared with placebo or low-dose active comparator medication in acutely agitated patients with schizophrenia (Andrezina et al. 2006; Breier et al. 2002; Brook et al. 2000). However, no studies have compared two or more of these agents with each other (Buchanan et al. 2010).

Some FGAs also can be administered intravenously. This practice is generally associated with a more rapid onset of action than occurs with IM preparations. However, intravenous antipsychotic use may increase the risk of cardiac arrhythmias and autonomic complications and consequently is a last treatment option (Allen et al. 2001). Long-acting formulations are seldom prescribed for acute psychotic episodes because they take several weeks to months to reach steady-state levels and are eliminated very slowly (Miyamoto et al. 2003a).

Maintenance Treatment

Therapeutic Goals

The goals of maintenance treatment are to make sure that symptom remission or control is sustained, that the patient is maintaining or improving his or her level of functioning and QOL, that increases in symptoms or relapses are successfully treated, and that monitoring for adverse treatment events continues (Lehman et al. 2004) (see Table 8–2). The main aim of pharmacological maintenance treatment is to prevent relapse and help keep a patient stable enough to live as normal a life as possible (Falkai et al. 2005). Managing treatment adherence is an important part of maintenance therapy treatment plans. Psychosocial interventions are recommended as an important adjunct to pharmacological treatment.

Selection of an Antipsychotic Agent

As mentioned earlier, patient preference and drug experience, including the patient's prior response and side effects, are key determinants of medication selection. Whether new-generation antipsychotics have advantages over traditional drugs in this respect remains an area of intense debate. A relapse prevention study comparing risperidone with haloperidol has found advantages of the newer drug over haloperidol in some but not all outcome criteria (Csernansky et al. 2002). In addition, three large long-term pragmatic studies have compared the effectiveness of SGAs with that of FGAs.

The Clinical Antipsychotic Trials of Intervention Effectiveness (CATIE) study compared the effectiveness of the FGA perphenazine with the SGAs olanzapine, quetiapine, risperidone, and ziprasidone in 1,493 chronic schizophrenic outpatients for up to 18 months of treatment (J.A. Lieberman et al. 2005). Results from the CATIE Phase I study indicated that olanzapine was superior to quetiapine and risperidone in terms of time to discontinuation for any cause, despite substantial metabolic side effects associated with olanzapine. All five medications showed comparable changes in Positive and Negative Syndrome Scale (PANSS) scores. Perphenazine was similar in efficacy, tolerability, cognition (Keefe et al. 2007a), cost (Rosenheck et al. 2006), QOL (Swartz et al. 2007), and psychosocial functioning (Swartz et al. 2007) to the SGAs, suggesting that certain FGAs remain viable treatment options in chronic schizophrenia.

In the Cost Utility of the Latest Antipsychotic Drugs in Schizophrenia Study (CUtLASS), in which FGAs and SGAs were compared as classes (most patients in the first group received sulpiride, and most in the second group received olanzapine), no significant differences in QOL, positive or negative symptoms, side effects, or patient satisfaction were observed between patients taking FGAs and those taking SGAs (Jones et al. 2006).

In a third large pragmatic trial, the European First Episode Schizophrenia Trial (EUFEST; Fleischhacker et al. 2005; Kahn et al. 2008), close to 500 first-episode patients were randomly allocated to treatment with either a low dose of haloperidol or one of four SGAs (amisulpride, olanzapine, quetiapine, or ziprasidone) for 1 year. Unlike CATIE and CUtLASS, EUFEST found a clear advantage of the four SGAs, both as a group and individually, over haloperidol in terms of the risk for any-cause discontinuation, Clinical Global Impressions Scale scores, Global Assessment of Functioning Scale scores (Kahn et al. 2008), and the proportions of response and remission (Boter et al. 2009). However, no group differences were found in PANSS total scores, Calgary Depression Scale for Schizophrenia scores, QOL scores, or the improvement of cognitive functions (Davidson et al. 2009).

In summary, CATIE, CUtLASS, and EUFEST did not provide unequivocal evidence to support the superiority of one antipsychotic over the other (Miyamoto et al., in press). However, a recent meta-analysis of RCTs in 1,055 patients with first-episode psychosis found that relapse rates were significantly lower with SGAs than with FGAs (Alvarez-Jimenez et al. 2011). Yet another meta-analysis (Leucht et al. 2009) corroborated these findings across numerous trials in chronically ill patients.

Antipsychotic Dosage

Deciding on the dose of an antipsychotic in the maintenance phase also remains under debate. For example, the practice guidelines by the American Psychiatric Association (APA) support the use of the "minimal effective dose," which means the lowest possible effective dose to minimize antipsychotic side effects (Lehman et al. 2004), whereas the "Expert Consensus Guidelines" generally recommend the continuous use of an antipsychotic dose that was effective in the acute phase to lower the risk of relapse (Kane et al. 2003). The 2009 Schizophrenia PORT treatment recommendations suggest that the maintenance dosage for FGAs should be in the range of 300–600 mg/day of chlorpromazine equivalents, and the dosage for aripiprazole, olanzapine, paliperidone, quetiapine, risperidone, and ziprasidone should be the dosage that was effective for reducing positive symptoms in the acute phase of treatment (Buchanan et al. 2010).

The recent first meta-analysis of the long-term efficacy of very-low-dose, low-dose, and standard-dose antipsychotic treatment for schizophrenia suggests that low-dose therapy may be as effective as standard-dose therapy in terms of efficacy and that less than half the standard dose may increase the risk of treatment failure (Uchida et al. 2011). However, further well-designed prospective clinical studies are warranted to draw firm conclusions on low- compared with standard-dose maintenance antipsychotic therapy.

Long-Acting Antipsychotic Formulations

Long-acting injectable antipsychotic medication should be offered as an alternative to oral antipsychotic medication for maintenance treatment when the long-acting injectable formulation is preferred to oral preparations (Buchanan et al. 2010). As of May 2010, several FGAs and three SGAs are available in long-acting injectable depot formulations (Fleischhacker 2009) (see Table 8–1). The long-acting injectable formulation of risperidone, which takes advantage of embedding the drug into slow-release microspheres, has been available for several years. Long-acting injectable paliperidone palmitate is the first once-monthly depot SGA available in the United States. Long-acting injectable olanzapine pamoate recently was approved by the European Registration Agency and the U.S. Food and Drug Administration. Its main safety concern is the risk of a postinjection syndrome of excessive sedation or delirium. Thus, after injecting long-acting injectable olanzapine pamoate, health care providers must monitor the patients for at least 3 hours.

Long-acting injectable formulations allow for stable concentrations of the active drug to remain at a therapeutic range for an extended period. Thus, they are especially advantageous in patients with adherence problems and those with a history of severe relapse after medication discontinuation (Davis and Andriukaitis 1986). They also simplify compliance monitoring because they are generally administered at scheduled intervals by a health care provider (Miyamoto et al., in press). This type of medication therefore may be particularly helpful in the maintenance phase of treatment.

Comparative studies of the efficacy and safety of long-acting injectable formulations of FGAs and SGAs have not been conducted. Thus, current evidence is insufficient to recommend a specific long-acting injectable antipsychotic drug over another.

Adjunctive Treatments

A broad variety of adjunctive medications have been used to enhance the response to antipsychotic drugs or to treat residual symptoms of chronic schizophrenia and comorbid conditions (Fleischhacker 2003). However, the evidence supporting the use of adjunctive therapies is relatively shallow and inconsistent.

Benzodiazepines

Benzodiazepines are generally used in agitation, anxiety, insomnia, and catatonia in schizophrenia (Fleischhacker 2003). Benzodiazepines also may allow the use of lower dosages of the concomitant antipsychotics. Volz et al. (2007) reviewed 31 RCTs comparing benzodiazepines with antipsychotics or placebo (or no intervention), whether as a sole treatment or as an adjunct to antipsychotic drugs, for the treatment of psychotic disorders. Most trials were small, of short duration, and inconsistently reported. They found significant effects of benzodiazepines on short-term sedation and antiparkinsonian medication to be less frequently used in the combination treatment group. Although the use of benzodiazepines is widespread, the evidence base supporting benzodiazepines either as a sole or as an adjunctive agent in schizophrenia is incomplete and inconclusive. Moreover, no evidence indicates that any one benzodiazepine is superior to another in the treatment of schizophrenia (Miyamoto et al., in press).

Lithium

Lithium has been studied both as a sole agent and as an adjunctive agent in schizophrenia. The current evidence shows that lithium as a sole drug is ineffective in the treatment of schizophrenia (Leucht et al. 2004). In a meta-analysis of 11 RCTs that examined the augmentation of antipsychotics with lithium (Leucht et al. 2007), participants with lithium augmentation had a marginally superior response. Its advantage was, however, not significant ($P=0.07$) when participants with schizoaffective disorders were excluded in a sensitivity analysis. Furthermore, significantly more patients receiving lithium left the trials early, suggesting a low acceptability of lithium augmentation. Lithium augmentation had no superior efficacy in any specific aspect of the mental state. In addition, no differences were found between groups for adverse events, although these results were based on very few data. Accordingly, lithium is not recommended as either monotherapy or adjunctive treatment in schizophrenia.

Anticonvulsants

Anticonvulsants have been considered a useful adjunctive treatment for specific subgroups of schizophrenic patients. Patients with manic, impulsive, and violent behavior or with abnormal electroencephalogram results may be more likely to show a beneficial response to the addition of an anticonvulsant (Siris 1993). Although numerous positive case reports and open-label trials of adjunctive anticonvulsants in the treatment of schizophrenia have been published, definitive controlled studies have not established a consistent benefit for adjunctive strategies in terms of increased efficacy or speed of response (Citrome 2009a).

Carbamazepine

The addition of carbamazepine to antipsychotics had controversial results. Carbamazepine augmentation of FGAs has been associated with modest reductions in persistent symptoms, including tension, aggression, and paranoia, in several controlled trials (Luchins 1984; Okuma et al. 1989), but the effects were small at best. Adverse effects such as disorientation and ataxia and interactions with antipsychotics induced by hepatic microsomal enzymes may limit the use of carbamazepine. A meta-analysis of 10 RCTs concluded that no evidence supports the efficacy of combining carbamazepine with antipsychotics in schizophrenia (Leucht et al. 2002a). The most promising targets for future studies may be patients with aggression, excitement, and schizoaffective disorder.

Valproic Acid (Sodium Valproate)

No evidence currently supports valproic acid (sodium valproate) as a sole agent for schizophrenia. Some evidence indicates positive effects of combining antipsychotics with valproic acid on aggression and tardive dyskinesia, but given that these results were based on only a single small study, they cannot be considered robust. The Cochrane Library systematic review of seven RCTs, published in 2008, which assessed the efficacy of valproic acid as an adjunct to antipsychotics for the treatment of schizophrenia, showed that it led to no significant benefit on Clinical Global Impressions Scale scores or the general mental state when compared with placebo (Schwarz et al. 2008). The overall lack of benefit of adjunctive divalproex has been further supported by the recent large 12-week double-blind trial of the combination of divalproex with olanzapine or risperidone in patients with acute exacerbations of schizophrenia (Casey et al. 2009). Antipsychotic monotherapy was actually superior to adjunctive valproate for negative symptoms at most of the time points at which these symptoms were assessed. Thus, adding valproic acid to antipsychotics must remain a last-resort treatment option.

Lamotrigine

In a recent meta-analysis of five RCTs of the combination of lamotrigine with clozapine in 161 patients with clozapine-refractory schizophrenia, lamotrigine augmentation was superior to placebo in ameliorating both positive and negative symptoms (Tiihonen et al. 2009), suggesting that the addition of lamotrigine may have some clinical benefits for patients with clozapine-resistant schizophrenia. However, few patients have been studied thus far in clozapine-lamotrigine augmentation trials, and the duration of trials was limited. Moreover, two large controlled studies in which most participants received SGAs other than clozapine did not support the use of lamotrigine as an adjunct to SGAs in patients with refractory psychosis (Glick et al. 2009; Goff et al. 2007). Therefore, further larger trials of longer duration are necessary to confirm its potential usefulness.

Antidepressants

Efficacy Against Depressive Symptoms

Patients with schizophrenia commonly complain of depression, which is associated with substantial morbidity and an increased risk of suicide. Antidepressants have no role as the sole treatment for schizophrenia. In general, when treating depressive symptoms in these patients, one must carefully evaluate whether they occur during the acute phase of the disorder or constitute postpsychotic depression (Hausmann and Fleischhacker 2002). The former usually subside after positive symptoms have been successfully treated with antipsychotics, but the latter may be an indication for antidepressant cotherapy (Hausmann and Fleischhacker 2000).

A meta-analysis was performed on results of 11 small RCTs that investigated the clinical efficacy of antidepressants in the treatment of depression in schizophrenic patients (Whitehead et al. 2003). In 5 trials that provided categorical outcome data, the proportion improved in the antidepressant group was 26% higher than in the placebo group. In 6 studies that gave the results for the Hamilton Rating Scale for Depression (Ham-D) total score at the trial end point, the standardized mean difference on the Ham-D was –0.27. No evidence indicated that antidepressant treatment given during the stable phase of illness induced a deterioration of psychotic symptoms. Earlier studies that used adjunctive tricyclic antidepressants generally provided favorable results (Hausmann and Fleischhacker 2000).

Among selective serotonin reuptake inhibitor (SSRI) antidepressants, only sertraline has been studied in schizophrenic patients with depression. One double-blind RCT led to positive results (Mulholland et al. 2003), but another trial showed no difference in efficacy between the sertraline and the placebo treatment groups (Addington et al. 2002). Taken together, results provide some evidence for the efficacy of antidepressants in patients with schizophrenia and depression, especially for postpsychotic depression.

Efficacy Against Negative Symptoms

Negative symptoms represent a core feature of schizophrenia and may be associated with long-term disability and prolonged hospitalization (Buchanan and Gold 1996). Negative symptoms can be divided into three subtypes that are often difficult to distinguish: 1) primary enduring (or deficit) negative symptoms, 2) primary nonenduring negative symptoms, and 3) secondary negative symptoms as a consequence of positive symptoms, depression, EPS or other iatrogenic effects, and substance misuse (Buchanan and Gold 1996; Murphy et al. 2006). These symptoms represent an important unmet treatment need. Even with the advent of SGAs and TGAs, primary negative symptoms remain a great treatment challenge.

In a meta-analysis of 7 trials examining antidepressants as add-on to antipsychotics in the treatment of negative symptoms of schizophrenia, augmentation with antidepressants was shown to improve these symptoms (Rummel et al. 2005). However, note that all included trials used FGAs, except for one study. Moreover, combined therapy with an antipsychotic and an antidepressant drug can result in higher plasma concentrations of both drugs than when either is given alone (Goff et al. 1995). A meta-analysis of 11 RCTs assessing SSRI add-on therapy for the negative symptoms of schizophrenia provided no general support for the improvement of negative symptoms with SSRI augmentation (Sepehry et al. 2007).

Beta-Blockers

A systematic review of five RCTs did not document clear evidence for any effect of adrenergic β-receptor antagonists (β-blockers) as an adjunct to FGAs in schizophrenia (Wahlbeck et al. 2000). At present, available data on the use of adjunctive β-blockers in schizophrenia appear to be too weak to support the utility of this treatment (Miyamoto et al., in press).

Combination Antipsychotic Therapy

The use of combinations of antipsychotic medications (antipsychotic polypharmacy) is not uncommon, with prevalence varying widely (4.1%–57.7%), depending on treatment setting and patient population (Pandurangi and Dalkilic 2008). However, the current literature has several shortcomings, including low numbers of participants, lack of adequate control of confounding variables, short durations of experimental follow-up, and inadequate monitoring of potential adverse effects (Tranulis et al. 2008). In a meta-analysis of 19 RCTs comparing antipsychotic monotherapy with polypharmacy, antipsychotic polypharmacy was superior to monotherapy regarding the two a priori–defined co-primary outcomes: less study-specific defined inefficacy and all-cause discontinuation (Correll et al. 2009). The interpretation of the results for specific psychopathology and adverse events was limited by the low numbers of studies and patients with available data. Moreover, because of the enormous heterogeneity of the trial data set and publication bias, the conclusions might be confounded. In another recent meta-analysis of 10 RCTs of antipsychotic augmentation of clozapine up to 16 weeks, only weak evidence of a therapeutic benefit was found (Taylor and Smith 2009). From an evidence-based perspective, further trials of antipsychotic polypharmacy with sufficient power to identify long-term effectiveness and safety issues, particularly regarding tardive dyskinesia and metabolic side effects, are required before recommending any antipsychotic combination (Miyamoto et al., in press). A recent report on the addition of aripiprazole to clozapine may serve as an example here (Fleischhacker et al. 2010).

Treatment of Nonpositive Symptoms

Negative Symptoms

In the most recent meta-analysis comparing SGAs with FGAs, four SGAs (clozapine, amisulpride, risperidone, and olanzapine) were more efficacious than FGAs against negative symptoms (Leucht et al. 2009). Other SGAs (sertindole, quetiapine, ziprasidone, and zotepine) and the TGA aripiprazole were not superior to FGAs in efficacy. Of the SGAs, amisulpride appears to have advantages in patients with predominantly negative symptoms, although experience in long-term treatment is limited (Falkai et al. 2006).

Whether the effects of antipsychotics on negative symptoms are related to a reduction in primary negative symptoms, secondary negative symptoms, or both has been debated (Murphy et al. 2006). Path analyses have suggested that risperidone and olanzapine exert direct effects on primary negative symptoms, independent of changes in positive, depressive, or extrapyramidal symptoms (Möller 1993; Tollefson and Sanger 1997), but the statistical approaches were performed post hoc, and only the most efficacious dosages of the SGAs were used.

The CATIE study provides a notable opportunity to compare the effectiveness of multiple SGAs in the treatment of negative symptoms. In Phase IIE of

Table 8–3. Strategies for treatment of negative symptoms in schizophrenia

Determine the most likely cause (primary, secondary?).

Change antipsychotic medication (preferably second-generation antipsychotics; best evidence for amisulpride).

Reduce the dosage of antipsychotic medication.

Try an anticholinergic.

Add treatment with antidepressants (no conclusive evidence).

Use psychosocial rehabilitation measures.

the study, no significant differences in PANSS negative symptom subscores were found either between or within groups receiving clozapine, olanzapine, quetiapine, or risperidone at baseline, 3 months, and 6 months (McEvoy et al. 2006). At 6 months, clozapine showed the greatest reduction in negative scores (–5.3); quetiapine (–1.1) and olanzapine (–0.7) performed less impressively, whereas risperidone achieved no reduction (0.0). For patients randomly assigned to receive olanzapine, quetiapine, risperidone, or ziprasidone in Phase IIT, no significant differences in PANSS negative symptom subscores again were reported among treatment groups at 12 months (Stroup et al. 2006). Thus, the results of CATIE Phase II suggested only modest efficacy for SGAs in the treatment of general negative symptoms of chronic schizophrenia, with a probable small advantage for clozapine.

More encouraging is that growing evidence suggests that adding certain augmentation agents to FGAs or SGAs may improve negative symptoms (Table 8–3). Some glycine site agonists of N-methyl-D-aspartate (NMDA) receptors (e.g., glycine, D-cycloserine, and D-serine) and glycine transporter-1 inhibitors (e.g., sarcosine) appear to be effective in reducing negative symptoms when they are added to nonclozapine antipsychotic treatment (Evins et al. 2002; Goff et al. 1999; Heresco-Levy et al. 2004; Javitt et al. 1994; Tsai et al. 2004). Double-blind, controlled trials that used the neurosteroid dehydro-epiandrosterone (DHEA) (Strous et al. 2003), selegiline (Bodkin et al. 2005; Jungerman et al. 1999), extract of *Ginkgo biloba* (Zhang et al. 2001), naltrexone (Marchesi et al. 1995), or pergolide (Roesch-Ely et al. 2006) as augmenters of antipsychotic medication also have suggested efficacy in the treatment of negative symptoms of schizophrenia. These studies, however, require replication.

Cognitive Symptoms

Cognitive impairment is also recognized as a core component of schizophrenia, and patients typically perform 1–2 standard deviations below normal on a variety of neuropsychological measures, particularly those that assess attention, verbal skills, processing speed, and executive function (Woodward et al. 2005). Cognitive deficits are usually present by the time of the first psychotic episode and tend to remain relatively stable or to worsen slowly after the onset (Aleman et al. 1999; Gold et al. 1999; Harvey et al. 1999). They are more strongly related to social and vocational functioning than to psychotic symptoms and may substantially impair activities of daily living and QOL (M. F. Green 1996; Harvey et al. 1998). Thus, cognitive deficits have become a major target of treatment.

As a class, FGAs have only modest effects on cognitive deficits in schizophrenia (Mishara and Goldberg 2004). In some cases, FGAs may aggravate preexisting cognitive impairments as a result of EPS, anticholinergic effects, or sedation (M. F. Green and Braff 2001; Velligan and Miller 1999). Cognitive functioning, particularly attention and memory, also may be worsened by anticholinergic agents, which are frequently required to treat FGA-induced EPS (Tollefson 1996). Such variables should be taken into account when assessing clinical studies of the effect of antipsychotics on cognitive symptoms. Excessive dosing of FGAs also can impair performance on time-sensitive tasks via EPS, sedation, and anticholinergic activity.

Many studies have investigated the efficacy of SGAs on cognitive impairments in schizophrenia. Earlier quantitative reviews reported a significant advantage for SGAs over FGAs in several cognitive domains (Harvey and Keefe 2001; Keefe et al. 1999), although these reviews have been criticized for the small number of studies they included (Woodward et al. 2005). Woodward and colleagues (2005) conducted a meta-analysis of 27 open-label and 14 double-blind studies (many of which involved a switch from prior treatments) comparing FGAs and SGAs. The analysis found somewhat greater cognitive improvement for SGAs (effect sizes = 0.17–0.46) compared with FGAs (effect sizes = 0.00–0.24). It is, however, difficult to draw firm conclusions from "switch" studies, in which patients who have been maintained on FGAs are tested before and after switching to an SGA (Hill et al. 2010). It is also unclear whether the improvements observed with SGAs represent true cognitive enhancement or only a relative reduction in EPS- and anticholinergic-related cognitive effects (Carpenter and Gold 2002; Harvey and Keefe 2001). This has led to discussions as to whether lower dosages of FGAs might show efficacy comparable to that of SGAs for cognitive symptoms of schizophrenia (Mishara and Goldberg 2004).

Recent studies with improved methodology suggest that low dosages of haloperidol may have a less deleterious effect on cognitive function (M. F. Green et al. 2002; Keefe et al. 2004, 2006a, 2006b). Moreover, several studies in first-episode patients with schizophrenia reported moderate improvement in the cognitive test performance after long-term (several months to 2 years) treatment with SGAs or low-dose haloperidol, but the magnitude of improvement did not differ between and among them (Crespo-Facorro et al. 2009; Davidson et al. 2009; Keefe et al. 2006b). Numerous cognitive-enhancing drugs have been developed and investigated in clinical trials. However, evidence is currently insufficient to support the use of any adjunctive agent for the treatment of cognitive deficits (Buchanan et al. 2010).

In summary, the observed differences in cognitive improvement between SGAs and FGAs might not be as large as initially reported if both classes of medication are dosed appropriately (Keefe et al. 1999; Purdon et al. 2000). In addition, SGAs generally do not show differential effects when compared with one another (Davidson et al. 2009; Keefe et al. 2007a, 2007b). Strategies for treatment of cognitive symptoms in schizophrenia are shown in Table 8–4.

Table 8–4. Strategies for treatment of cognitive symptoms in schizophrenia

Reduce the dosage of the first-generation antipsychotic.

Discontinue the use of anticholinergic drugs or reduce the dosage.

Switch antipsychotic medication to a second-generation antipsychotic.

Use cognitive remediation.

Add cognitive-enhancing drugs (no conclusive evidence).

Safety and Tolerability of Antipsychotics

All antipsychotic drugs carry the risk of a wide range of adverse effects (see Table 8–2). These can cause distress to patients and impair QOL, cause physical morbidity and mortality, cause stigma, and contribute to poor adherence, which may lead to an increased relapse rate (Haddad and Sharma 2007).

Acute Extrapyramidal Symptoms (Dystonia, Parkinsonism, and Akathisia)

All antipsychotics can produce EPS after acute or chronic treatment. In general, this propensity is more pronounced with FGAs than with SGAs (see Table 8–2). Among FGAs, drugs that possess a high potency with respect to the D_2 receptor such as haloperidol carry the highest risk of EPS even at very low dosages (Kahn et al. 2008; Schooler et al. 2005). However, at low to moderate dosages, mid- and low-potency FGAs may cause no more EPS than most SGAs (Jones et al. 2006; Leucht et al. 2003, 2009; J.A. Lieberman et al. 2005).

A recent meta-analysis determined that all SGAs induced fewer EPS than did haloperidol, even when the haloperidol dosage was lower than 7.5 mg/day (Leucht et al. 2009). Among SGAs, clozapine and quetiapine carry almost no risk of EPS (Dev and Raniwalla 2000; Kane et al. 1988; Small et al. 1997). In contrast, risperidone produces dose-dependent EPS (Gasquet et al. 2005; Lehman et al. 2004). EPS with aripiprazole, olanzapine, and ziprasidone appear to be less common than with risperidone but more common than with clozapine or quetiapine (Lehman et al. 2004). Asenapine has a lower propensity for EPS compared with haloperidol (Citrome 2009b). Iloperidone is reported to be essentially free of EPS (Citrome 2009c). Amisulpride and paliperidone may cause EPS in a dose-dependent manner (Haddad and Sharma 2007; Spina and Cavallaro 2007).

Acute EPS, including parkinsonism, dystonia, and akathisia, are dose-dependent and almost always reversible with medication dosage reduction or discontinuation (Casey et al. 1995; Lehman et al. 2004) (Table 8–5). More than 60% of the patients who receive acute treatment with FGAs may develop some form of clinically significant EPS (Lehman et al. 2004), although this evidence comes primarily from studies of high-potency FGAs administered at higher dosages. The increasing use of SGAs is thought to have substantially

Table 8–5. Strategies for management of acute extrapyramidal symptoms

Reduce dosage.

Change antipsychotic medication to a second-generation antipsychotic.

Use anticholinergic drug.

Use β-blocker or benzodiazepines for akathisia.

reduced the burden of acute EPS. In fact, a meta-analysis suggested that clozapine and olanzapine may induce fewer EPS than do FGAs despite prophylactic anticholinergic medication with the latter (Leucht et al. 2009).

Medication-induced parkinsonism occurs most commonly with high-potency antipsychotics, especially when anticholinergic medication is not administered concurrently. Its risk factors include older age, higher dosage, a history of parkinsonism, and underlying basal ganglia damage (Marder 1997). The initial treatment of parkinsonism is to reduce the antipsychotic dosage. If symptoms persist, switching to an antipsychotic with less EPS risk should be considered. If an adequate response is still not achieved, adding antiparkinsonian drugs may be efficacious, although they have their own risk of adverse effects and so should be used carefully (Lehman et al. 2004).

Dystonia usually occurs within the first few days of the antipsychotic administration and is often dramatic in presentation (see Table 8–5). Its risk factors include a history of dystonia, young age, male gender, use of high-potency antipsychotics, higher dosage, and intramuscular administration (Lehman et al. 2004). Acute dystonia is rapidly and effectively treated with an anticholinergic agent, particularly when administered parenterally. Short-term oral anticholinergic medication then should be continued to prevent a recurrence of dystonia.

Akathisia can occur in 21%–75% of patients taking antipsychotics (Kane et al. 2009), the incidence being consistently higher with FGAs than with newer antipsychotics. Patients may complain of anxiety or severe discomfort, which may contribute to medication nonadherence or self-injurious behavior. Initial treatment options for akathisia include lowering the dosage or switching to a lower risk antipsychotic. If symptoms persist, or if psychotic symptoms require a higher antipsychotic dosage, individual trials of β-blockers or benzodiazepines may be attempted; anticholinergic agents, in contrast, are generally less effective for akathisia (Casey 1993; Lehman et al. 2004; Miller and Fleischhacker 2000) (see Table 8–5).

Patients should be closely monitored for EPS during antipsychotic initiation and until their medication dosage has been stable for at least 2 weeks (Marder et al. 2004). At present, guidelines generally do not recommend the prophylactic use of anticholinergic agents (Lehman et al. 2004). A disadvantage of anticholinergic drugs is that they may themselves cause distressing side effects, such as dry mouth, constipation, and cognitive impairment, as well as potential abuse.

Chronic Extrapyramidal Symptoms (Tardive Dyskinesia and Related Syndromes)

Tardive dyskinesia is a potentially irreversible abnormal involuntary movement disorder. It begins either while the patient is receiving an antipsychotic drug or within a few weeks of discontinuing it. Among the predictors of tardive dyskinesia are older age, a history of EPS, substance abuse, duration of antipsychotic exposure, and possibly antipsychotic dosage (Casey 1999; Miller et al. 2005).

Tardive dyskinesia has been observed with all antipsychotic drugs except clozapine. Given that acute EPS represent a risk factor for later development of tardive dyskinesia, and in light of the relatively lower liability of SGAs to cause EPS, it is reasonable to expect that SGAs should cause less tardive dyskinesia than FGAs, at least as compared with high-potency FGAs. In a recent meta-analysis of 12 trials, the incidence and the prevalence of tardive dyskinesia were significantly lower for SGAs than for FGAs (Correll and Schenk 2008). However, note that the incidence of tardive dyskinesia might differ among the antipsychotics and even within the group of SGAs; the nature of the D_2 blockage may have an influence. Carefully designed, long-term, prospective comparison studies are needed to clarify the relative risks of tardive dyskinesia among the available antipsychotic drugs, although all evidence available to date speaks to a clear advantage of SGAs over FGAs.

Management of tardive dyskinesia begins with monitoring (Table 8–6). Clinicians should evaluate for signs of tardive dyskinesia before beginning antipsychotic treatment and every 3 months during treatment (Lehman et al. 2004). If dyskinetic movements appear, a neurological evaluation should be

Table 8–6. Strategies for management of tardive dyskinesia

Monitor involuntary movements; prophylaxis is the most effective option.

Change antipsychotic medication to second-generation antipsychotic (preferably clozapine).

Try supplementing with vitamin E (insufficient evidence).

considered to exclude other etiologies. If tardive dyskinesia develops in the context of FGA treatment, clinicians may consider lowering the dosage or switching to an SGA. Switching to an SGA soon after tardive dyskinesia develops may be advisable because the possibility of tardive dyskinesia reversibility declines with sustained exposure to the offending FGA. Although most SGAs have been observed to reverse FGA-induced tardive dyskinesia, clozapine is the best supported of these, with reported efficacy against tardive dyskinesia (Casey 1999). Although many other adjunctive agents have been evaluated for their potential therapeutic effects on tardive dyskinesia, evidence is insufficient to support a recommendation for the use of any specific agent to treat tardive dyskinesia (Buchanan et al. 2010).

Neuroleptic Malignant Syndrome

Neuroleptic malignant syndrome (NMS) is a potentially life-threatening complication of antipsychotic use and is characterized by the triad of rigidity, hyperthermia, and autonomic instability. NMS has been attributed to blockade of D_2 receptors in the hypothalamus and striatum, but the pathophysiology remains unclear (Haddad and Sharma 2007).

NMS is relatively rare, occurring in fewer than 1% of patients taking FGAs (Caroff et al. 1998). The relative risk of NMS among SGAs is likely to be even lower, but conclusive data are not yet available. Proposed risk factors include a prior episode of NMS, younger age, male gender, acute agitation, physical illness, dehydration, use of high-potency antipsychotics, rapid dosage titration, use of intramuscular preparations, and preexisting neurological disability (Lehman et al. 2004).

If NMS occurs, antipsychotic treatment should be terminated immediately, and the patient needs intensive care management with monitoring of vital signs (Falkai et al. 2006). Small studies suggest that dantrolene and dopaminergic agonists such as bromocriptine and amantadine may decrease NMS-associated mortality, compared with supportive treatment alone (Caroff et al. 1998). Electroconvulsive therapy also has been reported to be effective in treatment-refractory NMS, but it should be used with caution given the occurrence of several cases of cardiac arrhythmia (Caroff et al. 1998). After several weeks of recovery, an antipsychotic agent may be gradually reintroduced. An SGA or lower-potency FGA should be selected, and the dosage should be titrated slowly while observing for signs of NMS recurrence (Lehman et al. 2004).

Endocrine and Sexual Effects

All FGAs can elevate serum prolactin levels by the tonic blockade of pituitary D_2 receptors on lactotrophic cells (Hummer and Huber 2004). Among SGAs, amisulpride and risperidone can increase serum prolactin levels to an extent comparable to that of FGAs (Grunder et al. 1999; Haddad and Wieck 2004; Yasui-Furukori et al. 2002). In contrast, clozapine and quetiapine do not elevate serum prolactin levels across their full dosage range, and olanzapine causes hyperprolactinemia only at high dosages (Haddad and Wieck 2004; Turrone et al. 2002; Worrel et al. 2000). Ziprasidone is uncommonly associated with prolactin elevation. Aripiprazole can lower prolactin levels even below the antipsychotic-free baseline (Correll and Carlson 2006). Paliperidone appears to be as likely to elevate prolactin levels as risperidone in a dose-dependent manner (Kane et al. 2007; Marder et al. 2007). Asenapine's effect on prolactin is similar to that observed with olanzapine (Citrome 2009b). Iloperidone decreased prolactin levels in the pooled analysis of the three 6-week trials (Weiden et al. 2008). Although some patients develop partial tolerance to the pituitary effect of antipsychotics after several weeks, most have chronic serum prolactin elevation so long as antipsychotic treatment is continued (Haddad and Wieck 2004).

Women experience, on average, significantly greater elevation in prolactin than do men during long-term treatment with the same antipsychotic dosage (Haddad and Wieck 2004). Hyperprolactinemia may manifest differently in men and women, and individuals vary greatly as to the serum prolactin level at which symptoms appear (Haddad and Wieck 2004). In women, prolactin elevation not uncommonly leads to menstrual disturbances. Women also may experience decreased libido, impaired arousal, anorgasmia, and increased long-term risk of osteoporosis. Approximately 20% of women develop galactorrhea during treatment with an FGA (Windgassen et al. 1996), and one large retrospective study found dopamine antagonist use to be associated with a small increase in the risk of breast cancer (Wang et al. 2002). The major effects of hyperprolactinemia in men are loss of libido, hypospermatogenesis, erectile or ejaculatory deficits, and occasionally galactorrhea or gynecomastia.

Clinicians should assess for clinical signs and symptoms of hyperprolactinemia prior to and during treatment with antipsychotics (Marder et al. 2004). Presence of symptomatic hyperprolactinemia should trigger consideration of dosage reduction, switch to a lower-risk antipsychotic, or cotreatment with a full or partial dopamine agonist, although these medications carry a small risk of psychotic relapse (Correll 2007).

Glucose and Lipid Metabolism

Weight gain is a serious adverse event for patients taking antipsychotics, particularly with some SGAs (see Table 8–2). It has increasingly been a focus of research because of its significant influence on medication adherence and possible long-term physical complications, such as obesity, type 2 diabetes mellitus, metabolic syndromes, sleep apnea, and cardiovascular disease (Marder et al. 2004). Approximately half of all schizophrenic patients meet criteria for obesity, representing a relative risk of nearly 2 when compared with the general population (Newcomer 2007). Genetic and lifestyle factors may contribute to obesity. First-episode patients appear to be especially prone to gain weight (Fraguas et al. 2008; Kahn et al. 2008).

Up to 40% of patients taking FGAs can gain weight, with low-potency agents posing the greatest risk (Lehman et al. 2004). Marked differences in the liability for weight gain also have been discovered among SGAs (see Table 8–2). The most recent meta-analysis found that most SGAs (amisulpride, clozapine, olanzapine, quetiapine, risperidone, sertindole, and zotepine) induced more weight gain than did haloperidol in various degrees but not more than low-potency FGAs (Leucht et al. 2009). Aripiprazole and ziprasidone appear to be weight neutral (Leucht et al. 2009; Newcomer and Haupt 2006). Several short-term trials of paliperidone showed minimal weight gain (Fowler et al. 2008). Clinical trial data for iloperidone indicated a modest short- and long-term weight gain (Kane et al. 2008; Weiden et al. 2008). A short-term trial of asenapine showed that weight gain was comparable to that of placebo (Potkin et al. 2007).

The mechanisms of antipsychotic-induced weight gain have been hypothesized to involve changes in appetite and satiety mediated by histamine type 1 (H_1) and/or serotonin type 2C (5-HT_{2C}) receptor antagonism (Newcomer 2007). Antipsychotic dosage, at least within the therapeutic dosage range, does not have a significant effect on weight gain (Haddad and Sharma 2007).

Expert consensus guidelines recommend frequent monitoring of body mass index (BMI) for every patient with schizophrenia (American Diabetes Association et al. 2004; Marder et al. 2004) (Table 8–7). Most experts agree that the relative weight gain potential of the various antipsychotics must be considered in medication selection (Marder et al. 2004), and some have advocated avoiding the SGAs with the greatest weight gain propensity as first-line treatment (Sernyak 2007). Various pharmacological and nonpharmacological interventions to reduce body weight have been proposed and studied (Tschoner et al. 2007), and although the evidence concerning their success is modest, clinicians should encourage patients to participate in weight loss efforts that include dietary measures and exercise.

The prevalence of type 2 diabetes mellitus is twice as high among schizophrenia patients as in the general population (Dixon et al. 2000). The risk for type 2 diabetes mellitus is highest for clozapine and olanzapine, intermediate with quetiapine and risperidone, and lowest for aripiprazole and ziprasidone (American Diabetes Association et al. 2004; Newcomer and Haupt 2006). Several short- and long-term studies of paliperidone reported no clinically meaningful change in glucidic profiles (Fowler et al. 2008). Iloperidone produced only slight increases in blood glucose levels (Kane et al. 2008; Weiden et al. 2008). Asenapine showed limited effects on glucose-related laboratory parameters (Citrome 2009b). It is unclear whether the risk of type 2 diabetes mellitus with clozapine and olanzapine is entirely accounted for by the relatively greater increase in adiposity associated with these agents or whether an additional mechanism is partially responsible, such as a direct effect of the drugs on insulin-sensitive target tissues (Engl et al. 2005).

Expert consensus guidelines recommend measurement of baseline plasma glucose level before starting a new antipsychotic; a fasting glucose level is preferred, but a hemoglobin A_{1c} level is acceptable (Marder et al. 2004). Fasting plasma glucose or hemoglobin A_{1c} measurement should be repeated 3 to

Table 8–7. Strategies for management of antipsychotic-induced weight gain

Monitor repeatedly.

Incorporate psychoeducation.

Begin lifestyle intervention (exercise, modification of dietary habits).

Switch to another antipsychotic.

Use cognitive-behavioral treatment.

Add weight-reducing medication (e.g., sibutramine, metformin; limited evidence).

4 months after antipsychotic initiation, at least annually thereafter, and whenever a patient endorses symptoms of new-onset diabetes (American Diabetes Association et al. 2004; Marder et al. 2004).

Elevated lipid levels, particularly low-density lipoprotein (LDL) and triglyceride levels, are associated with cardiovascular diseases. Clozapine and olanzapine increase total cholesterol, LDL, and triglyceride levels significantly, as compared with FGAs and other SGAs (American Diabetes Association et al. 2004; J.A. Lieberman et al. 2005; Marder et al. 2004; McEvoy et al. 2006; Newcomer and Haupt 2006). Quetiapine and risperidone appear to raise cholesterol levels modestly, whereas aripiprazole, asenapine, iloperidone, paliperidone, and ziprasidone appear to be cholesterol neutral (American Diabetes Association et al. 2004; Citrome 2009c; Fowler et al. 2008; Tschoner et al. 2009).

Lipid levels should be assessed at treatment initiation and monitored more frequently than in the general population. If lipid abnormalities are present, clinicians should refer the patient to a specialist or primary care provider. If this is not possible, the patient should be advised to reduce dietary fat intake and to exercise. If this is unsuccessful, a switch to a lipid-neutral antipsychotic should be considered. Alternatively, a lipid-lowering drug can be prescribed (De Hert et al. 2006).

Cardiovascular Effects

Orthostatic hypotension occurs most frequently with low potency FGAs and clozapine, as a result of antagonism at α_1-adrenoceptors, but may be seen with other agents as well. It is most likely to occur early in treatment, particularly with rapid dosage titration (Haddad and Sharma 2007). Elderly individuals are more prone to this side effect, which may predispose to falls and related injuries. Gradual dosage titration often reduces its risk. Management strategies include reducing or dividing the medication dosage or switching to an antipsychotic with a lower α_1-adrenergic affinity (Miyamoto et al. 2008).

Sinus tachycardia can occur with any antipsychotic agent but is particularly common with clozapine (J.A. Lieberman 1998). It may result from the anticholinergic activity of antipsychotics or be secondary to orthostatic hypotension. In the absence of hypotension, tachycardia can be managed with low doses of a peripherally acting β-blocker (J.A. Lieberman 1998).

QTc prolongation, especially beyond 500 ms, is a serious cardiovascular adverse event because it increases the risk of torsades de pointes, a ventricular tachyarrhythmia that can lead to sudden death (Glassman and Bigger 2001). Women are more prone than men to develop QTc prolongation when taking antipsychotics (Haddad and Sharma 2007). Modest, dose-dependent QTc prolongation has been reported with many antipsychotics, but several FGAs (e.g., haloperidol, mesoridazine, pimozide, thioridazine) and SGAs (e.g., sertindole, ziprasidone) can increase the QTc interval considerably, and all of these have been associated with cases of fatal or potentially fatal arrhythmias (Glassman and Bigger 2001; Yap and Camm 2000). Aripiprazole, fluphenazine, and chlorpromazine do not appreciably prolong the QTc interval (Buchanan et al. 2010). A recent large retrospective cohort study reported that current users of FGAs and of SGAs had a similar dose-related increased risk of sudden cardiac death (Ray et al. 2009). Although ziprasidone increases the QTc interval, torsades de pointes has been reported only once (Heinrich et al. 2006).

Two large-scale Phase IV studies have been conducted with sertindole (Thomas et al. 2010) and ziprasidone (Strom et al. 2010). Although the latter study found no increased risk for non-suicide-related mortality in patients taking ziprasidone compared with olanzapine, patients taking sertindole were at higher risk for cardiac mortality than a control group taking risperidone.

Expert consensus guidelines recommend that mesoridazine, pimozide, and thioridazine should not be prescribed to patients with known heart disease, a personal history of syncope, a family history of sudden death before age 40 years, or congenital long QT syndrome (Marder et al. 2004). A baseline electrocardiogram (ECG) is appropriate prior to treatment with other QTc-prolonging antipsychotics (e.g., sertindole) in patients with any of the afore-mentioned risk factors, in elderly patients, and in those who are taking other drugs known to prolong the QTc interval (Glassman and Bigger 2001; Marder et al. 2004). It is mandatory to obtain baseline ECGs and to monitor ECGs in patients taking sertindole. The risk of QTc prolongation may be decreased by correcting hypokalemia and hypomagnesemia and by minimizing concomitant exposure to other QTc-prolonging drugs.

Other possible cardiovascular adverse events induced by antipsychotics are myocarditis and cardiomyopathy (Miyamoto et al. 2008). Clozapine is probably the most cardiotoxic SGA; however, its risk of potentially fatal myocarditis or cardiomyopathy is relatively low (0.015%–0.188%) (Merrill et al. 2005). Only a few case reports are available regarding associations between other SGAs (e.g., amisulpride, quetiapine, olanzapine, and risperidone) and cardiotoxicity (Krebs et al. 2006).

Gastrointestinal Effects

The gastrointestinal anticholinergic effects of antipsychotic medications include xerostomia (dry mouth) and constipation. These effects are relatively commonly encountered with clozapine and low-potency FGAs and less often with olanzapine and quetiapine (Lehman et al. 2004). They are frequently dose-related and thus may improve with antipsychotic dosage reduction. Constipation usually can be treated with stool softeners and laxatives. In rare instances, paralytic ileus occurs, in which case antipsychotic medication should be discontinued and medical or surgical consultation sought promptly. Clozapine also may cause sialorrhea (excess salivation).

Hepatic Effects

Asymptomatic elevations of liver enzyme levels occur with both FGAs and SGAs, usually during the first 3 months of treatment (Burns 2001). These abnormalities may be present in more than 20% of the patients receiving some antipsychotics, although they are often transient (Rettenbacher et al. 2006). The relative liabilities of individual agents have yet to be elucidated.

More severe antipsychotic-induced hepatic effects are infrequent. Approximately 0.1%–0.5% of the patients taking chlorpromazine develop cholestatic jaundice, and some of these cases progress to cirrhosis (Lehman et al. 2004). Occasionally, symptomatic hepatotoxicity (cholestatic or hepatitic) may be associated with SGAs (Burns 2001). If elevated liver transaminase levels persist, a hepatologist should be consulted. Should this not be possible, switching to a different antipsychotic is probably advisable. Patients taking an antipsychotic who develop nausea, abdominal pain, and jaundice should have their liver function evaluated to exclude hepatotoxicity. Because antipsychotic-induced jaundice is rare, other etiologies should be ruled out before antipsychotic medication is judged to be the cause.

Hematological Effects

Antipsychotic medications may cause blood dyscrasias, including leukopenia, neutropenia, agranulocytosis, and eosinophilia. Many of these effects have been found to be transient phenomena, so blood counts should be reevaluated before considering consequences (Hummer et al. 1994). Clozapine-induced agranulocytosis (defined as an absolute neutrophil count $<500/\text{mm}^3$) is a potentially fatal side effect. Agranulocytosis is more than twice as frequent in Asians as in Caucasians, and its risk increases with age and is higher among women (Haddad and Sharma 2007). With the advent of mandatory systematic blood count monitoring, the reported rate of clozapine-induced agranulocytosis has fallen below 0.4% in the United States (Lehman et al. 2004). Fewer than 2% of these cases now result in mortality, in part because clozapine-induced agranulocytosis is usually reversible if clozapine is withdrawn immediately. If agranulocytosis does occur, clinicians should discontinue clozapine, monitor for signs of infection, and consider bone marrow aspiration; if granulopoiesis is deficient, protective isolation is advisable. Monitoring and treatment guidelines on the use of clozapine vary between countries but usually include weekly white blood cell monitoring during the first 16 weeks of treatment, the period of highest risk for agranulocytosis. FGAs and nonclozapine SGAs pose a significantly lower risk of agranulocytosis, although cases have been reported, some involving patients with a history of this adverse event during previous clozapine exposure (Ruhe et al. 2001).

Other Side Effects

Sedation can occur with virtually any antipsychotic, but clozapine, quetiapine, and zotepine are more sedating, like low-potency FGAs (Leucht et al. 2009). Sedation is typically most pronounced when initiating medication, and most patients develop some tolerance with continued administration. The sedation that accompanies antipsychotic initiation may be beneficial in agitated patients, but persistent sedation can be associated with a decrease in functioning, impaired cognition, and treatment nonadherence. Sedation can sometimes be mitigated by lowering the antipsychotic dosage, by consolidating divided doses into a single evening dose, or by switching to a less-sedating agent.

Antipsychotic medications, particularly clozapine, zotepine, and low-potency FGAs, can lower the seizure threshold in a dose-dependent fashion (Lehman et al. 2004). Because the seizure rate rises with rapid dosage increases, antipsychotics should be titrated gradually.

Conclusion

Although SGAs and TGAs have some advantages over FGAs with regard to a broader spectrum of efficacy and a lower liability for inducing EPS and tardive dyskinesia (Leucht et al. 2009), these drugs have not fulfilled the high initial expectations after their introduction into clinical practice. Thus, medication regimens must be carefully tailored to the needs or preferences of individual patients, although more research is required to establish reliable predictors of antipsychotic response that may be applied to the individual. Until such data are available, we should make every effort to select the regimen with the highest benefit-risk balance in association with psychosocial interventions to improve patients' QOL and long-term outcome.

References

Addington D, Addington J, Patten S, et al: Double-blind, placebo-controlled comparison of the efficacy of sertraline as treatment for a major depressive episode in patients with remitted schizophrenia. J Clin Psychopharmacol 22:20–25, 2002

Aleman A, Hijman R, de Haan EH, et al: Memory impairment in schizophrenia: a meta-analysis. Am J Psychiatry 156:1358–1366, 1999

Allen MH, Currier GW, Hughes DH, et al: The Expert Consensus Guideline Series. Treatment of behavioral emergencies. Postgrad Med (Spec No):1–90, 2001

Alvarez-Jimenez M, Parker AG, Hetrick SE, et al: Preventing the second episode: a systematic review and meta-analysis of psychosocial and pharmacological trials in first-episode psychosis. Schizophr Bull 37:619–630, 2011

American Diabetes Association, American Psychiatric Association, American Association of Clinical Endocrinologists, North American Association for the Study of Obesity: Consensus development conference on antipsychotic drugs and obesity and diabetes. Diabetes Care 27:596–601, 2004

Andrezina R, Josiassen RC, Marcus RN, et al: Intramuscular aripiprazole for the treatment of acute agitation in patients with schizophrenia or schizoaffective disorder: a double-blind, placebo-controlled comparison with intramuscular haloperidol. Psychopharmacology (Berl) 188:281–292, 2006

Biedermann F, Fleischhacker WW: Antipsychotics in the early stage of development. Curr Opin Psychiatry 22:326–330, 2009

Bodkin JA, Siris SG, Bermanzohn PC, et al: Double-blind, placebo-controlled, multicenter trial of selegiline augmentation of antipsychotic medication to treat negative symptoms in outpatients with schizophrenia. Am J Psychiatry 162:388–390, 2005

Boter H, Peuskens J, Libiger J, et al: Effectiveness of antipsychotics in first-episode schizophrenia and schizophreniform disorder on response and remission: an open randomized clinical trial (EUFEST). Schizophr Res 115:97–103, 2009

Breier A, Meehan K, Birkett M, et al: A double-blind, placebo-controlled dose-response comparison of intramuscular olanzapine and haloperidol in the treatment of acute agitation in schizophrenia. Arch Gen Psychiatry 59:441–448, 2002

Brook S, Lucey JV, Gunn KP: Intramuscular ziprasidone compared with intramuscular haloperidol in the treatment of acute psychosis. Ziprasidone I.M. Study Group. J Clin Psychiatry 61:933–941, 2000

Buchanan RW, Gold JM: Negative symptoms: diagnosis, treatment and prognosis. Int Clin Psychopharmacol 11 (suppl 2):3–11, 1996

Buchanan RW, Kreyenbuhl J, Kelly DL, et al: The 2009 schizophrenia PORT psychopharmacological treatment recommendations and summary statements. Schizophr Bull 36:71–93, 2010

Buckley PF, Correll CU: Strategies for dosing and switching antipsychotics for optimal clinical management. J Clin Psychiatry 69 (suppl 1):4–17, 2008

Burns MJ: The pharmacology and toxicology of atypical antipsychotic agents. J Toxicol Clin Toxicol 39:1–14, 2001

Caroff SN, Mann SC, Keck PE Jr: Specific treatment of the neuroleptic malignant syndrome. Biol Psychiatry 44:378–381, 1998

Carpenter WT, Gold JM: Another view of therapy for cognition in schizophrenia. Biol Psychiatry 51:969–971, 2002

Casey DE: Neuroleptic-induced acute extrapyramidal syndromes and tardive dyskinesia. Psychiatr Clin North Am 16:589–610, 1993

Casey DE: Tardive dyskinesia and atypical antipsychotic drugs. Schizophr Res 35(suppl):S61–S66, 1999

Casey DE, Hirsch SR, Weinberger DR: Neuroleptic-induced extrapyramidal syndromes and tardive dyskinesia, in Schizophrenia. Edited by Hirsch SR, Weinberger DR. Oxford, UK, Blackwell, 1995, pp 546–565

Casey DE, Daniel DG, Tamminga C, et al: Divalproex ER combined with olanzapine or risperidone for treatment of acute exacerbations of schizophrenia. Neuropsychopharmacology 34:1330–1338, 2009

Citrome L: Adjunctive lithium and anticonvulsants for the treatment of schizophrenia: what is the evidence? Expert Rev Neurother 9:55–71, 2009a

Citrome L: Asenapine for schizophrenia and bipolar disorder: a review of the efficacy and safety profile for this newly approved sublingually absorbed second-generation antipsychotic. Int J Clin Pract 63:1762–1784, 2009b

Citrome L: Iloperidone for schizophrenia: a review of the efficacy and safety profile for this newly commercialised second-generation antipsychotic. Int J Clin Pract 63:1237–1248, 2009c

Correll CU: Balancing efficacy and safety in treatment with antipsychotics. CNS Spectr 12 (suppl 17):12–20, 35, 2007

Correll CU, Carlson HE: Endocrine and metabolic adverse effects of psychotropic medications in children and adolescents. J Am Acad Child Adolesc Psychiatry 45:771–791, 2006

Correll CU, Schenk EM: Tardive dyskinesia and new antipsychotics. Curr Opin Psychiatry 21:151–156, 2008

Correll CU, Rummel-Kluge C, Corves C, et al: Antipsychotic combinations vs monotherapy in schizophrenia: a meta-analysis of randomized controlled trials. Schizophr Bull 35:443–457, 2009

Crespo-Facorro B, Rodriguez-Sanchez JM, Perez-Iglesias R, et al: Neurocognitive effectiveness of haloperidol, risperidone, and olanzapine in first-episode psychosis: a randomized, controlled 1-year follow-up comparison. J Clin Psychiatry 70:717–729, 2009

Csernansky JG, Mahmoud R, Brenner R: A comparison of risperidone and haloperidol for the prevention of relapse in patients with schizophrenia. N Engl J Med 346:16–22, 2002

Davidson M, Galderisi S, Weiser M, et al: Cognitive effects of antipsychotic drugs in first-episode schizophrenia and schizophreniform disorder: a randomized, open-label clinical trial (EUFEST). Am J Psychiatry 166:675–682, 2009

Davis JM, Andriukaitis S: The natural course of schizophrenia and effective maintenance drug treatment. J Clin Psychopharmacol 6(suppl):2S–10S, 1986

Davis JM, Chen N: Dose response and dose equivalence of antipsychotics. J Clin Psychopharmacol 24:192–208, 2004

Davis JM, Chen N: Old versus new: weighing the evidence between the first- and second-generation antipsychotics. Eur Psychiatry 20:7–14, 2005

Davis JM, Chen N, Glick ID: A meta-analysis of the efficacy of second-generation
antipsychotics. Arch Gen Psychiatry 60:553–564, 2003

De Hert M, Kalnicka D, van Winkel R, et al: Treatment with rosuvastatin for severe
dyslipidemia in patients with schizophrenia and schizoaffective disorder. J Clin
Psychiatry 67:1889–1896, 2006

Dev V, Raniwalla J: Quetiapine: a review of its safety in the management of schizophrenia. Drug Saf 23:295–307, 2000

Dixon L, Weiden P, Delahanty J, et al: Prevalence and correlates of diabetes in national
schizophrenia samples. Schizophr Bull 26:903–912, 2000

Engl J, Laimer M, Niederwanger A, et al: Olanzapine impairs glycogen synthesis and
insulin signaling in L6 skeletal muscle cells. Mol Psychiatry 10:1089–1096, 2005

Evins AE, Amico E, Posever TA, et al: D-Cycloserine added to risperidone in patients
with primary negative symptoms of schizophrenia. Schizophr Res 56:19–23,
2002

Falkai P, Wobrock T, Lieberman J, et al: World Federation of Societies of Biological
Psychiatry (WFSBP) guidelines for biological treatment of schizophrenia, part 1:
acute treatment of schizophrenia. World J Biol Psychiatry 6:132–191, 2005

Falkai P, Wobrock T, Lieberman J, et al: World Federation of Societies of Biological
Psychiatry (WFSBP) guidelines for biological treatment of schizophrenia, part 2:
long-term treatment of schizophrenia. World J Biol Psychiatry 7:5–40, 2006

Fleischhacker WW: New developments in the pharmacotherapy of schizophrenia.
J Neural Transm Suppl 64:105–117, 2003

Fleischhacker WW: Second-generation antipsychotic long-acting injections: systematic review. Br J Psychiatry Suppl 195:S29–S36, 2009

Fleischhacker WW, Keet IP, Kahn RS: The European First Episode Schizophrenia Trial
(EUFEST): rationale and design of the trial. Schizophr Res 78:147–156, 2005

Fleischhacker WW, Heikkinen ME, Olie JP, et al: Effects of adjunctive treatment with
aripiprazole on body weight and clinical efficacy in schizophrenia patients treated
with clozapine: a randomized, double-blind, placebo-controlled trial. Int J Neuropsychopharmacol 13:1115–1125, 2010

Fowler JA, Bettinger TL, Argo TR: Paliperidone extended-release tablets for the acute
and maintenance treatment of schizophrenia. Clin Ther 30:231–248, 2008

Fraguas D, Merchan-Naranjo J, Laita P, et al: Metabolic and hormonal side effects in children and adolescents treated with second-generation antipsychotics. J Clin Psychiatry 69:1166–1175, 2008

Gasquet I, Haro JM, Novick D, et al: Pharmacological treatment and other predictors of treatment outcomes in previously untreated patients with schizophrenia: results from the European Schizophrenia Outpatient Health Outcomes (SOHO) study. Int Clin Psychopharmacol 20:199–205, 2005

Geddes J, Freemantle N, Harrison P, et al: Atypical antipsychotics in the treatment of schizophrenia: systematic overview and meta-regression analysis. BMJ 321:1371–1376, 2000

Glassman AH, Bigger JT Jr: Antipsychotic drugs: prolonged QTc interval, torsade de pointes, and sudden death. Am J Psychiatry 158:1774–1782, 2001

Glick ID, Bosch J, Casey DE: A double-blind randomized trial of mood stabilizer augmentation using lamotrigine and valproate for patients with schizophrenia who are stabilized and partially responsive. J Clin Psychopharmacol 29:267–271, 2009

Goff DC, Midha KK, Sarid-Segal O, et al: A placebo-controlled trial of fluoxetine added to neuroleptic in patients with schizophrenia. Psychopharmacology (Berl) 117:417–423, 1995

Goff DC, Tsai G, Levitt J, et al: A placebo-controlled trial of D-cycloserine added to conventional neuroleptics in patients with schizophrenia. Arch Gen Psychiatry 56:21–27, 1999

Goff DC, Keefe R, Citrome L, et al: Lamotrigine as add-on therapy in schizophrenia: results of 2 placebo-controlled trials. J Clin Psychopharmacol 27:582–589, 2007

Gold S, Arndt S, Nopoulos P, et al: Longitudinal study of cognitive function in first-episode and recent-onset schizophrenia. Am J Psychiatry 156:1342–1348, 1999

Green AI, Lieberman JA, Hamer RM, et al: Olanzapine and haloperidol in first episode psychosis: two-year data. Schizophr Res 86:234–243, 2006

Green MF: What are the functional consequences of neurocognitive deficits in schizophrenia? Am J Psychiatry 153:321–330, 1996

Green MF, Braff DL: Translating the basic and clinical cognitive neuroscience of schizophrenia to drug development and clinical trials of antipsychotic medications. Biol Psychiatry 49:374–384, 2001

Green MF, Marder SR, Glynn SM, et al: The neurocognitive effects of low-dose haloperidol: a two-year comparison with risperidone. Biol Psychiatry 51:972–978, 2002

Grunder G, Wetzel H, Schlosser R, et al: Neuroendocrine response to antipsychotics: effects of drug type and gender. Biol Psychiatry 45:89–97, 1999

Haddad PM, Sharma SG: Adverse effects of atypical antipsychotics: differential risk and clinical implications. CNS Drugs 21:911–936, 2007

Haddad PM, Wieck A: Antipsychotic-induced hyperprolactinaemia: mechanisms, clinical features and management. Drugs 64:2291–2314, 2004

Harvey PD, Keefe RS: Studies of cognitive change in patients with schizophrenia following novel antipsychotic treatment. Am J Psychiatry 158:176–184, 2001

Harvey PD, Howanitz E, Parrella M, et al: Symptoms, cognitive functioning, and adaptive skills in geriatric patients with lifelong schizophrenia: a comparison across treatment sites. Am J Psychiatry 155:1080–1086, 1998

Harvey PD, Silverman JM, Mohs RC, et al: Cognitive decline in late-life schizophrenia: a longitudinal study of geriatric chronically hospitalized patients. Biol Psychiatry 45:32–40, 1999

Hausmann A, Fleischhacker WW: Depression in patients with schizophrenia: prevalence, and diagnostic and treatment considerations. CNS Drugs 14:289–300, 2000

Hausmann A, Fleischhacker WW: Differential diagnosis of depressed mood in patients with schizophrenia: a diagnostic algorithm based on a review. Acta Psychiatr Scand 106:83–96, 2002

Heinrich TW, Biblo LA, Schneider J: Torsades de pointes associated with ziprasidone. Psychosomatics 47:264–268, 2006

Heresco-Levy U, Ermilov M, Lichtenberg P, et al: High-dose glycine added to olanzapine and risperidone for the treatment of schizophrenia. Biol Psychiatry 55:165–171, 2004

Hill SK, Bishop JR, Palumbo D, et al: Effect of second-generation antipsychotics on cognition: current issues and future challenges. Expert Rev Neurother 10:43–57, 2010

Hummer M, Huber J: Hyperprolactinaemia and antipsychotic therapy in schizophrenia. Curr Med Res Opin 20:189–197, 2004

Hummer M, Kurz M, Barnas C, et al: Clozapine-induced transient white blood count disorders. J Clin Psychiatry 55:429–432, 1994

Janicak PG, Davis JM: Antipsychotic dosing strategies in acute schizophrenia. Int Clin Psychopharmacol 11 (suppl 2):35–40, 1996

Javitt DC, Zylberman I, Zukin SR, et al: Amelioration of negative symptoms in schizophrenia by glycine. Am J Psychiatry 151:1234–1236, 1994

Jones PB, Barnes TR, Davies L, et al: Randomized controlled trial of the effect on Quality of Life of second- vs first-generation antipsychotic drugs in schizophrenia: Cost Utility of the Latest Antipsychotic Drugs in Schizophrenia Study (CUtLASS 1). Arch Gen Psychiatry 63:1079–1087, 2006

Jungerman T, Rabinowitz D, Klein E: Deprenyl augmentation for treating negative symptoms of schizophrenia: a double-blind, controlled study. J Clin Psychopharmacol 19:522–525, 1999

Kahn RS, Fleischhacker WW, Boter H, et al: Effectiveness of antipsychotic drugs in first-episode schizophrenia and schizophreniform disorder: an open randomised clinical trial. Lancet 371:1085–1097, 2008

Kane J[M], Honigfeld G, Singer J, et al: Clozapine for the treatment-resistant schizophrenic: a double-blind comparison with chlorpromazine. Arch Gen Psychiatry 45:789–796, 1988

Kane JM, Leucht S, Carpenter D, et al: Expert consensus guideline series. Optimizing pharmacologic treatment of psychotic disorders. Introduction: methods, commentary, and summary. J Clin Psychiatry 64 (suppl 12):5–19, 2003

Kane J[M], Canas F, Kramer M, et al: Treatment of schizophrenia with paliperidone extended-release tablets: a 6-week placebo-controlled trial. Schizophr Res 90:147–161, 2007

Kane JM, Lauriello J, Laska E, et al: Long-term efficacy and safety of iloperidone: results from 3 clinical trials for the treatment of schizophrenia. J Clin Psychopharmacol 28 (suppl 1):S29–S35, 2008

Kane JM, Fleischhacker WW, Hansen L, et al: Akathisia: an updated review focusing on second-generation antipsychotics. J Clin Psychiatry 70:627–643, 2009

Kapur S, Remington G, Jones C, et al: High levels of dopamine D2 receptor occupancy with low-dose haloperidol treatment: a PET study. Am J Psychiatry 153:948–950, 1996

Kapur S, Zipursky R, Jones C, et al: Relationship between dopamine D(2) occupancy, clinical response, and side effects: a double-blind PET study of first-episode schizophrenia. Am J Psychiatry 157:514–520, 2000

Kapur S, Arenovich T, Agid O, et al: Evidence for onset of antipsychotic effects within the first 24 hours of treatment. Am J Psychiatry 162:939–946, 2005

Keefe RS, Silva SG, Perkins DO, et al: The effects of atypical antipsychotic drugs on neurocognitive impairment in schizophrenia: a review and meta-analysis. Schizophr Bull 25:201–222, 1999

Keefe RS, Seidman LJ, Christensen BK, et al: Comparative effect of atypical and conventional antipsychotic drugs on neurocognition in first-episode psychosis: a randomized, double-blind trial of olanzapine versus low doses of haloperidol. Am J Psychiatry 161:985–995, 2004

Keefe RS, Seidman LJ, Christensen BK, et al: Long-term neurocognitive effects of olanzapine or low-dose haloperidol in first-episode psychosis. Biol Psychiatry 59:97–105, 2006a

Keefe RS, Young CA, Rock SL, et al: One-year double-blind study of the neurocognitive efficacy of olanzapine, risperidone, and haloperidol in schizophrenia. Schizophr Res 81:1–15, 2006b

Keefe RS, Bilder RM, Davis SM, et al: Neurocognitive effects of antipsychotic medications in patients with chronic schizophrenia in the CATIE Trial. Arch Gen Psychiatry 64:633–647, 2007a

Keefe RS, Sweeney JA, Gu H, et al: Effects of olanzapine, quetiapine, and risperidone on neurocognitive function in early psychosis: a randomized, double-blind 52-week comparison. Am J Psychiatry 164:1061–1071, 2007b

Kinon BJ, Volavka J, Stauffer V, et al: Standard and higher dose of olanzapine in patients with schizophrenia or schizoaffective disorder: a randomized, double-blind, fixed-dose study. J Clin Psychopharmacol 28:392–400, 2008

Krebs M, Leopold K, Hinzpeter A, et al: Current schizophrenia drugs: efficacy and side effects. Expert Opin Pharmacother 7:1005–1016, 2006

Lehman AF, Lieberman JA, Dixon LB, et al: Practice guideline for the treatment of patients with schizophrenia, second edition. Am J Psychiatry 161(suppl):1–56, 2004

Leucht S, McGrath J, White P, et al: Carbamazepine augmentation for schizophrenia: how good is the evidence? J Clin Psychiatry 63:218–224, 2002a

Leucht S, Pitschel-Walz G, Engel RR, et al: Amisulpride, an unusual "atypical" antipsychotic: a meta-analysis of randomized controlled trials. Am J Psychiatry 159:180–190, 2002b

Leucht S, Wahlbeck K, Hamann J, et al: New generation antipsychotics versus low-potency conventional antipsychotics: a systematic review and meta-analysis. Lancet 361:1581–1589, 2003

Leucht S, Kissling W, McGrath J. Lithium for schizophrenia revisited: a systematic review and meta-analysis of randomized controlled trials. J Clin Psychiatry 65:177–186, 2004

Leucht S, Kissling W, McGrath J: Lithium for schizophrenia. Cochrane Database of Systematic Reviews 2007, Issue 3. Art. No.: CD003834. DOI: 10.1002/14651858.CD003834.pub2.

Leucht S, Corves C, Arbter D, et al: Second-generation versus first-generation antipsychotic drugs for schizophrenia: a meta-analysis. Lancet 373:31–41, 2009

Lewis SW, Barnes TR, Davies L, et al: Randomized controlled trial of effect of prescription of clozapine versus other second-generation antipsychotic drugs in resistant schizophrenia. Schizophr Bull 32:715–723, 2006

Liberman RP, Kopelowicz A: Basic elements in biobehavioral treatment and rehabilitation of schizophrenia. Int Clin Psychopharmacol 9 (suppl 5):51–58, 1995

Lieberman JA: Maximizing clozapine therapy: managing side effects. J Clin Psychiatry 59 (suppl 3):38–43, 1998

Lieberman JA: Is schizophrenia a neurodegenerative disorder? A clinical and pathophysiological perspective. Biol Psychiatry 46:729–739, 1999

Lieberman JA, Stroup TS, McEvoy JP, et al: Effectiveness of antipsychotic drugs in patients with chronic schizophrenia. N Engl J Med 353:1209–1223, 2005

Luchins DJ: Carbamazepine in violent non-epileptic schizophrenics. Psychopharmacol Bull 20:569–571, 1984

Marchesi GF, Santone G, Cotani P, et al: The therapeutic role of naltrexone in negative symptom schizophrenia. Prog Neuropsychopharmacol Biol Psychiatry 19:1239–1249, 1995

Marder SR: Pharmacological treatment strategies in acute schizophrenia. Int Clin Psychopharmacol 11 (suppl 2):29–34, 1996

Marder SR: Antipsychotic drugs, in Psychiatry. Edited by Tasman A, Kay J, Lieberman JA. Philadelphia, PA, WB Saunders, 1997, pp 1569–1585

Marder SR, Essock SM, Miller AL, et al: Physical health monitoring of patients with schizophrenia. Am J Psychiatry 161:1334–1349, 2004

Marder SR, Kramer M, Ford L, et al: Efficacy and safety of paliperidone extended-release tablets: results of a 6-week, randomized, placebo-controlled study. Biol Psychiatry 62:1363–1370, 2007

McEvoy JP, Lieberman JA, Stroup TS, et al: Effectiveness of clozapine versus olanzapine, quetiapine, and risperidone in patients with chronic schizophrenia who did not respond to prior atypical antipsychotic treatment. Am J Psychiatry 163:600–610, 2006

Meltzer HY: Suicide in schizophrenia: risk factors and clozapine treatment. J Clin Psychiatry 59 (suppl 3):15–20, 1998

Meltzer HY, Bobo WV, Roy A, et al: A randomized, double-blind comparison of clozapine and high-dose olanzapine in treatment-resistant patients with schizophrenia. J Clin Psychiatry 69:274–285, 2008

Merrill DB, Dec GW, Goff DC: Adverse cardiac effects associated with clozapine. J Clin Psychopharmacol 25:32–41, 2005

Miller CH, Fleischhacker WW: Managing antipsychotic-induced acute and chronic akathisia. Drug Saf 22:73–81, 2000

Miller DD, McEvoy JP, Davis SM, et al: Clinical correlates of tardive dyskinesia in schizophrenia: baseline data from the CATIE schizophrenia trial. Schizophr Res 80:33–43, 2005

Mishara AL, Goldberg TE: A meta-analysis and critical review of the effects of conventional neuroleptic treatment on cognition in schizophrenia: opening a closed book. Biol Psychiatry 55:1013–1022, 2004

Miyamoto S, Lieberman JA, Fleischhacker WW, et al: Antipsychotic drugs, in Psychiatry, 2nd Edition, Vol 2. Edited by Tasman A, Kay J, Lieberman JA. Chichester, UK, Wiley, 2003a, pp 1928–1964

Miyamoto S, Stroup TS, Duncan GE, et al: Acute pharmacologic treatment of schizophrenia, in Schizophrenia, 2nd Edition. Edited by Hirsch SR, Weinberger DR. Oxford, UK, Blackwell Science, 2003b, pp 442–473

Miyamoto S, Merrill DB, Lieberman JA, et al: Antipsychotic drugs, in Psychiatry, 3rd Edition. Edited by Tasman A, Maj M, First MB, et al. Chichester, UK, Wiley, 2008, pp 2161–2201

Miyamoto S, Fleischhacker WW, Lieberman JA: Pharmacologic treatment of schizophrenia, in Comprehensive Care of Schizophrenia, 2nd Edition. Edited by Murray R, Lieberman JA. New York, Oxford University Press (in press)

Möller HJ: Neuroleptic treatment of negative symptoms in schizophrenic patients: efficacy problems and methodological difficulties. Eur Neuropsychopharmacol 3:1–11, 1993

Moore TA, Buchanan RW, Buckley PF, et al: The Texas Medication Algorithm Project antipsychotic algorithm for schizophrenia: 2006 update. J Clin Psychiatry 68:1751–1762, 2007

Mulholland C, Lynch G, King DJ, et al: A double-blind, placebo-controlled trial of sertraline for depressive symptoms in patients with stable, chronic schizophrenia. J Psychopharmacol 17:107–112, 2003

Murphy BP, Chung YC, Park TW, et al: Pharmacological treatment of primary negative symptoms in schizophrenia: a systematic review. Schizophr Res 88:5–25, 2006

Newcomer JW: Antipsychotic medications: metabolic and cardiovascular risk. J Clin Psychiatry 68 (suppl 4):8–13, 2007

Newcomer JW, Haupt DW: The metabolic effects of antipsychotic medications. Can J Psychiatry 51:480–491, 2006

Okuma T, Yamashita I, Takahashi R, et al: A double-blind study of adjunctive carbamazepine versus placebo on excited states of schizophrenic and schizoaffective disorders. Acta Psychiatr Scand 80:250–259, 1989

Pandurangi AK, Dalkilic A: Polypharmacy with second-generation antipsychotics: a review of evidence. J Psychiatr Pract 14:345–367, 2008

Pani L: The need for individualised antipsychotic drug therapy in patients with schizophrenia. Eur Rev Med Pharmacol Sci 13:453–459, 2009

Pereira S, Fleischhacker W, Allen M: Management of behavioural emergencies. J Psychiatr Inten Care 2:71–83, 2006

Peuskens J: Risperidone in the treatment of patients with chronic schizophrenia: a multi-national, multi-centre, double-blind, parallel-group study versus haloperidol. Risperidone Study Group. Br J Psychiatry 166:712–726, 1995

Pollack S, Lieberman JA, Fleischhacker WW, et al: A comparison of European and American dosing regimens of schizophrenic patients on clozapine: efficacy and side effects. Psychopharmacol Bull 31:315–320, 1995

Potkin SG, Cohen M, Panagides J: Efficacy and tolerability of asenapine in acute schizophrenia: a placebo- and risperidone-controlled trial. J Clin Psychiatry 68:1492–1500, 2007

Purdon SE, Jones BD, Stip E, et al: Neuropsychological change in early phase schizophrenia during 12 months of treatment with olanzapine, risperidone, or haloperidol. The Canadian Collaborative Group for research in schizophrenia. Arch Gen Psychiatry 57:249–258, 2000

Ray WA, Chung CP, Murray KT, et al: Atypical antipsychotic drugs and the risk of sudden cardiac death. N Engl J Med 360:225–235, 2009

Rettenbacher MA, Baumgartner S, Eder-Ischia U, et al: Association between antipsychotic-induced elevation of liver enzymes and weight gain: a prospective study. J Clin Psychopharmacol 26:500–503, 2006

Robinson DG, Woerner MG, Delman HM, et al: Pharmacological treatments for first-episode schizophrenia. Schizophr Bull 31:705–722, 2005

Roesch-Ely D, Gohring K, Gruschka P, et al: Pergolide as adjuvant therapy to amisulpride in the treatment of negative and depressive symptoms in schizophrenia. Pharmacopsychiatry 39:115–116, 2006

Rosenheck RA, Leslie DL, Sindelar J, et al: Cost-effectiveness of second-generation antipsychotics and perphenazine in a randomized trial of treatment for chronic schizophrenia. Am J Psychiatry 163:2080–2089, 2006

Ruhe HG, Becker HE, Jessurun P, et al: Agranulocytosis and granulocytopenia associated with quetiapine. Acta Psychiatr Scand 104:311–313, 2001

Rummel C, Kissling W, Leucht S: Antidepressants as add-on treatment to antipsychotics for people with schizophrenia and pronounced negative symptoms: a systematic review of randomized trials. Schizophr Res 80:85–97, 2005

Schooler N, Rabinowitz J, Davidson M, et al: Risperidone and haloperidol in first-episode psychosis: a long-term randomized trial. Am J Psychiatry 162:947–953, 2005

Schwarz C, Volz A, Li C, et al: Valproate for schizophrenia. Cochrane Database of Systematic Reviews 2008, Issue 3. Art. No.: CD004028. DOI: 10.1002/14651858.CD004028.pub3.

Sepehry AA, Potvin S, Elie R, et al: Selective serotonin reuptake inhibitor (SSRI) add-on therapy for the negative symptoms of schizophrenia: a meta-analysis. J Clin Psychiatry 68:604–610, 2007

Sernyak MJ: Implementation of monitoring and management guidelines for second-generation antipsychotics. J Clin Psychiatry 68 (suppl 4):14–18, 2007

Siris SG: Adjunctive medication in the maintenance treatment of schizophrenia and its conceptual implications. Br J Psychiatry Suppl 22:66–78, 1993

Small JG, Hirsch SR, Arvanitis LA, et al: Quetiapine in patients with schizophrenia: a high- and low-dose double-blind comparison with placebo. Seroquel Study Group. Arch Gen Psychiatry 54:549–557, 1997

Spina E, Cavallaro R: The pharmacology and safety of paliperidone extended-release in the treatment of schizophrenia. Expert Opin Drug Saf 6:651–662, 2007

Strom BL, Eng SM, Faich G, et al: The Ziprasidone Observational Study of Cardiac Outcomes (ZODIAC): findings from a large simple trial of ziprasidone vs. olanzapine in real-world use among 18,154 patients with schizophrenia. Schizophr Res 117:311, 2010

Stroup TS, Lieberman JA, McEvoy JP, et al: Effectiveness of olanzapine, quetiapine, risperidone, and ziprasidone in patients with chronic schizophrenia following discontinuation of a previous atypical antipsychotic. Am J Psychiatry 163:611–622, 2006

Strous RD, Maayan R, Lapidus R, et al: Dehydroepiandrosterone augmentation in the management of negative, depressive, and anxiety symptoms in schizophrenia. Arch Gen Psychiatry 60:133–141, 2003

Swartz MS, Perkins DO, Stroup TS, et al: Effects of antipsychotic medications on psychosocial functioning in patients with chronic schizophrenia: findings from the NIMH CATIE study. Am J Psychiatry 164:428–436, 2007

Tandon R, Belmaker RH, Gattaz WF, et al: World Psychiatric Association Pharmacopsychiatry Section statement on comparative effectiveness of antipsychotics in the treatment of schizophrenia. Schizophr Res 100:20–38, 2008

Taylor DM, Smith L: Augmentation of clozapine with a second antipsychotic—a meta-analysis of randomized, placebo-controlled studies. Acta Psychiatr Scand 119:419–425, 2009

Thomas SH, Drici MD, Hall GC, et al: Safety of sertindole versus risperidone in schizophrenia: principal results of the sertindole cohort prospective study (SCoP). Acta Psychiatr Scand 122:345–355, 2010

Tiihonen J, Wahlbeck K, Kiviniemi V: The efficacy of lamotrigine in clozapine-resistant schizophrenia: a systematic review and meta-analysis. Schizophr Res 109:10–14, 2009

Tollefson GD: Cognitive function in schizophrenic patients. J Clin Psychiatry 57 (suppl 11):31–39, 1996

Tollefson GD, Sanger TM: Negative symptoms: a path analytic approach to a double-blind, placebo- and haloperidol-controlled clinical trial with olanzapine. Am J Psychiatry 154:466–474, 1997

Tranulis C, Skalli L, Lalonde P, et al: Benefits and risks of antipsychotic polypharmacy: an evidence-based review of the literature. Drug Saf 31:7–20, 2008

Tsai G, Lane HY, Yang P, et al: Glycine transporter I inhibitor, N-methylglycine (sarcosine), added to antipsychotics for the treatment of schizophrenia. Biol Psychiatry 55:452–456, 2004

Tschoner A, Engl J, Laimer M, et al: Metabolic side effects of antipsychotic medication. Int J Clin Pract 61:1356–1370, 2007

Tschoner A, Fleischhacker WW, Ebenbichler CF: Experimental antipsychotics and metabolic adverse effects—findings from clinical trials. Curr Opin Investig Drugs 10:1041–1048, 2009

Turrone P, Kapur S, Seeman MV, et al: Elevation of prolactin levels by atypical antipsychotics. Am J Psychiatry 159:133–135, 2002

Uchida H, Suzuki T, Takeuchi H, et al: Low dose vs standard dose of antipsychotics for relapse prevention in schizophrenia: meta-analysis. Schizophr Bull 37:788–799, 2011

Van Putten T, Marder SR, Mintz J, et al: Haloperidol plasma levels and clinical response: a therapeutic window relationship. Am J Psychiatry 149:500–505, 1992

Velligan DI, Miller AL: Cognitive dysfunction in schizophrenia and its importance to outcome: the place of atypical antipsychotics in treatment. J Clin Psychiatry 60 (suppl 23):25–28, 1999

Volavka J, Cooper T, Czobor P, et al: Haloperidol blood levels and clinical effects. Arch Gen Psychiatry 49:354–361, 1992

Volz A, Khorsand V, Gillies D, et al: Benzodiazepines for schizophrenia. Cochrane Database of Systematic Reviews 2007, Issue 1. Art. No.: CD006391. DOI: 10.1002/14651858.CD006391.

Wahlbeck K, Cheine MV, Gilbody S, et al: Efficacy of beta-blocker supplementation for schizophrenia: a systematic review of randomized trials. Schizophr Res 41:341–347, 2000

Wang PS, Walker AM, Tsuang MT, et al: Dopamine antagonists and the development of breast cancer. Arch Gen Psychiatry 59:1147–1154, 2002

Weiden PJ, Cutler AJ, Polymeropoulos MH, et al: Safety profile of iloperidone: a pooled analysis of 6-week acute-phase pivotal trials. J Clin Psychopharmacol 28 (suppl 1):S12–S19, 2008

Whitehead C, Moss S, Cardno A, et al: Antidepressants for the treatment of depression in people with schizophrenia: a systematic review. Psychol Med 33:589–599, 2003

Windgassen K, Wesselmann U, Schulze MH: Galactorrhea and hyperprolactinemia in schizophrenic patients on neuroleptics: frequency and etiology. Neuropsychobiology 33:142–146, 1996

Woodward ND, Purdon SE, Meltzer HY, et al: A meta-analysis of neuropsychological change to clozapine, olanzapine, quetiapine, and risperidone in schizophrenia. Int J Neuropsychopharmacol 8:457–472, 2005

Worrel JA, Marken PA, Beckman SE, et al: Atypical antipsychotic agents: a critical review. Am J Health Syst Pharm 57:238–255, 2000

Yap YG, Camm J: Risk of torsades de pointes with non-cardiac drugs: doctors need to be aware that many drugs can cause QT prolongation. BMJ 320:1158–1159, 2000

Yasui-Furukori N, Kondo T, Suzuki A, et al: Comparison of prolactin concentrations between haloperidol and risperidone treatments in the same female patients with schizophrenia. Psychopharmacology (Berl) 162:63–66, 2002

Zhang XY, Zhou DF, Zhang PY, et al: A double-blind, placebo-controlled trial of extract of Ginkgo biloba added to haloperidol in treatment-resistant patients with schizophrenia. J Clin Psychiatry 62:878–883, 2001

9

Treatment-Resistant Schizophrenia

Kazuyuki Nakagome, M.D., Ph.D.

Tamiko Mogami, Ph.D.

Although antipsychotic medications show effectiveness in reducing psychotic symptom severity, they are not equally effective in improving functional outcomes of patients with schizophrenia. They are relatively ineffective for alleviating negative symptoms and cognitive impairment, which are closely related to functional outcomes. Approximately 5%–25% of patients are considered unresponsive to medication and do not show clinically significant improvement of symptomatology, especially positive symptoms (Brenner et al. 1990). Similarly, approximately 5%–20% of patients are intolerant of therapeutic dosages of antipsychotic drugs because of extrapyramidal side effects (EPS), including akathisia, parkinsonism, and tardive dyskinesia (Meltzer 1992). However, these figures reflect the treatment outcome of first-generation antipsychotic drugs (FGAs). Although second generation antipsychotic drugs

(SGAs) were initially considered to be more efficacious than FGAs, clinicians became increasingly skeptical about this purported advantage, except in the case of the SGAs' lower risk of EPS (Meltzer 1992). Moreover, if treatment outcome is evaluated in broader domains that include negative symptoms, cognitive functioning, and functional outcome, the proportion of patients with treatment-resistant schizophrenia would be expected to increase.

Definition and Assessment

Defining treatment-resistant schizophrenia is a complicated undertaking, especially because refractoriness to treatment in schizophrenia is best viewed as a continuum rather than a discrete category. Treatment-resistant patients may be generally defined as patients who do not respond well enough to standard treatment (Table 9–1). Therefore, determining how we *expect* patients to benefit from standard treatment is critical. We must consider which outcome measures should be used for patient assessment and determine what threshold level should be used for the definition of treatment resistance.

In clinical settings, there has been a trend to broaden the treatment goal to include the concept of *recovery,* which encompasses symptom alleviation in addition to improvement in functional outcome and subjective well-being. By contrast, Andreasen et al. (2005) took a novel approach by proposing operational criteria for symptomatic *remission* in schizophrenia that were based on reaching and maintaining distinct thresholds of improvement, rather than on percentage improvement from a particular baseline. Andreasen and colleagues chose not to develop consensus criteria for recovery "because more research is needed on this topic." Cognitive deficits are known to be relatively unresponsive to medication treatment and to persist even with successful pharmacotherapy, and their association with symptomatology is still being actively investigated; thus, it may be premature to incorporate cognitive functioning and functional outcome in the definition of treatment-resistant schizophrenia. On the other hand, it seems impractical to consider as treatment resistant all patients who fail to meet the criteria for symptomatic remission defined by Andreasen et al. (2005), because that threshold appears too high in light of the finding of Helldin et al. (2006) that only about one-third of patients in their cohort fulfilled the criteria for remission. Interestingly, Helldin et al. (2006, 2007) reported that the patients who met criteria for symptomatic remission

Table 9–1.   Overview of treatment-resistant schizophrenia

• Treatment-resistant patients are defined as patients who do not respond well enough to standard treatment.

• Outcome measures should encompass not only symptom severity but also functional outcomes.

• Refractoriness to treatment is better viewed as a continuum than as a discrete category.

• When defining standard treatment protocols, one should be cautious about prematurely including psychosocial approaches whose clinical feasibility has not yet been well demonstrated.

• Patients who have intolerable side effects with pharmacological treatment also should be regarded as having treatment-resistant schizophrenia.

showed higher cognitive abilities and functional outcomes compared with those who did not, suggesting that the concept of remission has important implications for the treatment of schizophrenia.

Another issue pertains to whether psychosocial treatment should be included in standard treatment. Although the primary treatment modality for schizophrenia has been pharmacological since the 1950s, many patients did not show adequate improvements in occupational, social, or independent living skills. In the 1960s, behavioral interventions emerged, followed by psychoeducation and family intervention. More recently, psychosocial treatments have made progress, as evidenced by positive outcomes of social skills training (SST), cognitive-behavioral therapy (CBT), cognitive remediation, and vocational rehabilitation in areas such as symptom alleviation as well as broader psychosocial improvement. These psychosocial approaches are widely accepted and have been incorporated in comprehensive treatment programs for patients with schizophrenia along with pharmacological treatment. Should these approaches be considered as standard treatment or as optional methods for treating specific symptoms and improving functional outcome? Despite recent progress in this area, when one considers that psychosocial treatment generally requires well-trained clinicians with specific expertise, and that there are wide variations in the types of psychosocial treatment recommended in schizophrenia guidelines (Gaebel et al. 2005), at least in part because of cross-cultural differences, we may also be cautious about prematurely including, in the definition of standard treatment, psychosocial approaches with insufficient evidence of clinical feasibility.

Finally, we also should include those patients for whom pharmacological treatment is associated with intolerable side effects in the category of treatment-resistant schizophrenia, because they may be equally regarded as having a treatment-resistant form of illness.

Original Concept of Treatment Resistance (Kane et al. 1988) and Subsequent Revisions

In their 6-week double-blind, randomized study of 268 patients with treatment-resistant schizophrenia, Kane et al. (1988) found that 30% of the patients improved following treatment with clozapine, compared with 4% of those who received chlorpromazine. Kane et al. (1988) defined *treatment resistance* according to both historical criteria and severity criteria (Table 9–2). Since this seminal study, the core principles used in defining treatment resistance have not been changed, despite reductions in the threshold of dosage level, number of trials, and period of assessment, presumably in accordance with the movement toward earlier institution of clozapine (see Table 9–3).

Table 9–2. Kane et al. (1988) criteria for treatment-resistant schizophrenia

Historical criteria

1. At least three periods of treatment in the preceding 5 years with neuroleptic agents (from at least two different chemical classes) at dosages ≥1,000 mg/day of chlorpromazine for a period of 6 weeks, each without significant symptomatic relief

2. No period of good functioning within the preceding 5 years

Severity criteria

1. Total Brief Psychiatric Rating Scale (BPRS) score of at least 45 (18-item version) plus a minimum Clinical Global Impressions (CGI) Scale rating of 4 (moderately ill)

2. Item scores of at least 4 (moderate) on two of the following four BPRS items: conceptual disorganization, suspiciousness, hallucinatory behavior, and unusual thought content

Source. Adapted from Kane et al. 1988.

Table 9–3. Commonly used criteria for treatment-resistant schizophrenia

- Developed to determine a patient's eligibility for clozapine treatment
- Exclude patients with refractory symptoms who are not candidates for clozapine treatment
- Originally incorporated a narrow definition of eligibility but are now moving toward more relaxed definitions, with earlier institution of clozapine

It has been suggested that the onset of antipsychotic drug action is rapid and that responders and nonresponders can be identified as early as 2 weeks after beginning treatment (Leucht et al. 2007). Despite clozapine's great promise in treatment-resistant schizophrenia (Juarez-Reyes et al. 1995; Kane et al. 1988), use of this medication has been limited because of its unfamiliar side-effect profile, need for hematological monitoring, and substantial costs. These disadvantages have led to the use of stringent criteria to determine who is eligible for clozapine treatment.

Juarez-Reyes et al. (1995) examined the effects of using a less restrictive definition of treatment-resistant schizophrenia in determining patient eligibility for clozapine. Data abstracted from clinical records of a stratified random-cluster sample of 293 patients with schizophrenia served by the San Francisco, California, city and county mental health system during 1991 were used to estimate clozapine eligibility by applying the broadest defensible criteria (BDC) suggested by the medication package insert. These BDC were defined as follows:

1. A diagnosis of schizophrenia or schizoaffective disorder;
2. Age 16 years or older;
3. Two previous antipsychotic trials at a minimum dosage of 600 mg/day in chlorpromazine equivalents for at least 4 weeks *or* a documented diagnosis of tardive dyskinesia;
4. Severe illness, as indicated by an average yearly Global Assessment of Functioning (GAF) Scale score of less than 61; and
5. Absence of contraindications described in the package insert.

Patients with schizoaffective disorder were included in the sample because they were expected to benefit from antipsychotic medications. Medication dosage and duration criteria were changed to 600 mg/day in chlorpromazine equivalents for 4 weeks, as opposed to 1,000 mg/day in chlorpromazine equivalents for 6 weeks, as proposed by Kane et al. (1988). Moreover, two instead of three prior antipsychotic medication trials were required. As for the severity criteria, a 12-month GAF Scale score of less than 61, which indicates "moderate symptoms and/or moderate difficulty in social, occupational, or school functioning," was considered to correspond to "severe mental illness" in the U.S. Food and Drug Administration (FDA) requirements. Patients with tardive dyskinesia were considered eligible for clozapine regardless of medication trial history, because clozapine may help relieve tardive dyskinesia, which could prevent them from receiving adequate medication trials. Intolerance of antipsychotic medications was also incorporated in the definition of treatment-resistant schizophrenia.

Juarez-Reyes et al. (1995) found that when the BDC were used, 43% of the patients qualified for clozapine. By contrast, when the most stringent criteria—similar to those of Kane et al. (1988), which excluded patients with tardive dyskinesia and patients with schizoaffective disorder and required three previous medication trials of 6 weeks each—were applied, only 13% of the sample were eligible for clozapine.

From the viewpoint of clozapine eligibility, Essock et al. (1996) adopted criteria that fell somewhat between the criteria used by Kane et al. (1988) and the BDC in their single-day screening study of inpatients in Connecticut State psychiatric hospitals. Essock and colleagues included any patients with a current diagnosis of schizophrenia or schizoaffective disorder and required at least two adequate trials with different antipsychotic medications as the criteria for clozapine eligibility, which was similar to the BDC. However, similar to Kane et al. (1988), they defined an adequate trial as at least 6 weeks of treatment at a dosage of at least 1,000 mg/day in chlorpromazine equivalents. Essock et al. (1996) also considered patients who were intolerant of therapeutic dosages of antipsychotic medications because of side effects such as tardive dyskinesia or neuroleptic malignant syndrome as being eligible for clozapine treatment. They found that among the inpatients screened, 60% met the criteria for clozapine eligibility. Although no improvements in discharge rates were associated with clozapine treatment, once discharged, patients assigned to clozapine were less likely to be readmitted compared with patients assigned to usual care. Hence, Essock et al. (1996) concluded that clozapine might be more cost-effective than usual care for those patients who fulfilled the eligibility criteria.

Clozapine was approved in Japan in April 2009. A strict regimen of regular monitoring of blood cell counts, blood sugar levels, hemoglobin A_{1c}, and electrocardiogram is required to prevent serious side effects such as agranulocytosis, myocarditis, or diabetic acidosis. Psychiatrists and pharmacologists who administer clozapine must be registered with the Clozapine Patient Monitoring Service (CPMS) system. Clozapine can be used only at institutions where at least two registered psychiatrists and pharmacologists are present and where hematologists, cardiologists, and experts in diabetology are available for consultation whenever serious physical side effects occur. "Guidelines for Adequate Usage of Clozaril" ("Clozapine Committee" of the Japanese Society of Clinical Neuropsychopharmacology 2009) were formulated to guide selection of patients eligible for clozapine treatment (Table 9–4). The guidelines include criteria for both treatment nonresponse and treatment intolerance and address issues associated with polypharmacy, which is not unusual in clinical practice in Japan.

Because the criteria in Table 9–4 were developed to assess the eligibility of patients for clozapine treatment, they exclude patients with refractory symptoms who (for various reasons) are not candidates for clozapine treatment. Expanding the concept of treatment resistance would have significant clinical importance because it would open up additional treatment possibilities for those patients who currently do not optimally benefit from antipsychotic drugs and are unable to function well in the community.

Assessment of Clinical Domains Relevant to Treatment Resistance: Positive and Negative Symptoms, Behavior Problems, Cognitive Deficits, and Functional Outcomes

Considering the significance of expanding the concept of treatment resistance, assessment of patients with schizophrenia should optimally encompass a variety of aspects of the illness, including positive, negative, extrapyramidal, cognitive, affective, suicidality, behavioral, functional, and quality of life. These parameters are usually unconsciously integrated into the clinician's assessment. However, not all of these parameters can be assessed with standard rating scales with good validity, and interrelations among the parameters are not clarified. Moreover, scant data are available to determine the severity levels that imply treatment resistance.

Table 9–4.   Proposed criteria for clozapine treatment eligibility: "Clozapine Committee" of the Japanese Society of Clinical Neuropsychopharmacology

Criteria for poor treatment response

Failure to respond[c] to a sufficient term (≥4 weeks) of treatment with a sufficient dosage of at least two well-tolerated antipsychotics[a,b] (i.e., including at least one atypical antipsychotic [risperidone, perospirone, olanzapine, quetiapine, or aripiprazole]) at ≥600 mg/day chlorpromazine equivalents). Drug compliance should be carefully checked.

[a]In patients receiving concomitant atypical antipsychotics, the antipsychotics administered at the highest chlorpromazine equivalent dose among the others.

[b]Typical antipsychotics: a history of at least 1-year treatment.

[c]Fail to respond to treatment: patients have never been in a state equivalent to Global Assessment of Functioning (GAF) score of 41 points or higher.

Criteria for poor treatment tolerance

Failure to adequately respond to monotherapy with at least two atypical antipsychotics (including risperidone, perospirone, olanzapine, quetiapine, and aripiprazole) due to failure to increase the dose to a necessary level for any of the following reasons:

• Occurrence or worsening of moderate or more severe tardive dyskinesia,[a] tardive dystonia,[b] or other tardive extrapyramidal symptoms

• Occurrence of uncontrolled parkinsonian symptoms,[c] akathisia,[d] or acute dystonia[e]

[a]Drug-Induced Extrapyramidal Symptoms Scale (DIEPSS) with "dyskinesia" score of ≥3 points.

[b]Tardive extrapyramidal symptoms corresponding to DIEPSS "dystonia" score ≥3 points.

[c]Among four DIEPSS items ("gait," "bradykinesia," "muscle rigidity," and "tremor"), the score of an item ≥3 points or the scores of 2 or more items ≥2 points despite treatment with an antiparkinsonian drug at the highest of the usual dose range.

[d]DIEPSS "akathisia" score ≥3 points despite various treatments including an antiparkinsonian drug at the highest of the usual dose range.

[e]The patient is severely suffering due to frequent occurrence of acute dystonia that corresponds to DIEPSS dystonia ≥3 points despite various treatments including an antiparkinsonian drug at the highest of the usual dose range.

Source.   Adapted from Clozaril Package Insert (Novartis Pharma KK 2009) and from Inagaki A: "Treatment-resistant schizophrenia and its treatment," in *Treatment Strategies for Treatment-Refractory Psychiatric Disorders* ("Lumière" Series for Specialists of Clinical Psychiatry no. 15). Edited by Nakagome K. Tokyo, Japan, Nakayama Shoten Co., Ltd., 2010, pp. 14–33. Used with permission.

Several objective rating scales are available for monitoring positive and negative symptoms as well as EPS. They include the Brief Psychiatric Rating Scale (BPRS; Overall and Gorham 1962; Ventura et al. 1993) and the Positive and Negative Syndrome Scale (PANSS; Kay et al. 1987) for monitoring psychopathology and the Drug-Induced Extrapyramidal Symptoms Scales (DIEPSS; Inada 2009) and Abnormal Involuntary Movement Scale (AIMS; Guy 1976) for monitoring EPS. However, most of these scales are time-consuming to administer and are more frequently used in the research field than in clinical settings. The Clinical Global Impressions (CGI) Scale is another tool that is widely accepted for its ease of administration and established correspondence to PANSS total scores (Leucht et al. 2005; Levine et al. 2008) (Table 9–5).

To address functional outcome, which may well be involved in the concept of treatment-resistant schizophrenia, cognitive functioning should be assessed. A variety of neuropsychological test batteries are used for the measurement of cognitive functioning, leading to some difficulty in directly comparing findings across studies. One candidate for a globally standardized test battery to assess outcomes of cognitive changes in clinical trials is the Measurement and Treatment Research to Improve Cognition in Schizophrenia (MATRICS) Consensus Cognitive Battery (MCCB), developed by the U.S. National Institute of Mental Health (NIMH) and FDA. MCCB focuses on key cognitive domains relevant to schizophrenia and related disorders and takes approximately 70 minutes to administer. A less time-consuming test battery is the Brief Assessment of Cognition in Schizophrenia (BACS; Keefe et al. 2004), which takes only 30 minutes to administer, can much more feasibly be used in everyday clinical practice, and demonstrates sound reliability and validity. Unfortunately, BACS does not measure social cognition, which is another key determinant of functional outcome.

Although neuropsychological test batteries have been widely accepted for the assessment of cognitive functioning in psychiatric populations, a tool that can assess cognitive skills directly associated with a patient's daily functioning is also warranted. To address this need, interview-based measures of cognition, such as Clinical Global Impression of Cognition in Schizophrenia (Ventura et al. 2008) and Schizophrenia Cognition Rating Scale (Keefe et al. 2006), have been designed. These measures also may help avoid practical limitations associated with neuropsychological tests, including differences in the amount of prior training of the testers, administration and scoring time, prac-

Table 9–5.   Linkage of Clinical Global Impressions–Severity (CGI-S) Scale score and Positive and Negative Syndrome Scale (PANSS) total score

CGI-S	PANSS (Levine et al. 2008)	PANSS (Leucht et al. 2005)
Not ill	31–32	
Mild	55–62	58
Moderate	71–77	75
Marked	88–94	95
Severe	105–110	116
Extreme	126–134	—

tice effects, and validity issues associated with interpretation. These measures assess cognitive deficits and the degree to which they affect daily functioning by obtaining the patient's report, a caregiver's report, and a clinical evaluation of both sources of information by the clinician. Both measures fulfilled the criteria for psychometric property, including sound test-retest reliability, associations with cognitive performance measures, and associations with real-world functioning. It may require further studies to determine whether a combination of both neuropsychological tests and interview-based measures is necessary for the assessment of cognitive functioning or whether administering either of these measures is sufficient.

Several functional outcome measures have been used for the assessment of social and occupational functioning (Bryson et al. 1997; McGurk et al. 2003), activities of daily living, and ability to live independently (Buchanan et al. 2005; Matza et al. 2006). It has been pointed out that the measures do not tap into the cognitive abilities underlying these functions. For example, the Independent Living Scale was primarily designed to help clinicians make decisions regarding treatment choice (Loeb 1996) and not to evaluate the changes in cognitive deficits and functioning by intervention.

Functional outcome measures that are more sensitive to identifying changes in functioning and underlying cognitive abilities are now being introduced. The University of California, San Diego, Performance-Based Skills Assessment (UPSA) is a performance-based measure of the functional capacity, which was developed to assess the capacity of persons with schizophrenia

Table 9–6.   Assessment of treatment-resistant schizophrenia

- Patients with schizophrenia should be assessed on various aspects of the illness, particularly those related to functional outcome.

- Assessment tools with adequate feasibility and validity are needed for measuring cognitive skills and functional outcome.

- Interview-based measures that can assess cognitive skills directly associated with daily functioning may well be widely accepted in clinical settings.

- Use of functional outcome measures that are sensitive to changes in function and underlying cognitive abilities are warranted for assessing treatment response.

to adequately perform skills necessary for daily functioning (Patterson et al. 2001). The UPSA has shown high correlations with measures of cognitive function, activities of daily living, interpersonal skills, community activities, and level of independence in living (Bowie et al. 2006; Mausbach et al. 2008; Twamley et al. 2002). A short version, the UPSA-Brief, has been developed that requires only 10–15 minutes to administer (Mausbach et al. 2007). The UPSA-Brief was found to have adequate psychometric properties, predict residential independence, and be sensitive to the changes by intervention.

Some may argue that performance-based functional outcome measures do not fully capture the activities and level of real-life functioning in the community. An interview-based scale such as the Schizophrenia Outcomes Functioning Interview (SOFI) may address this concern by measuring community functioning related to cognitive impairment and psychopathology (Kleinman et al. 2008). The SOFI consists of two versions, one to be completed by the patient (SOFI-P) and the other to be completed by a caregiver informant (SOFI-I). The SOFI has demonstrated strong reliability and validity and is expected to be a useful measure of functional outcomes in schizophrenia. Further studies, particularly longitudinal research tracking the effects of interventions, are necessary to make definitive recommendations for interview-based measures that evaluate a broader range of functional domains (Table 9–6).

Standard Treatment for Schizophrenia

Standard Pharmacological Treatment

Determining what constitutes standard pharmacological treatment for schizophrenia is mandatory before defining the criteria for treatment resistance. It is critical to note that deterioration of psychiatric symptoms, cognitive abilities, and functioning may emerge secondary to inappropriate pharmacological interventions.

Several existing guidelines for schizophrenia share commonalities in their recommendations for pharmacological treatment. Compared with older FGAs, SGAs are considered to have a lower risk for EPS and to be more effective, as evidenced by a broader spectrum of efficacy—namely, negative, cognitive, and mood symptoms. As a result, many guidelines recommended the use of SGAs in preference to FGAs (Table 9–7). However, data from two large government-sponsored trials, Clinical Antipsychotic Trials of Intervention Effectiveness (CATIE) in schizophrenia and Cost Utility of the Latest Antipsychotic Drugs in Schizophrenia Study (CUtLASS), overturned the view that SGAs were vastly superior to FGAs (Jones et al. 2006; Lieberman et al. 2005). It should, however, be noted that both studies were criticized for their sampling methods and overall methodology, suggesting the need for caution in interpreting their findings (Naber and Lambert 2009).

To clarify the confusing findings, the World Psychiatric Association Pharmacopsychiatry Section reviewed literature on the comparative effectiveness of different antipsychotic treatments for schizophrenia (Tandon et al. 2008). The researchers concluded that SGAs and FGAs were similarly effective in terms of positive symptoms, but that SGAs were consistently more effective than FGAs in alleviating negative, cognitive, and depressive symptoms and had a lower risk for tardive dyskinesia. Although FGAs and SGAs appeared similar in their efficacy in treating psychotic symptoms, substantial differences were seen in terms of side effects. For instance, SGAs generally have a lower risk for EPS and a higher risk for metabolic side effects. In treating schizophrenia, it may be more clinically meaningful to focus on selecting drugs to minimize side effects in a customized manner rather than selecting drugs based on equivocal findings regarding superiority hypotheses for SGAs.

Because the subjects participating in the CUtLASS and CATIE studies were mostly chronically ill patients, great caution is warranted in extrapolating effectiveness findings from these studies to first-episode patients. Results of the European First Episode Schizophrenia Trial h ave recently been published (Kahn et al. 2008). This pragmatic open randomized controlled trial (RCT) was conducted at multiple sites and included 498 patients. The investigators examined the clinical effectiveness of SGAs and FGAs in a broad

Table 9–7.   Standard pharmacological treatment of schizophrenia

- Second-generation antipsychotics (SGAs) are generally recommended rather than first-generation antipsychotics (FGAs) for the treatment of first-episode schizophrenia.

- SGAs are more effective than FGAs in alleviating negative, cognitive, and depressive symptoms, whereas SGAs and FGAs are similarly effective in terms of positive symptoms.

- SGAs have a lower risk for extrapyramidal side effects and tardive dyskinesia but a higher risk for metabolic side effects.

- The dosage level should be expeditiously titrated to the target therapeutic dose (approximately 300–1,000 mg/day in chlorpromazine equivalents) while monitoring for intolerance.

- Nonadherence should be continuously monitored; patients with recurrent relapse as a result of nonadherence are candidates for depot medication.

range of patients in the early stages of schizophrenia. Most SGAs were found to be superior to haloperidol in low doses in terms of the proportion of patients who achieved treatment response and remission within 12 months. In addition, the discontinuation rate within 12 months was greater in the patients receiving haloperidol than in those receiving SGAs (Kahn et al. 2008). Although these findings may generally support the use of SGAs rather than FGAs for patients with first-episode schizophrenia, the history of sensitivity to side effects such as weight gain, hyperglycemia, or hyperlipidemia should be taken into consideration. Cost-effectiveness also should be weighed, because it varies according to the resources available in different countries.

Clinical guidelines for the treatment of schizophrenia in developed countries include those developed by the National Institute for Health and Clinical Excellence (2009) in England, the Texas Medication Algorithm Project (TMAP; Miller et al. 1999; Moore et al. 2007) and the American Psychiatric Association (Lehman et al. 2004) in the United States, and the Royal Australian and New Zealand College of Psychiatrists (RANZCP) Clinical Practice Guidelines Team for the Treatment of Schizophrenia and Related Disorders (2005) in Australia. All of these guidelines recommend SGAs rather than FGAs for the treatment of first-episode schizophrenia on the basis of the SGAs' better tolerability and reduced risk of tardive dyskinesia. It is important to select the antipsychotic drug and a dose level that is effective and unlikely to cause side effects that are subjectively distressful. Optimal antipsychotic dosage ranges recommended for first-episode patients are relatively lower than those recommended for patients with multiepisode illness, because first-episode patients are more sensitive to the therapeutic effects and medication side effects.

Determining the optimal dosage level for antipsychotic medication in the acute phase, regardless of whether in the first episode, is complicated because therapeutic response is usually delayed from the time of treatment initiation. It may take approximately 2–4 weeks before initial response can be seen and up to 6 months for full response to be observed. Therefore, the dosage level should be expeditiously titrated to the target therapeutic range (considered to be approximately 300–1,000 mg/day in chlorpromazine equivalents, depending on the patient's previous experience with antipsychotic medication), while monitoring for intolerance. Unless the patient has uncomfortable side effects, the patient's clinical status then should be monitored for 2–4 weeks before increasing the dose or changing medication. During these weeks, it is important for the clinician to avoid the temptation to prematurely elevate the dose of patients who may be showing improvement at only a limited rate.

If the patient shows no improvement, the clinician first must consider whether the lack of response can be explained by medication nonadherence. If nonadherence is the problem, then the patient's symptoms should not be considered treatment resistant, and behavioral tailoring (i.e., incorporating medication into daily routine), motivational interviewing, and other cognitive-behavioral techniques may be introduced to improve the patient's understanding of the potential benefits of medication (Kemp et al. 1998). Although many patients prefer oral medication, patients with recurrent relapses because of nonadherence are candidates for a long-acting injectable (depot) antipsychotic medication, which has the practical clinical advantage of avoiding covert nonadherence. Plasma concentration is clinically relevant when clozapine and haloperidol are used to confirm the adherence level. Depot preparations guarantee consistent drug delivery and overcome the bioavailability problems that occur with oral preparations. Despite these advantages, some patients may experience depot injection as controlling, limiting of their autonomy, and painful. Nevertheless, more than a few patients receiving depot medication prefer depot to oral medication because of the convenience (Heres et al. 2007; Walburn et al. 2001). If the patient is adhering to treatment but still is not responding to treatment within 2–4 weeks of attaining the target therapeutic dose, another medication—preferably one from a different chemical class—should be considered.

In the acute phase of schizophrenia, other psychoactive medications are commonly added to antipsychotic medications to treat comorbid conditions or associated symptoms such as agitation, aggression, affective symptoms, sleep disturbances, and drug side effects. For example, benzodiazepines are commonly used to manage anxiety and agitation. Mood stabilizers and β-blockers are considered effective in reducing the severity of hostility and aggression. Major depression and obsessive-compulsive disorder are common comorbid conditions in patients with schizophrenia and may respond to antidepressants. Sleep disturbances are also very common in the acute phase, and benzodiazepines and sedating antidepressants are reported to be helpful. The decision to use antiparkinsonian medications to treat EPS is driven by the severity and by whether other potential strategies are available, including reducing the dosage of the antipsychotic medication or switching to a different antipsychotic drug. The propensity of the antipsychotic drug to induce EPS, the patient's preferences, the patient's history of EPS, other risk factors for EPS, and potential consequences of anticholinergic side effects must be considered in the decision. Careful attention must be paid to potential drug interactions, especially those related to the cytochrome P450 enzymes, in using these adjunctive medications.

Standard Psychosocial Treatment

It seems reasonable to state that standard psychosocial treatments have not yet been established, gauging from variability among psychosocial treatments recommended in the guidelines. Some basic psychosocial approaches are available that are feasible and essential for the treatment of schizophrenia (Table 9–8). Schizophrenia should not be defined as treatment resistant until these approaches have been administered, even if the patient failed to attain an adequate level of functioning. We briefly refer to these approaches in this subsection.

Above all, establishing a good therapeutic alliance helps the patient to participate actively in treatment in partnership with the clinician. Identifying the patient's goals and relating them to treatment outcomes fosters the patient's motivation for treatment, which ultimately improves treatment adherence. The clinician also may identify factors that could hamper the patient's ability to participate in treatment, such as cognitive deficits, disorganization, lack of

Table 9–8. Standard psychosocial treatment of schizophrenia

- Basic psychosocial approaches should be appropriately administered before the patient is labeled treatment resistant due to suboptimal treatment response.

- Establishing and maintaining a good therapeutic alliance throughout the treatment course is essential for good outcomes.

- Psychoeducation, family intervention, and social skills training are recommended as standard psychosocial approaches, considering their feasibility and effectiveness across broad clinical domains.

insight, and inadequate social resources. Engagement of the family and other significant caregivers is recommended to further strengthen the patient's adherence to treatment. The social circumstances, including living situation, family involvement, relationships with significant others, and available social services, are all areas that may be periodically explored by clinicians. The psychiatrist should work with team members, the patient, and the family to ensure that such concerns are attended to.

At the very least, all patients with schizophrenia should receive education that provides reliable and accurate information about their illness. In mental health care, the delivery of information to clarify the goals of treatment and to help patients or their caregivers change their behavior, skills, and attitudes, with the aim of improving their cognitive, affective, and psychomotor processes, has been termed *psychoeducation.* Psychoeducation has been developed as an aspect of treatment in schizophrenia with a variety of goals beyond the provision of accurate information.

Another standard psychosocial approach is family intervention, which has several aims, including developing an alliance with caregivers, reducing emotional distress, creating or re-creating a positive home atmosphere, recovering a healthy family relationship, problem solving, maintaining realistic expectations of patient performance, and helping to set limits and appropriate relationship boundaries. Family interventions have evolved from studies of the family environment and its possible role in the course of schizophrenia (Bebbington and Kuipers 1994; Brown et al. 1962, 1972). Family interventions usually have three components: 1) alliance formation, 2) didactic instruction, and 3) more specialized family therapy, such as problem solving and crisis management. A given family's needs are assessed, followed by didactics on a range of topics, such as community resources; clinical features, treatment, and etiology of schizophrenia; and the family's role in promoting recovery. The intended goal is to prevent relapse when the treatment program is provided over 6 months or longer or for more than 10 sessions, especially when the patient is included in the sessions. Families, especially those with high expressed emotion, have been known to benefit from the approach, as indicated by reduced relapse rates. Favorable effects on patient employment and independent living skills also have been reported. Effects of the intervention on families have included lower burden of illness, increased knowledge, and decreased expressed emotion.

Social skills training (SST) was developed as a more sophisticated treatment strategy derived from behavioral and social learning traditions (Wallace et al. 1980), given the complex and debilitating behavioral and social effects of schizophrenia. SST was designed to help people with schizophrenia regain their social skills and confidence, improve their ability to cope in social situations, reduce social distress, improve their quality of life, and aid symptom reduction and relapse prevention.

SST has been thoroughly disseminated in many countries. For example, the modules of the UCLA Social and Independent Living Skills Program have been translated into 23 languages and are used on six continents (Kopelowicz et al. 2006). However, the review used for the National Institute for Health and Clinical Excellence (2009) guidelines found insufficient evidence to determine whether SST as a discrete intervention improved outcomes in schizophrenia. A Cochrane review also failed to find conclusive evidence of benefit (Tungpunkom and Nicol 2008). Nonetheless, the APA guidelines (Lehman et al. 2004) noted the benefit of SST in improving knowledge, social skills, and symptom and medication management when offered with adequate pharmacological treatments. More research is needed to determine whether patients transfer the skills learned in these programs to real-world settings. To enhance generalization of skills to everyday life, social skills training must be tailored to the patient's specific circumstances and integrated with other therapies and treatments, and must also seek to foster supportive relationships with nonprofessional helpers in the patient's environment (Kopelowicz et al. 2006).

Other effective psychosocial treatments, including CBT, supported employment, Assertive Community Treatment (ACT), and intensive case management, are available but may not be the best fit in certain settings because of impracticality and may not be considered standard treatment. Therefore, these treatments are best regarded as optional according to the patients' needs and social context.

Definitions of Treatment Resistance Beyond the Concept of Clozapine Eligibility

The appropriate definition of *treatment resistance* depends on the circumstances in which the definition is to be applied. For example, a narrow definition is suitable for research purposes relating to an antipsychotic drug for which the indication will be treatment-resistant schizophrenia, whereas a broader definition that incorporates assessment of psychosocial functioning, cognitive deficits, affective symptoms, and behavior problems may be appropriate for clinical practice (Table 9–9).

Narrower definitions primarily focused on suboptimal response of positive symptoms to medication treatment. Persistent psychotic symptomatology gained much interest, largely as a result of lack of valid outcome assessment or standard treatment in other domains such as psychosocial functioning, cognitive deficits, affective symptoms, and behavior problems. A trend in the field has been a movement away from the rigorous criteria of Kane et al. (1988) and toward a broader definition of treatment resistance from the viewpoint of expanding the group of patients who were considered to be clinically eligible for treatment with clozapine. For example, the historical criteria of Kane et al. (1988) required suboptimal response in at least three trials of antipsychotic medication at dosages equivalent to or greater than 1,000 mg/day in chlorpromazine equivalents in order to be categorized as treatment resistant; however, more recent guidelines suggest that two adequate trials at dosages equivalent to 300–1,000 mg/day of chlorpromazine are sufficient.

Additional domains to be used in the broader definition are particularly important for systems of care worldwide, with their growing emphasis on community-based treatment and recovery-oriented practice, although standard criteria for assessment of outcome measures are not yet available. As early as 1990, Brenner et al. clearly stated that "treatment refractoriness is defined as continuing psychotic symptoms with substantial functional disability and/or behavioral deviances that persist in well-diagnosed persons with schizophrenia despite reasonable and customary pharmacological and psychosocial treatment

Table 9–9.   Definitions of treatment resistance

- At least two definitions of treatment resistance are proposed: a narrow definition suitable for research purposes and a broader definition appropriate for clinical practice.

- Narrower definitions primarily focused on suboptimal response of positive symptoms to medication treatment.

- A broader definition includes not only medication effects but also psychosocial treatment effects and assessment of psychosocial functioning, cognitive deficits, affective symptoms, and behavior problems.

- A broader definition is appropriate for clinical practice, although standard criteria for assessment of outcome measures are not yet available.

- Both definitions of treatment resistance using a continuum and those using dichotomous cutoff thresholds are of practical use, according to the circumstances.

that has been provided continuously for an adequate time period" (pp. 552–553). Brenner and colleagues noted that it would be premature to label suboptimal response as treatment resistance before providing adequate exposure to well-administered psychosocial treatment. Moreover, they included functional disability and/or behavioral deviances as outcome measures in their definition of treatment resistance (Brenner et al. 1990). It was recognized that accuracy of the clinical history of a patient's exposure to adequate drug and psychosocial treatments might be limited because such information often relies on self-report. With all other complexities, such as the patient's adherence level and side effects that obviate use of appropriate dose levels, further screening for treatment responsiveness under a well-controlled trial may be required before the schizophrenia is categorized as treatment resistant.

The criteria proposed by Brenner et al. (1990) incorporated a construct reflecting a multidimensional continuum of treatment resistance–treatment response (Table 9–10). This method of depicting treatment resistance arose from the view that most patients with schizophrenia who are considered unresponsive to treatment are, in fact, suboptimal responders of various degrees. Meanwhile, dichotomous cutoff thresholds along the continuum also might be relevant in determining "treatment resistance" for referring patients to intensive treatment programs, including psychosocial and pharmacological interventions.

Table 9–10.   Global Rating Scale of Treatment Response and Resistance in Schizophrenia

Level 1—Clinical remission	Rapid and substantial response when antipsychotic medication given in recommended dosage, but the patient might manifest some anhedonic traits and other negative symptoms. CGI: normal, not mentally ill. Any of the BPRS psychotic scale items score ≤2. Able to function without supervision.
Level 2—Partial remission	Rapid reduction of schizophrenic symptoms with mild signs of residual psychotic symptomatology. CGI: score of 2=borderline mentally ill. None of the BPRS psychotic scale items score ≥3. Able to function with only occasional supervision in one domain of social and vocational activities.
Level 3—Slight resistance	Slow and incomplete symptom reduction and residual positive and negative symptoms have adverse effects on two or more areas of personal and social adjustment requiring occasional supervision. CGI: score of 3=mildly ill. Not more than one BPRS psychotic scale item score ≥4.
Level 4—Moderate resistance	Some symptom reduction, but persistent and obvious symptoms adversely affect four or more areas of personal and social adjustment requiring frequent supervision. CGI: score of 4=moderately ill. Two of the BPRS psychotic scale items scores=4. Total BPRS score is at least 45 on the 18-item version and at least 60 on the 24-item expanded BPRS.
Level 5—Severe resistance	Some symptom reduction, but persistent symptoms adversely affect six or more areas of personal and social adjustment requiring frequent supervision. CGI: score of 5=markedly ill. One BPRS psychotic scale item score =5, or at least three of the items =4. Total BPRS score of at least 50 on the 18-item version and at least 67 on the 24-item expanded version.

Table 9–10. Global Rating Scale of Treatment Response and Resistance in Schizophrenia *(continued)*

Level 6—Refractory	Slight or no obvious symptom reduction, and persistent positive and negative symptoms markedly disrupt all areas of personal and social adjustment. CGI: score of 6 = severely ill. At least one BPRS psychotic scale item score = 6, or two items score ≥5. Total BPRS scores are at least as high as in level 5.
Level 7—Severely refractory	No symptom reduction, with high levels of positive and negative psychotic symptoms associated with behavior observed to be helpless, disturbing, or dangerous. All areas of personal and social adjustment are seriously impaired and require constant supervision. CGI: score of 7 = among the most extremely ill patients. At least one BPRS psychotic scale item score = 7. Total BPRS scores are at least as high as in level 5.

Note. The scale levels consist of an index of values from the Clinical Global Impressions (CGI) Scale, the psychotic items from the Brief Psychiatric Rating Scale (BPRS), and a determination of independent functioning from a scale such as the Independent Living Skills Survey. "Rapid" reduction of symptoms is defined by relief in the first 6 weeks of treatment. To permit initial treatments to have their effect, no patient should be classified as level 5 or higher before 2 years of persisting symptoms and disability have elapsed following the first admission to hospital. For convenience, the Global Rating Scale can be collapsed into three levels: 1 and 2 reflect "remission"; 3 and 4 reflect "suboptimal response"; and 5, 6, and 7 reflect "treatment refractory."

Source. Reprinted from Brenner HD, Dencker SJ, Goldstein MJ, et al: "Defining Treatment Refractoriness in Schizophrenia." *Schizophrenia Bulletin* 16(4):558, 1990. Used by permission of Oxford University Press.

The Japanese Society of Psychiatry and Neurology is currently in the process of developing clinical guidelines for the treatment of schizophrenia. In the preliminary guidelines, tentative definition criteria for treatment-resistant schizophrenia were developed by combining responses to the survey of expert opinions and the proposals in other previously reported international guidelines (Table 9–11). Although most experts in Japan recognized the need to include domains other than positive and negative symptomatology, such as cognitive and psychosocial functioning, in the criteria, they decided against

Table 9–11.   Proposed criteria for treatment resistance in schizophrenia: Japanese Society of Psychiatry and Neurology

Moderate level

1.   With appropriate psychoeducation providing information about the illness and monitoring medication adherence, at least two trials of different antipsychotic medications with adequate daily dosage levels (≥600 mg/day of chlorpromazine equivalents) for a period of at least 6 weeks should be administered, along with other appropriate psychosocial approaches.

2.   With appropriate psychoeducation providing information about the illness and monitoring medication adherence, and if adequate daily dosage levels (≥600 mg/day of chlorpromazine equivalents) could not be attained because of severe side effects, the eligible upper limit of dosage levels should be administered, along with other appropriate psychosocial approaches.

3.   Positive or negative symptoms that may adversely affect the patient's activities of daily living (score of at least 3 in at least two items of Positive and Negative Syndrome Scale [PANSS] positive or negative symptom scales and PANSS total scores of at least 80) should last for at least 1 year.

Severe level

1.   With appropriate psychoeducation providing information about the illness and monitoring medication adherence, at least two trials of different antipsychotic medications with adequate daily dosage levels (≥1,000 mg/day of chlorpromazine equivalents) for a period of at least 6 weeks should be administered, along with other appropriate psychosocial approaches.

2.   With appropriate psychoeducation providing information about the illness and monitoring medication adherence, and if adequate daily dosage levels (≥1,000 mg/day of chlorpromazine equivalents) could not be attained because of severe side effects, the eligible upper limit of dosage levels should be administered, along with other appropriate psychosocial approaches.

3.   Prominent positive or negative symptoms that may seriously affect the patient's activities of daily living (score of at least 4 in at least two items of PANSS positive or negative symptom scales and PANSS total scores of at least 100) should last for at least 1 year.

Source.   Reprinted from Nakagome K: "Treatment refractory, treatment resistant?" in *Treatment Strategies for Treatment-Refractory Psychiatric Disorders* ("Lumière" Series for Specialists of Clinical Psychiatry no. 15). Edited by Nakagome K. Tokyo, Japan, Nakayama Shoten Co., Ltd., 2010, pp. 2–11. Used with permission.

including them at this time because they were unable to reach a consensus on the standard cutoff thresholds for defining "treatment resistant" in these domains. They also refrained from rigorously defining the standard psychosocial treatments for a similar reason, considering the great variance in the range and level of available treatments. Finally, they agreed that the definition of treatment resistance should reflect a continuum of responsiveness-unresponsiveness, and thus, two-stage models—including both a moderate level and a severe level—were adopted. The proposed guidelines have many limitations that must be overcome in the future. For example, what are the appropriate psychosocial treatments? We need more evidence to support which psychosocial approach is most effective for a particular patient and more clinicians in the field who could implement the psychosocial treatment optimally by promoting a process of dissemination.

Before moving to the topic of methods to treat schizophrenia that is labeled as treatment resistant, we need to explore other confounding factors relevant in forming a clinical picture as observed in a treatment-resistant patient. The patient factors include illicit substance misuse, physical comorbidity, and poor quality of the social environment, and the treatment factors include noncompliance, drug-drug interactions, delay in initiating treatment, drug bioavailability problems, and poor therapeutic alliance between physician and patient, all of which should be addressed before undergoing various interventions noted in the next section.

Treatment of Resistant Schizophrenia

Recommendations for Physical Treatment

Clozapine

Strong evidence suggests that clozapine is more efficacious than other antipsychotic drugs in treatment-resistant schizophrenia (Table 9–12). However, clozapine's potential for agranulocytosis and other serious side effects has generally limited its use to patients with treatment-resistant schizophrenia (Tandon et al. 2008). Clozapine has shown benefits over other antipsychotic drugs not only for positive symptoms but also for suicidality (Meltzer et al. 2003), violent behaviors (Krakowski et al. 2006), and comorbid substance misuse (Green 2006). Clozapine also was found to be associated with a remarkably

Table 9–12.   Physical intervention strategies for treatment-resistant schizophrenia

- Clozapine shows superiority in treatment-unresponsive and -intolerant schizophrenia.

- Clozapine shows benefits not only in terms of positive symptoms but also suicidality, violent behaviors, or comorbid substance misuse.

- Clozapine is associated with low incidence of tardive dyskinesia and plasma prolactin elevation.

- Clozapine has been underused for various reasons, including occurrence of agranulocytosis, restriction of the providers, costs, and complexities of clozapine treatment.

- Besides clozapine, limited treatment options with scarce evidence are often used in a trial-and-error process, including augmentation or adjunctive strategies with various types of drugs.

- Efficacy of electroconvulsive therapy (ECT), maintenance ECT, and repetitive transcranial magnetic stimulation (rTMS) adjunctive to antipsychotic medications is supported by several studies.

- Recently, development of novel drugs that target unmet treatment needs, including cognitive deficits, has been in progress with the hope that they may show efficacy against treatment-resistant schizophrenia of broader definition.

low incidence of tardive dyskinesia and plasma prolactin elevation, which may be the result of its weak dopamine type 2 (D_2) receptor blockade. In contrast to clozapine's superiority in treatment-unresponsive and -intolerant schizophrenia, no such evidence of its greater efficacy is found in first-episode schizophrenia (Lieberman et al. 2003) or among other patient populations, raising the question of exactly when in the course of the illness clozapine's benefits for treatment-resistant schizophrenia begin to appear.

Several studies suggested that clozapine serum concentrations can be useful to help guide dosing (Perry et al. 1991; VanderZwaag et al. 1996). Dosage levels of 300–600 mg/day are generally needed to achieve the plasma concentrations for good response (≥ 350 ng/mL), although care is needed because nicotine lowers the concentrations (Chung and Remington 2005). The dosage levels should be increased gradually—not exceeding 600 mg/day—to avoid serious side effects (e.g., the risk of seizures is dose-dependent).

Although many researchers strongly recommend clozapine as the agent of choice for treatment-resistant schizophrenia, and progression to clozapine use in the treatment course is explicitly encouraged, reluctance to use clozapine in the clinical field is apparent. For example, Phase II results of CATIE showed that many participants chose the tolerability pathway ($n=444$) over the efficacy pathway ($n=99$) (Swartz et al. 2008), presumably to avoid being assigned to clozapine treatment (clozapine was an option in the efficacy pathway of Phase II but not in the tolerability pathway). The provider restrictions, high costs, and complexities of clozapine treatment are necessary for treatment safety and efficiency but may have had the unintended consequence of reducing training opportunities for many residents and leading to underuse of clozapine for patients who might otherwise gain benefit from the drug.

Augmentation and Adjunctive Strategies

Besides clozapine, options are limited for the many patients with treatment-resistant schizophrenia, and none has been supported by systematic evidence. Various augmentation strategies that have limited or no evidence supporting their efficacy are often used. Overall effectiveness in a certain patient group does not always translate into effectiveness in each individual patient. No best drug or best dose of any drug exists for all patients. Predicting which antipsychotic medication might be optimal for a given patient is impossible. Decisions about antipsychotic therapy consequently entail a trial-and-error process with careful monitoring of clinical response and side effects and an ongoing risk-benefit assessment. Therefore, clinicians may consider a time-limited trial of a drug to determine whether it may offer any benefit exceeding risk to an individual patient.

It is recommended that patients with treatment-resistant schizophrenia be given a trial of clozapine monotherapy for up to 6 months insofar as no serious side effects occur. If optimal response is not attained after an adequate trial of clozapine, adjunctive agents such as mood stabilizers (e.g., lithium, valproate, lamotrigine), benzodiazepines (e.g., clonazepam), propranolol, antidepressants, or antipsychotic drugs may be tried, depending on the residual symptom profile. It should be noted that these augmentation strategies for clozapine are not supported by evidence. For example, the TMAP algorithm recommends clozapine augmentation with an SGA or FGA for patients whose symptoms do not respond to clozapine alone, although a review of the TMAP documentation suggests that the evidence favoring either risperidone or lamotrigine is weak (Moore et al. 2007). In one study, the placebo group actually showed greater improvement than the risperidone group on PANSS positive syndrome scale scores (Anil Yaciolu et al. 2005). RANZCP guidelines, by contrast, recommend the use of the most effective prior drug and an appropriate adjunctive therapy, such as lithium (Royal Australian and New Zealand College of Psychiatrists Clinical Practice Guidelines Team for the Treatment of Schizophrenia and Related Disorders 2005). Such adjunctive strategies should be considered on an individual basis, with goals of treatment carefully defined and subsequently monitored so that ineffective polypharmacy is not sustained.

Adjunctive Brain Stimulation Therapies

Patients with schizophrenia who are not eligible for clozapine treatment because of intolerable side effects or physical comorbidity may respond to electroconvulsive therapy (ECT) in combination with different antipsychotic medications (Tharyan and Adams 2005). Even though this initial beneficial effect may not last long, several studies suggest the sustained effectiveness of maintenance ECT adjunctive to antipsychotic medications (Chanpattana et al. 1999; Shimizu et al. 2007). Efficacy of adjunctive ECT with clozapine also was supported by several case series and open studies, which did not present any serious side effects of coadministration (Braga and Petrides 2005).

Several studies indicated the efficacy of slow repetitive transcranial magnetic stimulation (rTMS) adjunctive to antipsychotic medications, targeting the left temporoparietal cortex at a frequency of 1 Hz, for treatment-resistant auditory hallucinations. In a meta-analytic review of 10 sham-controlled trials (involving 212 patients), a significant mean weighted effect size for rTMS versus sham—$d = 0.76$ (95% confidence interval = 0.36–1.17)—was observed for treatment gain on hallucination ratings across the studies, but no significant effect was seen on a composite index of general psychotic symptoms (Aleman et al. 2007). Although more studies are needed to confirm its efficacy, slow rTMS may well be a treatment option for resistant auditory hallucinations. Only one small controlled study compared the efficacy of active rTMS with sham for clozapine nonresponders; it concluded that rTMS could be administered safely to patients taking clozapine, although no significant benefit was found for rTMS in this population (Rosa et al. 2007).

Novel Pharmacological Approaches

Although scarcely any evidence favors antipsychotic combination therapy, which also increases the side-effect burden, an alternative paradigm has been proposed (Carpenter 2004; Webber and Marder 2008). In this paradigm, the relative independence of reality distortion, disorganization, negative pathology, and cognition deficits is stressed. Monotherapy with antipsychotic drugs does not address all of these problems. These unmet treatment needs are clinical targets for drug discovery involving novel therapeutic strategies including combination therapy. Considering the unique properties of clozapine's mechanism of action, clozapine's major active metabolite N-desmethylclozapine (NDMC), which has glycine reuptake inhibition properties and cholinergic muscarinic-1 receptor agonistic function, is a candidate for an adjunct to existing antipsychotic medications for patients with treatment-resistant positive symptoms (Natesan et al. 2007). In regard to persistent negative symptoms, the effectiveness of adjunctive antidepressants has been reported in several studies, although findings remain inconsistent. Augmentation of antipsychotic medications with mirtazapine, paroxetine, fluvoxamine, or the selective monoamine oxidase type B inhibitor selegiline has shown benefit in respective controlled studies that have isolated the effect on negative symptoms from the effect on secondary factors, including positive symptoms, depression, and EPS (Webber and Marder 2008). The MATRICS project identified nine promising molecular targets for cognition-enhancing agents with a potential for pronounced efficacy in cognitive deficits in schizophrenia, which has been unfulfilled by atypical antipsychotic drugs (Green 2007; Webber and Marder 2008):

1. α_7-Nicotinic receptor agonists

   - Partial α_7-nicotinic cholinergic agonist (3-[(2,4-dimethoxy)benzylidene]-anabaseine, DMXB-A)
   - Acetylcholinesterase inhibitor (galantamine)

2. D_1 receptor agonists

   - Full D_1 agonist (dihydrexidine, DAR-0100)

3. AMPA (α-amino-3-hydroxy-5-methyl-4-isoxazolepropionic acid) glutamatergic receptor agonists

   - Positive allosteric modulators of AMPA receptors, AMPAkines (CX-516)

4. α_2-Adrenergic receptor agonists
   - α_2 Receptor stimulators, antihypertensive drugs (clonidine, guanfacine)

5. N-methyl-D-aspartate glutamatergic receptor agonists
   - D-Cycloserine, glycine, D-serine

6. Metabotropic glutamate receptor agonists
   - mGlu2/3 agonist (LY2140023)

7. Glycine reuptake inhibitors
   - Sarcosine

8. M_1 muscarinic receptor agonists
   - NDMC (ACP-104)

9. γ-Aminobutyric acid$_A$ receptor subtype selective agonists
   - α_2-Subunit specific stimulator, positive allosteric modulators

Recommendations for Psychosocial Treatment

Psychosocial treatments may play an important role in improving outcomes in treatment-resistant schizophrenia. In the same way that pharmacological treatment must be individually tailored to the needs and preferences of the patient, so, too, must psychosocial treatment (Table 9–13). The selection of appropriate and effective psychosocial interventions for patients with treatment-resistant schizophrenia must be driven by the individual patient's needs and his or her social circumstances. Most patients will benefit from at least some of the recommended psychosocial interventions. However, because patients' health and social needs may vary at different points in their illness course, it would be rare for all of these psychosocial interventions to be used during any one phase of illness for an individual patient.

The contribution of pharmacological treatment in enabling patients to fully benefit from participation in psychosocial treatment programs is noteworthy. Rosenheck et al. (1998) monitored the use of different levels of psychosocial treatments and rehabilitation in patients assigned to a comparison of clozapine and haloperidol. Patients receiving clozapine were more likely to use higher levels of psychosocial treatment. Moreover, the use of these higher

Table 9–13. Psychosocial intervention strategies for treatment-resistant schizophrenia

The selection of appropriate and effective psychosocial treatments needs to be driven by the individual patient's needs and his or her social circumstances.

• **Cognitive-behavioral therapy (CBT)** is focused on patients with persistent delusions and hallucinations based on a cognitive model of psychopathology. Cognitive-behavioral approaches have small to medium effect sizes on positive symptoms, negative symptoms, community functioning, hopelessness, and social anxiety.

• **Cognitive remediation** aims to improve cognitive functioning through stimulation of impaired areas of cognition and teach patients strategies to compensate for deficits. Cognitive remediation approaches are associated with small to medium effect sizes for cognitive performance (medium), psychosocial functioning (slightly lower), and symptoms (small). Cognitive remediation yields greater benefits in functional outcomes when combined with adjunctive psychiatric rehabilitation than when provided alone.

• **Case management** is the coordination, integration, and allocation of care according to the needs of each individual. **Assertive Community Treatment (ACT)** is a multidisciplinary approach to community-based care that delivers treatment and care for patients with serious mental health problems in the community.

  – Whereas case management reduces the number of hospital days but increases the number of total admissions, ACT reduces both.

  – Case management and ACT have shown some efficacy in reducing family burden, cost of care, symptoms, and dropout rates; increasing family and patients' satisfaction with services and patients' contacts with services; and improving social functioning.

levels was associated with greater improvements in quality of life. This suggests that patients who experience more improvement in symptoms with a better pharmacological treatment have a greater potential to benefit from psychosocial treatments.

Cognitive-Behavioral Therapy

It is well documented that psychotic symptoms are only weakly correlated with psychosocial functioning, given that they respond to antipsychotic medications and that their severity can vary dramatically throughout the illness course. However, some evidence indicates that worsening of psychotic symptoms (Angell and Test 2002) and persistence of psychotic symptoms (Racenstein et al. 2002) can reduce social and work functioning. Alternative approaches to treatment-resistant psychotic symptoms are needed that can ameliorate both the distress caused by the symptoms and the functional impairment that accompanies them.

CBT initially was focused on patients with persistent delusions and hallucinations based on a cognitive model of psychopathology. According to the model, current psychotic symptoms are seen as resulting from misattributions of perceptions of events prompted by viewing them through the prism of a faulty developmental belief structure, exacerbated by ongoing logical errors. These faulty attributional styles are also enhanced by a tendency to "jump to conclusions" and personalizing bias. More recently, greater attention has been paid to applying the cognitive model of psychosis to negative symptoms (Kern et al. 2009). In schizophrenia, the development of positive symptoms and underlying cognitive deficits results in many experiences that might be taken as disgraceful failures, such as being unable to attend in school, follow conversations with friends, succeed at a job, or manage hygiene. Negative symptoms are conceptualized as understandable, but maladaptive, responses to these circumstances. The behaviors and attitudes that are related to negative symptoms likely reflect, at least in part, negative self-beliefs.

Although some variability exists within the school of CBT, Garety et al. (2000) noted that all CBT includes the following components: 1) engagement and assessment; 2) coping enhancement; 3) developing a shared understanding of the experience of psychosis; 4) working on delusions and hallucinations, often using gentle challenging; 5) addressing mood and negative self-evaluations; and 6) managing the risk of relapse and social disability.

A review of CBT concluded that although more studies are needed, the evidence to date supports adjunctive use of CBT with antipsychotic medications for persistent psychotic symptoms of schizophrenia (Turkington et al. 2006). A more recent meta-analysis of RCTs comparing CBT with a control group, including primarily patients with schizophrenia and some who were treatment resistant, found that CBT had small to medium effect sizes (d=0.19–0.44) on positive symptoms, negative symptoms, community functioning, hopelessness, and social anxiety, whereas the number of cited studies ranged from 2 (for social anxiety) to 32 (for positive symptoms) (Wykes et al. 2008). NICE guidelines recommend the use of CBT for the treatment of persistent psychotic symptoms rather than for acute symptoms (National Institute for Clinical Excellence 2002). These guidelines suggest that the benefits of CBT are most marked when treatment is continued for more than 6 months and involves more than 10 treatment sessions. Finally, CBT is highly manualized and is designed to be independently mastered by practicing clinical psychiatrists, psychologists, and community mental health professionals, in contrast to other psychosocial treatments with requirements for expertise or supervision.

Cognitive Remediation

Cognitive deficits are now recognized as a core feature of schizophrenia that is strongly related to functioning in the community and also a strong predictor of response to psychiatric rehabilitation. Because the effects of pharmacological approaches targeting cognitive deficits have been rather more limited than initially expected, cognition-enhancing agents or psychosocial treatments are urgently needed for patients with severe mental illnesses and poor functioning. Cognitive-enhancing psychosocial approaches aim to improve cognitive functioning through stimulation of impaired areas of cognition, such as attention, memory, and problem solving. The approach is based on the neuroplasticity model of brain development, in which it is believed that engaging in tasks that challenge particular neural processes will enhance those functions. The goal of these cognitive remediation programs is to improve cognitive functioning and teach patients strategies to compensate for deficits. The different approaches of cognitive remediation include personal or small-group sessions; computer-based programs or paper-and-pencil exercises; teaching strategies to improve cognitive functioning; compensatory strategies to reduce the burden of cognitive capacities; group discussions; bridging the exercises in the program to daily living activities; and emphasizing meta-cognitive processes such as learning styles.

Results of a meta-analysis of 26 RCTs of cognitive remediation in schizophrenia including 1,151 patients were reported by McGurk et al. (2007). The investigators suggested that cognitive remediation was associated with significant improvements across all three outcomes, with a medium effect size for cognitive performance (0.41), a slightly lower effect size for psychosocial functioning (0.36), and a small effect size for symptoms (0.28). The effects of cognitive remediation on psychosocial functioning were significantly stronger in studies that provided adjunctive psychiatric rehabilitation than in those that provided cognitive remediation alone.

Case Management and Assertive Community Treatment

Since the 1960s, the movement toward deinstitutionalization pushed large psychiatric hospitals to close down and to treat patients in outpatient clinics, day centers, or community mental health centers. However, readmission rates were such that this type of community was thought to be less effective than expected. In the 1970s, case management along with ACT arose as a new means of community-based care of severely mentally ill patients.

Case management.   Many patients with schizophrenia have a broad range of needs for health and social care. Case management is the coordination, integration, and allocation of care according to the needs of each individual. Case management includes the following components: 1) psychosocial needs assessment, 2) individual care planning, 3) referral and linking to appropriate services or supports, 4) ongoing monitoring of the care plan, 5) advocacy, 6) monitoring the patient's mental state, 7) compliance with medication and possible side effects, 8) establishment and maintenance of a therapeutic relationship, and 9) supportive counseling.

Assertive Community Treatment.   ACT is a specific model of community-based care that delivers treatment and care for patients with serious mental health problems in the community who are at risk for hospital readmission and whose symptoms cannot be maintained by more conventional community-based treatment. ACT involves a multidisciplinary approach in which a team of social workers, nurses, psychiatrists, and other health professionals work together to provide all psychiatric and social care for the patient. ACT is provided exclusively for a group of patients defined as having "serious mental illness." Care is provided at home or in the workplace and involves assertiveness with patients who are uncooperative and reluctant service users. The specific goals of the treatment are 1) monitoring patients who are unwell but do not require hospital admission; 2) reducing the number of hospital admissions; and 3) improving patients' social functioning and quality of life within the community in which they reside.

Efficacy of ACT and case management.   In regard to ACT, a Cochrane review (Marshall and Lockwood 1998) indicated that, compared with patients receiving standard community care, those receiving ACT were more likely to remain in contact with services and less likely to be admitted to the hospital;

they also spent less time in the hospital. In addition, ACT showed a better outcome than standard community care In the domains of accommodation, employment, and patient satisfaction, whereas no differences were seen between ACT and control treatments on mental state or social functioning. Therefore, it was implied that ACT is an effective approach for the care of severely mentally ill patients in the community, especially for the high users of inpatient care.

Evidence on the effects of case management has been contradictory. A Cochrane review (Marshall et al. 1998) presented a negative view of the effectiveness of case management other than ACT on several domains. The review found indications that case management retained more people in contact with psychiatric services and also increased hospital admission rates. However, except for a positive finding on compliance from one study, case management showed no significant advantages over standard care on any psychiatric or social variables.

A meta-analytic review by Ziguras and Stuart (2000) proposed an alternative view of the effectiveness of case management. These investigators analyzed 44 studies (compared with 11 in the Cochrane review); 35 compared ACT or clinical case management with usual treatment, and 9 directly compared ACT with clinical case management. Because Ziguras and colleagues believed that ACT and case management share common features to a great extent, they referred to those studies on ACT and case management collectively rather than separately, unlike the Cochrane review. Moreover, they included quasi-experimental studies in addition to RCTs, whereas the Cochrane reviewers used RCTs only. Furthermore, Ziguras and Stuart included domains measured with nonpublished scales and also parametric analysis of skewed data, both of which were excluded in the Cochrane review. These differences resulted in greater statistical power with a larger data set (Ziguras and Stuart 2000; Ziguras et al. 2002); consequently, both types of case management were found to be more effective than usual treatment in three outcome domains: family burden, family satisfaction with services, and cost of care. The total number of admissions and the proportion of patients hospitalized were reduced in ACT and increased in case management. The number of hospital days was reduced in both programs, but ACT was significantly more effective than case management. Although patients in case management had more admissions than did those in usual treatment, the admissions were shorter, which reduced the total number of hospital days. The two types of case management were equally effective in reducing symptoms, increasing patients' contacts with services, reducing dropout rates, improving social functioning, and increasing patients' satisfaction (Ziguras et al. 2002).

Although these two reviews of case management appear to contradict each other, the results were curiously the same for the two domains common to both analyses. Both studies found that case management was effective in preventing patients from dropping out of services and led to a greater proportion of patients being hospitalized. However, Ziguras and Stuart (2000) found a range of other domains in which case management showed benefit and concluded that it produced small to moderate improvements in care provided to people with a serious mental illness. In a conflictual relationship between increasing statistical power and adherence to rigorous methodology, the partial overlap in the results of the Cochrane review (Marshall et al. 1998) and the meta-analytic reviews of Ziguras and colleagues (Ziguras and Stuart 2000; Ziguras et al. 2002) implies that methodologies other than randomized controlled designs do not necessarily provide a lower level of evidence when reviewing valid psychosocial interventions.

Conclusion

Refining the definition of treatment resistance holds both advantages and disadvantages. Consensually developed definitions may yield good criteria to guide the use of specialized treatment agents such as clozapine. Broader definitions may provide more chances for patients to receive trials of such treatments. But what if those trials end up in failure? Because we have few pharmacological options beyond the step of using clozapine, definition may lead to additional serious stigma. The definitions of treatment resistance widely accepted today actually represent "drug resistance," to the extent that psychosocial approaches are ignored or inadequately implemented. Now that we have more resources in terms of psychosocial treatments, we surely need to take these approaches into consideration in future efforts to define true treatment resistance. We should keep in mind that our ultimate goal is not merely to broaden the criteria; rather, it is to ensure that no patient remains in a state of treatment nonresponse.

References

Aleman A, Sommer IE, Kahn RS: Efficacy of slow repetitive transcranial magnetic stimulation in the treatment of resistant auditory hallucinations in schizophrenia: a meta-analysis. J Clin Psychiatry 68:416–421, 2007

Andreasen NC, Carpenter WT Jr, Kane JM, et al: Remission in schizophrenia: proposed criteria and rationale for consensus. Am J Psychiatry 162:441–449, 2005

Angell B, Test MA: The relationship of clinical factors and environmental opportunities to social functioning in young adults with schizophrenia. Schizophr Bull 28:259–271, 2002

Anil Yaciolu AE, Kivircik Akdede BB, Turgut TI, et al: A double-blind controlled study of adjunctive treatment with risperidone in schizophrenic patients partially responsive to clozapine: efficacy and safety. J Clin Psychiatry 66:63–72, 2005

Bebbington P, Kuipers L: The predictive utility of expressed emotion in schizophrenia: an aggregate analysis. Psychol Med 24:707–718, 1994

Bowie CR, Reichenberg A, Patterson TL, et al: Determinants of real-world functioning performance in schizophrenia: correlations with cognition, functional capacity, and symptoms. Am J Psychiatry163:418–425, 2006

Braga RJ, Petrides G: The combined use of electroconvulsive therapy and antipsychotics in patients with schizophrenia. J ECT 21:75–83, 2005

Brenner HD, Dencker SJ, Goldstein MJ, et al: Defining treatment refractoriness in schizophrenia. Schizophr Bull 16:551–561, 1990

Brown GW, Monck EM, Carstairs GM, et al: Influence of family life on the course of schizophrenic illness. Br J Prev Soc Med 16:55–68, 1962

Brown GW, Birley JL, Wing JK: Influence of family life on the course of schizophrenic disorders: a replication. Br J Psychiatry 121:241–258, 1972

Bryson GJ, Bell MD, Lysaker PH, et al: The Work Behavior Inventory: a scale for the assessment of work behavior for clients with severe mental illness. Psychiatr Rehabil J 20:47–55, 1997

Buchanan RW, Davis M, Goff D, et al: A summary of the FDA-NIMH-MATRICS workshop on clinical trial design for neurocognitive drugs for schizophrenia. Schizophr Bull 31:5–19, 2005

Carpenter WT Jr: Clinical constructs and therapeutic discovery. Schizophr Res 72:69–73, 2004

Chanpattana W, Chakrabhand ML, Sackeim HA, et al: Continuation ECT in treatment-resistant schizophrenia: a controlled study. J ECT 15:178–192, 1999

Chung C, Remington G: Predictors and markers of clozapine response. Psychopharmacology (Berl) 179:317–335, 2005

Clozapine Committee of the Japanese Society of Clinical Neuropsychopharmacology: Guidance for Adequate Usage of Clozaril (in Japanese). Kyowa-Kikaku, Tokyo, Japan, 2009

Essock SM, Hargreaves WA, Dohm FA, et al: Clozapine eligibility among state hospital patients. Schizophr Bull 22:15–25, 1996

Gaebel W, Weinmann S, Sartorius N, et al: Schizophrenia practice guidelines: international survey and comparison. Br J Psychiatry 187:248–255, 2005

Garety PA, Fowler D, Kuipers E: Cognitive-behavioral therapy for medication-resistant symptoms. Schizophr Bull 26:73–86, 2000

Green AI: Treatment of schizophrenia and comorbid substance abuse: pharmacologic approaches. J Clin Psychiatry 67 (suppl 7):S31–S35, 2006

Green MF: Stimulating the development of drug treatments to improve cognition in schizophrenia. Annu Rev Clin Psychol 3:159–180, 2007

Guy W: ECDEU Assessment Manual for Psychopharmacology—Revised (DHHS Publ No ADM 91-338). Rockville, MD, U.S. Department of Health and Human Services, 1976, pp 534–537

Helldin L, Kane JM, Karilampi U, et al: Remission and cognitive ability in a cohort of patients with schizophrenia. J Psychiatr Res 40:738–745, 2006

Helldin L, Kane JM, Karilampi U, et al: Remission in prognosis of functional outcome: a new dimension in the treatment of patients with psychotic disorders. Schizophr Res 93:160–168, 2007

Heres S, Schmitz FS, Leucht S, et al: The attitude of patients towards antipsychotic depot treatment. Int Clin Psychopharmacol 22:275–282, 2007

Inada T: A Second-Generation Rating Scale for Antipsychotic-Induced Extrapyramidal Symptoms: Drug-Induced Extrapyramidal Symptoms Scale. Tokyo, Japan, Seiwa Publishing, 2009

Jones PB, Barnes TR, Davies L, et al: Randomized controlled trial of the effect on Quality of Life of second- vs first-generation antipsychotic drugs in schizophrenia: Cost Utility of the Latest Antipsychotic Drugs in Schizophrenia Study (CUtLASS 1). Arch Gen Psychiatry 63:1079–1087, 2006

Juarez-Reyes MG, Shumway M, et al: Effects of stringent criteria on eligibility for clozapine among public mental health clients. Psychiatr Serv 46:801–806, 1995

Kahn RS, Fleischhacker WW, Boter H, et al: Effectiveness of antipsychotic drugs in first-episode schizophrenia and schizophreniform disorder: an open randomised clinical trial. Lancet 371:1085–1097, 2008

Kane J, Honigfeld G, Singer J, et al: Clozapine for the treatment-resistant schizophrenic: a double-blind comparison with chlorpromazine. Arch Gen Psychiatry 45:789–796, 1988

Kay SR, Fiszbein A, Opler LA: The Positive and Negative Syndrome Scale (PANSS) for schizophrenia. Schizophr Bull 13:261–276, 1987

Keefe RS, Goldberg TE, Harvey PD, et al: The Brief Assessment of Cognition in Schizophrenia: reliability, sensitivity, and comparison with a standard neurocognitive battery. Schizophr Res 68:283–297, 2004

Keefe RS, Poe M, Walker TM, et al: The Schizophrenia Cognition Rating Scale: an interview-based assessment and its relationship to cognition, real-world functioning, and functional capacity. Am J Psychiatry 163:426–432, 2006

Kemp R, Kirov G, Everitt B, et al: Randomised controlled trial of compliance therapy: 18-month follow-up. Br J Psychiatry 172:413–419, 1998

Kern RS, Glynn SM, Horan WP, et al: Psychosocial treatments to promote functional recovery in schizophrenia. Schizophr Bull 35:347–361, 2009

Kleinman L, Lieberman J, Dube S, et al: Development and psychometric performance of the schizophrenia objective functioning instrument: an interviewer administered measure of function. Schizophr Res 107:275–285, 2008

Kopelowicz A, Liberman RP, Zarate R: Recent advances in social skills training for schizophrenia. Schizophr Bull 32 (suppl 1):S12–S23, 2006

Krakowski MI, Czobor P, Citrome L, et al: Atypical antipsychotic agents in the treatment of violent patients with schizophrenia and schizoaffective disorder. Arch Gen Psychiatry 63:622–629, 2006

Lehman AF, Lieberman JA, Dixon LB, et al: Practice guideline for the treatment of patients with schizophrenia, second edition. Am J Psychiatry 161(suppl):1–56, 2004

Leucht S, Kane JM, Kissling W, et al: What does the PANSS mean? Schizophr Res 79:231–238, 2005

Leucht S, Busch R, Kissling W, et al: Early prediction of antipsychotic nonresponse among patients with schizophrenia. J Clin Psychiatry 68:352–360, 2007

Levine SZ, Rabinowitz J, Engel R, et al: Extrapolation between measures of symptom severity and change: an examination of the PANSS and CGI. Schizophr Res 98:318–322, 2008

Lieberman JA, Phillips M, Gu H, et al: Atypical and conventional antipsychotic drugs in treatment-naive first-episode schizophrenia: a 52-week randomized trial of clozapine vs chlorpromazine. Neuropsychopharmacology 28:995–1003, 2003

Lieberman JA, Stroup TS, McEvoy JP, et al: Effectiveness of antipsychotic drugs in patients with chronic schizophrenia. N Engl J Med 353:1209–1223, 2005

Loeb PA: Independent Living Scale Manual. San Antonio, TX, Psychological Corporation, 1996

Marshall M, Lockwood A: Assertive community treatment for people with severe mental disorders. Cochrane Database of Systematic Reviews 1998, Issue 2. Art. No.: CD001089. DOI: 10.1002/14651858.CD001089.

Marshall M, Gray A, Lockwood A, et al: Case management for people with severe mental disorders. Cochrane Database of Systematic Reviews 1998, Issue 2. Art. No.: CD000050. DOI: 10.1002/14651858.CD000050.

Matza LS, Buchanan R, Purdon S, et al: Measuring changes in functional status among patients with schizophrenia: the link with cognitive impairment. Schizophr Bull 32:666–678, 2006

Mausbach BT, Harvey PD, Goldman SR, et al: Development of a brief scale of everyday functioning in persons with serious mental illness. Schizophr Bull 33:1364–1372, 2007

Mausbach BT, Bowie CR, Harvey PD, et al: Usefulness of the UCSD Performance-Based Skills Assessment (UPSA) for predicting residential independence in patients with chronic schizophrenia. J Psychiatr Res 42:320–327, 2008

McGurk SR, Mueser KT, Harvey PD, et al: Cognitive and symptom predictors of work outcomes for clients with schizophrenia in supported employment. Psychiatr Serv 54:1129–1135, 2003

McGurk SR, Twamley EW, Sitzer DI, et al: A meta-analysis of cognitive remediation in schizophrenia. Am J Psychiatry 164:1791–1802, 2007

Meltzer HY: Treatment of the neuroleptic-nonresponsive schizophrenic patient. Schizophr Bull 18:515–542, 1992

Meltzer HY, Alphs L, Green AI, et al: Clozapine treatment for suicidality in schizophrenia: International Suicide Prevention Trial (InterSePT). Arch Gen Psychiatry 60:82–91, 2003

Miller AL, Chiles JA, Chiles JK, et al: The Texas Medication Algorithm Project (TMAP) schizophrenia algorithms. J Clin Psychiatry 60:649–657, 1999

Moore TA, Buchanan RW, Buckley PF, et al: The Texas Medication Algorithm Project antipsychotic algorithm for schizophrenia: 2006 update. J Clin Psychiatry 68:1751–1762, 2007

Naber D, Lambert M: The CATIE and CUtLASS studies in schizophrenia: results and implications for clinicians. CNS Drugs 23:649–659, 2009

Natesan S, Reckless GE, Barlow KB, et al: Evaluation of N-desmethylclozapine as a potential antipsychotic—preclinical studies. Neuropsychopharmacology 32:1540–1549, 2007

National Institute for Health and Clinical Excellence: Clinical Guideline 82. Schizophrenia. Care Interventions in the Treatment and Management of Schizophrenia in Adults in Primary and Secondary Care (Update). London, National Institute for Health and Clinical Excellence, 2009. Available at: http://www.nice.org.uk/cg82. Accessed October 1, 2011.

Novartis Pharma KK: Clozaril Package Insert (Japanese). 2009

Overall JE, Gorham DR: The Brief Psychiatric Rating Scale. Psychol Rep 10:799–812, 1962

Patterson TL, Goldman S, McKibbin CL, et al: UCSD Performance-Based Skills Assessment: development of a new measure of everyday functioning for severely mentally ill adults. Schizophr Bull 27:235–245, 2001

Perry PJ, Miller DD, Arndt SV, et al: Clozapine and norclozapine plasma concentrations and clinical response of treatment-refractory schizophrenic patients. Am J Psychiatry 148:231–235, 1991

Racenstein JM, Harrow M, Reed R, et al: The relationship between positive symptoms and instrumental work functioning in schizophrenia: a 10 year follow-up study. Schizophr Res 56:95–103, 2002

Rosa MO, Gattaz WF, Rosa MA, et al: Effects of repetitive transcranial magnetic stimulation on auditory hallucinations refractory to clozapine. J Clin Psychiatry 68:1528–1532, 2007

Rosenheck R, Tekell J, Peters J, et al: Does participation in psychosocial treatment augment the benefit of clozapine? Department of Veterans Affairs Cooperative Study Group on Clozapine in Refractory Schizophrenia. Arch Gen Psychiatry 55:618–625, 1998

Royal Australian and New Zealand College of Psychiatrists Clinical Practice Guidelines Team for the Treatment of Schizophrenia and Related Disorders: Royal Australian and New Zealand College of Psychiatrists clinical practice guidelines for the treatment of schizophrenia and related disorders. Aust N Z J Psychiatry 39:1–30, 2005

Shimizu E, Imai M, Fujisaki M, et al: Maintenance electroconvulsive therapy (ECT) for treatment-resistant disorganized schizophrenia. Prog Neuropsychopharmacol Biol Psychiatry 31:571–573, 2007

Swartz MS, Stroup TS, McEvoy JP, et al: What CATIE found: results from the schizophrenia trial. Psychiatr Serv 59:500–506, 2008

Tandon R, Belmaker RH, Gattaz WF, et al: World Psychiatric Association Pharmacopsychiatry Section statement on comparative effectiveness of antipsychotics in the treatment of schizophrenia. Schizophr Res 100:20–38, 2008

Tharyan P, Adams CE: Electroconvulsive therapy for schizophrenia. Cochrane Database of Systematic Reviews 2005, Issue 2. Art. No.: CD000076. DOI: 10.1002/14651858.CD000076.pub2

Tungpunkom P, Nicol M: Life skills programmes for chronic mental illnesses. Cochrane Database of Systematic Reviews 2008, Issue 2. Art. No.: CD000381. DOI: 10.1002/14651858.CD000381.pub2

Turkington D, Kingdon D, Weiden PJ: Cognitive behavior therapy for schizophrenia. Am J Psychiatry 163:365–373, 2006

Twamley EW, Doshi RR, Nayak GV, et al: Generalized cognitive impairments, ability to perform everyday tasks, and level of independence in community living situations of older patients with psychosis. Am J Psychiatry 159:2013–2020, 2002

VanderZwaag C, McGee M, McEvoy JP, et al: Response of patients with treatment-refractory schizophrenia to clozapine within three serum level ranges. Am J Psychiatry 153:1579–1584, 1996

Ventura J, Green MF, Shaner A, et al: Training and quality assurance in the use of the Brief Psychiatric Rating Scale: the "drift busters." Int L Methods Psychiatr Res 3:221–244, 1993

Ventura J, Cienfuegos A, Boxer O, et al: Clinical Global Impression of Cognition in Schizophrenia (CGI-CogS): reliability and validity of a co-primary measure of cognition. Schizophr Res 106:59–69, 2008

Walburn J, Gray R, Gournay K, Quraishi S, et al: Systematic review of patient and nurse attitudes to depot antipsychotic medication. Br J Psychiatry 179:300–307, 2001

Wallace CJ, Nelson CJ, Liberman RP, et al: A review and critique of social skills training with schizophrenic patients. Schizophr Bull 6:42–63, 1980

Webber MA, Marder SR: Better pharmacotherapy for schizophrenia: what does the future hold? Curr Psychiatry Rep 10:352–358, 2008

Wykes T, Steel C, Everitt B, et al: Cognitive behavior therapy for schizophrenia: effect sizes, clinical models, and methodological rigor. Schizophr Bull 34:523–537, 2008

Ziguras SJ, Stuart GW: A meta-analysis of the effectiveness of mental health case management over 20 years. Psychiatr Serv 51:1410–1421, 2000

Ziguras SJ, Stuart GW, Jackson AC: Assessing the evidence on case management. Br J Psychiatry 181:17–21, 2002

10

Psychological Interventions for Schizophrenia

Alessandro Rossi, M.D.

Paolo Stratta, M.D.

Ilaria Riccardi, Ph.D.

Psychosocial Treatment of Schizophrenia

Schizophrenia is one of the most disabling mental disorders because of its severe prognosis and need for continuous care and treatment. Impairment in social functioning is one of the hallmarks of schizophrenia in the DSM-IV-TR criteria (American Psychiatric Association 2000) and leads to important limitations in the realms of social interaction, work, and education. Because schizophrenia usually has an onset in late adolescence or early adulthood, during a key phase of socialization in terms of professional career and interpersonal relationships, this impairment is a considerable potential risk for an accumulation of complicating factors and future chronicity (Brekke et al. 2005)

Deficits in social functioning, although present in other clinical disorders (e.g., bipolar disorder), become more prominent in persons with schizophrenia throughout the course of the disorder. Such deficits are usually present in patients during the first episode, may persist despite antipsychotic treatment, and tend to remain stable in severity or even to worsen in subsequent phases of the illness. Deficits in social functioning are frequently present before the onset of psychosis and are also evident in relatives. Therefore, these deficits are likely to be premorbid and may be considered as vulnerability factors, implicated in the development of the disorder and contributing to the rate of relapse.

Impairments in social functioning appear to represent a core behavioral feature of schizophrenia. The importance of social dysfunction in the course of schizophrenia suggests that any interventions, psychosocial or pharmacological, must target social functioning if they are to positively influence long-term outcome. Despite the availability of new pharmacological treatments, psychosocial interventions are also needed to ensure the best psychosocial functioning achievable (Mueser and McGurk 2004).

Psychosocial rehabilitation seeks to enable patients with mental disease to live successfully in their environment with minimal intervention, helping in the development of the skills necessary to achieve personal goals and community integration and to establish a network of support and strategies to compensate for impaired abilities (Anthony 1996; Anthony and Liberman 1986).

Skills, different from *abilities,* are based on learning experiences and are the source of the full range of human social performance, such as accurate social perception and expression of empathy and other emotions, appropriate to the context and expectations of others. *Social skills* represent the topography of social interaction, whereas *social competence* reflects the accumulation of self-efficacy and real-world success through experiencing the favorable consequences of interactions. Learning social skills is the fundamental raw material of a large part of psychosocial treatment for patients with schizophrenia (Kopelowicz et al. 2006).

Psychosocial rehabilitation comprises training aimed at the acquisition of skills related to real-life settings, as opposed to skills taught through psycho-educational methods or applied in laboratory settings, which often do not generalize outside those settings. Sometimes this means determining whether it is preferable to help the patient develop a skill or, alternatively, to implement compensatory interventions, identifying and facilitating a comprehensive support network (Stip and Rialle 2005; Vallée 2001).

Psychosocial treatments for schizophrenia include the well-established social skills training but also other, newer interventions such as cognitive behavioral therapy (CBT), social cognition training, and cognitive remediation. These interventions differ in their selected treatment targets. *Social skills training* targets social and independent living skills; *CBT* targets symptoms that interfere with social functioning and reduce quality of life; *social cognition training* targets social cognitive components such as emotion perception, social perception, theory of mind, and social attribution that have been linked to successful social functioning; and *cognitive remediation* generally targets a range of cognitive impairments that affect work and social functioning (Kern et al. 2009).

Structured Psychosocial Interventions

Several structured psychosocial intervention protocols, heterogeneous in methods and approaches, have been developed, both in community and in hospital settings, although relatively few persons with schizophrenia have access to the full array of evidence-based psychosocial programs (Dixon et al. 2010). Psychosocial treatment is recommended chiefly for persons with disabling schizophrenia who are at risk for discontinuation of treatment or for repeated crises; treatment recommendations encompass an array of clinical, rehabilitation, and social services to address unmet needs of patients and ensure coordination, integration, and continuity of services among providers.

Assertive Community Treatment and Supported Employment

The Assertive Community Treatment (ACT) program emphasizes patients' adaptation to community life; it provides support and consultation to patients' natural networks—family members, employers, friends and peers, and community agencies—and assertive outreach to ensure that patients remain in treatment.

Evidence has consistently confirmed that supported employment is more effective than traditional vocational services in helping individuals with schizophrenia to achieve competitive jobs (Burns et al. 2007; Cook et al. 2005; Lehman et al. 2002; McFarlane et al. 2000). The key elements of supported employment are rapid search for an individually tailored job, provision of ongoing job supports, and integration of vocational and mental health services.

Social Skills Training

Social skills training is strongly recommended for patients with deficits in skills involved in everyday activities that affect community functioning. The scientific foundations of social skills training encompass operant conditioning, experimental analysis of behavior, social learning theory, social psychology, and social cognition. When acquisition of instrumental skills is reinforced by achievement of interpersonal goals, the likelihood of initiating future social communications is increased. Successful application of social skills in community life builds social competence, leading to improvement in self-efficacy, self-esteem, self-confidence, empowerment, optimism, and mood (Kopelowicz et al. 2006).

In the stress-vulnerability model of schizophrenia, social competence can be viewed as a protective factor (Liberman et al. 2005). Together with other evidence-based services, strengthened social competence can help compensate for the noxious effects of cognitive deficits, neurobiological vulnerability, stressful events, and social maladjustment, thus improving quality of life.

Skills training programs vary widely in content but typically share several key elements, including behaviorally based instruction, role modeling, rehearsal, corrective feedback, and positive reinforcement, supplemented with strategies for ensuring adequate practice in applying skills in the individual's environment (Table 10–1). Evidence indicates that social skills training produces significant effects on proximal measures of skill (as demonstrated in role-play tests) as well as more distal measures of community functioning (Kurtz and Mueser 2008). Several studies have reported retention of the trained skills over periods of even up to 1 year (Glynn et al. 2002; Xiang et al. 2007).

One emerging strategy for teaching social skills involves enlisting and training family members as "generalization agents" to participate in skills training efforts. Useful tools for teaching skills include trainers' materials, demonstration videos, and workbooks (Bellack et al. 2004).

Social skills training and family psychoeducation interventions (see discussion later in chapter) are typically delivered in small groups (6–10 participants maximum) with predefined curricula in terms of content and goals. These groups typically meet 2–3 times per week, with sessions lasting 45–90 minutes. In such groups, cotherapists are preferred but not required. Group structure can be closed or open; the duration of group interventions varies de-

Table 10–1. Social skills training procedures

Identify the problem: Identify together with the patient the actual obstacles to the personal goals in life.

Set the goal: Specify the suitable social behaviors required for successful attainment of short-term goals after a detailed description of what communication skills are to be learned.

Role-playing: Demonstrate the communication skills required for successful social interaction.

Feedback: Focus on the quality of the behaviors used in the role-play.

Social modeling: Teach, through demonstration, the desired interpersonal behaviors.

Behavioral practice: Repeat the target behavior until it reaches success in real life.

Positive social reinforcement: Reinforce contingently the improved skills.

Homework: Motivate the patient to use communication skills in real-life situations.

Problem solving: Provide reinforcement on the basis of the patient's experience in using the skills.

pending on the content and the level of training geared to participants (Bellack 2004).

Cognitive-Behavioral Therapy

Cognitive-behaviorally oriented psychotherapy should be offered to persons with schizophrenia who are experiencing persistent severe psychotic symptoms despite receiving adequate pharmacotherapy. Whether provided in group or individual format, the therapy should last approximately 4–9 months for optimal effects in reducing symptom severity.

Controlled studies have shown that CBT provided adjunctively to adequate pharmacotherapy is beneficial in reducing the severity of delusions, hallucinations, positive and negative symptoms, and overall symptoms (Durham et al. 2003; Gumley et al. 2003; Trower et al. 2004; Turkington et al. 2008) as well as in improving social functioning (Wykes et al. 2005). A meta-analysis of CBT found small to medium effect sizes for positive and negative symptoms, mood, community functioning, and quality of life (Tarrier and Wykes 2004; Wykes et al. 2008).

CBT interventions work through collaborative identification of target problems or symptoms and development of specific cognitive and behavioral coping strategies. Intervention components include the following:

- Build a collaborative, trusting relationship with mutual goals.
- Provide psychoeducation to help the patient understand the illness and reduce stigma.
- Teach the patient to process information more accurately (e.g., challenge assumptions underlying delusions; place voices inside head) and to use more effective coping strategies to reduce the frequency or effects of hallucinations and delusions.
- Apply problem-solving and relapse-prevention strategies to maintain improvement.

CBT strategies vary in their specific treatment elements. In some CBT interventions, the therapist and the patient identify the psychological precipitants of the patient's illness and develop a normalizing rationale as a first step in the therapeutic process (Sensky et al. 2000). In others, the psychological origins of the illness are not addressed; instead, the intervention focuses exclusively on cognitive and behavioral strategies combined with social skills training (Granholm et al. 2005). All CBT approaches focus on the patient's view of the symptoms or problems and on helping him or her to develop more rational or adaptive coping responses.

Although CBT approaches to psychosis differ somewhat, all include the following core components: 1) engagement and assessment; 2) coping enhancement; 3) developing a shared understanding of the experience of psychosis (i.e., case formulation); 4) working on delusions and hallucinations, often using gentle challenging; 5) addressing mood disturbance and negative self-evaluations; and 6) managing the risk of relapse and social disability (Garety et al. 2000).

Token Economy Interventions

A token economy is a psychosocial intervention used in residential or long-term inpatient settings that applies social learning principles to improve personal hygiene, social interactions, and other adaptive behaviors. In token economy behavioral interventions, immediate positive reinforcement is provided to patients in the form of tokens or points for their performance of specified target behaviors. The tokens or points may be exchanged at a later time for individually selected reinforcers (Dixon et al. 2010).

Family Psychoeducation Interventions

Another important element to be considered for psychosocial rehabilitation is family intervention for those patients who have contact with their relatives or significant others. Family interventions that last for at least 6–9 months have been found to significantly reduce relapse and rehospitalization rates. Research also has found other benefits for patients and families, such as increased medication adherence, reduced psychiatric symptoms, and decreased levels of perceived stress (Pfammatter et al. 2006; Pitschel-Walz et al. 2001). Family members also have been found to have lower levels of burden and distress, as well as improved family relationships. Key elements of effective family interventions include illness education, crisis intervention, emotional support, and training in how to cope with illness symptoms and related problems (Pilling et al. 2002).

Psychosocial Interventions for Comorbid Conditions

Psychosocial rehabilitation recently has focused on patients with schizophrenia who have a comorbid alcohol or drug use disorder and/or who are obese. The key elements of treatment for alcohol or drug use disorders in persons with schizophrenia include motivational enhancement and behavioral strategies that focus on engagement in treatment, coping skills training, relapse prevention training, and treatment delivery in a service model that is integrated with mental health care. The duration of the recommended substance abuse treatment cannot be specified at this time; both brief (1–6 meetings) and more extended (10 or more meetings) interventions have been found to be helpful in reducing substance use and improving psychiatric symptoms and functioning (Baker et al. 2006; Mangrum et al. 2006).

Psychosocial interventions for individuals with schizophrenia who are overweight or obese include psychoeducation focused on nutritional counseling, caloric expenditure, and portion control; and behavioral self-management including motivational enhancement, goal setting, regular weighing, self-monitoring of daily food and activity levels, and dietary and physical activity modifications (Álvarez-Jiménez et al. 2008; Weber and Wyne 2006).

Social Cognition Training

Persons with schizophrenia show substantial deficits in several aspects of social cognition (Mirabilio et al. 2006, Penn et al. 2006), with impairments most frequently documented in 1) affect perception, including the ability to recognize facial and vocal expressions of emotion (Cerroni et al. 2007); 2) social perception, including the ability to judge social cues from contextual information and nonverbal communicative gestures; 3) attributional style, including biases in how individuals characteristically explain the causes for positive and negative events in their lives (e.g., "jumping to conclusions"); and 4) theory of mind, which refers to the ability to understand that others have mental states that differ from one's own and the capacity to make correct inferences about the content of those mental states (e.g., understanding false beliefs and hints, irony, metaphors) (Lysaker and Buck 2008; Riccardi et al. 2007).

Growing evidence indicates that impairments in the domain of social cognition are important determinants of poor functioning in persons with schizophrenia (Stratta et al. 2007). Such findings have generated great interest in the potential benefits of targeting social cognitive disabilities. Recent studies have explored the possibility that deficits in one domain of metacognition, self-reflectivity, may be a barrier to effective work performance (Lysaker et al. 2010). An emerging body of research suggests that social cognitive impairments are amenable to a range of psychosocial interventions.

The modifiability of social cognitive impairments in schizophrenia is supported by two general types of studies (Horan et al. 2008): 1) "broad treatment" studies that are often grounded in basic neurocognitive remediation, with additional training components designed to generalize the benefits of improved neurocognition to different aspects of functioning; and 2) "targeted treatment" studies that specifically use social cognitive training, without other intervention components, to improve performance on measures of social cognition (Kayser et al. 2006; Russell et al. 2006).

Although psychosocial treatment of social cognitive deficits in schizophrenia is currently in an early stage, the initial efficacy results are encouraging. Results of studies employing a variety of treatment approaches indicate that individuals with schizophrenia can improve their performance on tasks measuring a range of social cognitive processes (mainly affect perception) that have been linked to successful social functioning (Kern et al. 2009).

Intervention Setting and Team Framework

The literature on psychosocial interventions targeting psychotic disorders, particularly those of recent onset, can be conceptualized as consisting of two broad categories: 1) studies evaluating integrated (multidimensional) interventions delivered in tandem with pharmacological treatment, typically including education to enhance recognition of early signs of crisis; individual, group, or family therapy during hospitalization or outpatient interventions; and case management; and 2) studies evaluating specific (one-dimensional) psychosocial interventions (e.g., individual cognitive-behavioral treatment).

Psychosocial interventions can be suitable for hospitalized persons as well as stabilized outpatients. Treatment for patients hospitalized in psychiatric wards tends to be oriented toward overcoming the immediate crisis, with the goal of controlling positive symptoms and discharging the patient as soon as possible to the appropriate community services. Also during the acute psychotic patient hospitalization, CBT groups can represent an innovative psychosocial intervention of great interest (Bazzoni et al. 2001). A CBT intervention tailored to the psychiatric inpatient environment may include discussion of alternative reactions to the situation that led to hospitalization, coping strategies and model of psychiatric disorders, definition of psychotic experiences, evaluation of individual targets, identification of early signs of crisis and relapse prevention, and education about the prescribed drugs and their side effects. Controlled studies of individual CBT for psychosis found short-term advantages compared with routine treatment: shorter durations of hospital stay, decrease in hospitalizations, reduced psychotic symptoms, improved insight, and greater adherence to psychopharmacological treatment (Penn et al. 2006). Moreover, recent studies showed particular improvements in illness adaptation, symptomatology, and quality of life.

General, nonspecific behavioral treatment interventions for improving social skills can be optimized for application to important areas such as living, working, and leisure. After discharge from the acute ward, passage toward community-based psychosocial rehabilitation can be arranged in a different setting, such as that of a day hospital (Anthony 1996). For persons admitted to a highly staffed day hospital, care can be provided for the full range of post-acute conditions, although patients who are suicidal or potentially violent are usually excluded. Psychiatric service interventions such as ACT and day hospital care are designed to reduce hospital admissions for people with poor functioning who are at high risk of future relapse and rehospitalization.

Regardless of the setting, a multidisciplinary team is necessary to deliver community-based psychosocial rehabilitation care. Community mental health teams provide the core of local specialized mental health services. Usually teams are composed of professionals from several disciplines, including nurses, occupational therapists, psychiatrists, psychologists, and social workers. Community mental health teams work to keep mentally ill people in contact with care, reducing hospital admissions and improving outcomes. Such teams provide the most suitable framework for implementing psychosocial interventions (Marshall and Lockwood 1998).

The link between mental health team members and their patients is crucial; team members work with different patients as required, and several members commonly work together with the same patient. This link permits the team to contact and offer services even to reluctant or uncooperative patients (as in the ACT practice of "assertive outreach"). Team members carry small caseloads and frequently see patients in their own homes, providing 24-hour coverage for the full range of acutely ill patients.

With active support and specialized services provided by well-structured professional teams, community or home-based psychosocial interventions can more directly address factors leading to improvement in the daily life environment of the person. For example, the growth of the self-help, peer support, and advocacy movements in communities could become an important source of nonprofessional, natural supporters for improving generalization of skills into patients' everyday lives. This will require bridges to be built between professionals and other organizations.

Communication technologies also can be tapped to extend the reach of therapists and trainers into patients' natural environments. Internet chat rooms can be used for purposes of education, social support, and consultation from professionals. Telemedicine, cell phones, and programmable hand-operated computers are suitable means for augmenting generalization of skills into the community (Stip and Rialle 2005). These electronic devices are becoming less expensive and, if shown to be effective in promoting generalization and improving quality of life, could be used by mental health organizations and their patients.

Summary of Structured Psychosocial Interventions

Current targets for the treatment of schizophrenia go beyond reduction of symptoms and prevention of psychotic exacerbations to encompass symptomatic remission, functional recovery, and psychosocial rehabilitation of patients. This expanded focus has contributed to several developments, including increased availability of nonpharmacological and pharmacological treatments, changes in contexts of care, and evidence supporting a more encouraging view of the outcomes possible in schizophrenia.

The optimism that these trends reflect, however, is not always supported by unequivocal empirical evidence. The enthusiasm for new drug treatments, for instance, is tempered by data from several studies and a meta-analysis showing no clear advantage of different drugs (Leucht et al. 2009) and by evidence that the problem of overcoming barriers to treatment remains one of the crucial factors in achieving therapeutic objectives. The growing number of studies on symptomatic remission shows that symptom improvement does not always coincide with improvement in the patient's social and occupational functioning. Several research groups have found various forms of integration of the main evidence-based psychosocial treatments (Cleary et al. 2008; Jones et al. 2004). Some controversial aspects remain to be clarified, such as persistence and generalization of improvements, characteristics of patients receiving these interventions, benefits of individualization of training programs, and the necessary elements to increase participants' motivation.

Future research should reveal whether the cognitive and psychosocial rehabilitation programs that are drawing the attention of many researchers and clinicians have a greater effect than other kinds of intervention.

Cognitive Remediation

Cognitive impairment is a core feature of schizophrenia predictive of poor functional adaptation in terms of successfully coping with everyday activities such as employment, social networks, and independent living. About 85% of persons with schizophrenia consistently show a relevant impairment from 1.5 to 2.5 standard deviations below the normal range, and the remaining have a performance below that predictable from the parental level. Cognitive impairment is often evident before illness onset, persisting during life regardless of remission periods (Keefe et al. 2005).

In the past few decades, cognitive impairment in schizophrenia has become an important target of therapeutic intervention. Efforts have been made not only to understand its underlying etiopathogenic mechanisms but also to develop treatments aimed at its amelioration.

Interventions aimed at improving cognitive functioning in schizophrenia evolved from cognitive rehabilitation methods developed for people with brain injury. Cognitive remediation interventions in psychiatry are becoming a promising treatment for cognitive impairment not only in persons with psychotic disorders but also in persons with other severe mental disorders (Marronaro et al. 2009; Stratta and Rossi 2004).

Cognitive remediation therapy for schizophrenia is an intervention based on behavioral training that seeks to improve cognitive processes (attention, memory, executive function, social cognition or metacognition), with the goals of durability and generalization to community functioning (Cognitive Remediation Therapy Expert Working Group [CREW], personal communication, 2010).

Cognitive remediation acts by modifying processes that are not an expression of a neurochemical dysfunction (the target of antipsychotics) or related to the content of thought (the target of psychotherapy). It uses strategies that attempt to enable individuals with impaired cognitive functions to more efficiently cope with environmental demand, improving functional outcome through the empowerment of coping abilities.

The challenge that the neurocognitive deficits could be modified by psychological remediation with benefits not exclusively confined to the cognitive domain has been accepted. Numerous studies indicate that cognitive remediation interventions are effective and durable, with a strong translational effect on social functioning, working abilities, self-esteem, and eventually symptomatology.

Meta-analyses of randomized controlled trials of remediation techniques performed in both laboratory and clinical settings have generally found moderate to large effect sizes, varying in accordance with the goals of treatment. When the studies had a highly proximal goal of improvement on a training task (e.g., the Wisconsin Card Sorting Test [WCST]), the effect size—not surprisingly—was large. When the goals of training became more distal and thus affected by a greater number of variables, the effect sizes diminished. Still, effect sizes in the moderate range were found both for studies that used neuropsychological test results as an outcome measure and for studies with the more distal goal of improving daily functioning. Taken together, this literature informs us that remediation effects persist after cognitive remediation stops and that the cognitive gains can generalize to improvements in social behaviors, real-world problem-solving ability, and occupational outcomes (Krabbendam and Aleman 2003; Kurtz et al. 2001; McGurk et al. 2007; Twamley et al. 2003; Wykes et al. 2011).

Cognitive Remediation Models and Intervention Strategies

Current models of remediation in psychiatry are borrowed from neurocognitive research in patients with deficits resulting from traumatic brain injury (TBI). Sohlberg and Mateer (1989) divided neurocognitive rehabilitation into two approaches: compensatory and restorative. The *compensatory* approach includes alternative methods—usually environmental interventions— to lead to effective coping with tasks involving impaired cognitive functions; the *restorative* approach focuses directly on the cognitive deficit, with the purpose of restoring the impaired cognitive skill; for instance, training the individual by using drill and practice exercises.

The compensatory approach is based on the *absence* model in Diller's (1987) classification of remediation models, which assumes an intrinsic and unchanging shortage or lack of function that must be compensated by "prosthetic" environmental facilities (see below). Initially used in patients with deficits in executive functions following TBI, the compensatory approach can also be used in persons with schizophrenia by providing structured activities in which the necessary behavioral planning, organizing, initiating, and controlling are largely supported by a "prosthetic environment" (Jaeger and Berns 1999).

An example is the use of "task cards" on which a subject faced with a problem can identify and arrange the steps of his or her response; the answer to the task is divided into concrete elements—"cards"—that can be organized and consistently used. Environmental manipulation is a technique that enacts compensatory changes to facilitate adequate cognitive functioning, which usually simplifies the task. Examples of "prostheses" from environmental manipulation include use of different key hooks to help distinguish the correct key and the door to be opened, and use of pill dispensers with alarms to help remember drug therapy. Other, more sophisticated prostheses are now available—for example, "smart houses" that apply the most recent technological products of home automation to improve and facilitate the daily life functioning of persons with cognitive impairment due to schizophrenia or other conditions (Stip and Rialle 2005).

However, most neurocognitive rehabilitation paradigms in psychiatry use a restorative approach based on Diller's (1987) remediation models of deficit and interference. *Deficit* models assume that the function is not irretrievably lost but rather is deficient as a result of lack of use secondary to a neurological problem. Remediation of a functional deficit involves enrichment of the functional domain through relearning and retraining methods. *Interference* models assume a permanent loss of function as a result of a neurocognitive deficit that directly interferes with normal functioning. Remediation of functional interference involves the teaching of methods to remove the interference by isolating and bypassing it and by developing alternative cognitive strategies to overcome the functional deficit (Table 10–2).

There is wide variability in how remediation interventions are administered. Commonly used cognitive rehabilitation exercises for persons with psychiatric disorders include paper-and-pencil or computerized tasks developed for training and rehabilitation of skills.

Remediation strategies can also be categorized as "bottom-up" versus "top-down" interventions. In "bottom-up" rehabilitative interventions (i.e., from the particular to the general), discrete brain functions are targeted in specific, usually computerized, exercises. This kind of training (i.e., drill and practice) typically employs repetitive tasks, often involving several cognitive functions, such as the presentation of information to consider, remember, or quickly respond to. Task-related intensive activation of specific hypofunctioning cognitive functions can lead to durable and generalized improvements. A "top-down" remediation (i.e., from the general to the particular) teaches problem-solving strategies to be applied in everyday life. This approach, based on strategy elaboration, characterizes many of the interventions used in rehabilitation of patients with psychotic disorders. These interventions can have a positive influence on basic cognitive skills, resulting in sustained improvements in attention, memory, and verbal fluency.

Table 10–2. Cognitive impairment models and associated remediation strategies

Absence model: intrinsic and unchanging shortage or lack of a cognitive function

- *Remediation:* compensation through "prosthetic" environmental facilities

Deficit model: impaired function resulting from lack of use secondary to a neurological problem or its treatment (e.g., iatrogenic consequences of a drug or neurosurgical treatment)

- *Remediation:* enrichment and training of the impaired functional domain

Interference model: loss of function caused by a neurocognitive deficit that directly interferes with normal functioning

- *Remediation:* teaching of methods to remove the interference by isolating it and bypassing it through development of alternative cognitive strategies

Remediation Methods

Following the initial studies examining whether improvement in learning capacity in schizophrenia was possible (Choi and Kurtz 2009) and observations that cognitive impairment was indeed malleable (Szoke et al. 2008), several remediation intervention techniques were developed. These methods, which are based on the kind of help experimentally offered to subjects engaged in laboratory cognitive tasks such as the WCST, usually fit into one, but occasionally more than one, of Sohlberg and Mateer's (1989) or Diller's (1987) strategies.

Step-by-Step Instructions

In step-by-step strategies, the task rules and didactic instructions are offered at each step. The elements to be considered and those to be ignored are repeated, allowing the examined person to respond accordingly. The examiner reports on the reasonableness and correctness of the response; any errors are corrected.

Didactic Education

In didactic interventions, the basic rules of the task are explained with examples. The subject experiments with each rule while the examiner provides encouragement, feedback, and error correction. The subject is reminded of the rules at predetermined times during the task. Didactic strategies differ from

step-by-step ones in that instructions are provided only at specific times during the task, and the subject performs more practice trials during instruction,
with correction of the errors.

Monetary Reinforcement

Given a lack of motivation to follow correct procedures or rehabilitation protocols, a tangible social reinforcement (e.g., money) may be effective. Use of
monetary reinforcement is common but sometimes has negative results or
positive results of short duration. Another problem with this method is that
the person may be distracted by the reinforcement itself or be overwhelmed by
information if other forms of remediation are associated.

Verbalization

In the verbalization method, the examined person is instructed to provide an
explicit verbal description of the task. For instance, in performance of the
WCST, the person is required to verbally express the criterion of matching
(color, shape, or number) before the card sorting. Difficulties in reaching the
correct categorization by extracting the essential characteristics of the stimuli
and in elaborating a cognitive "set" that allows the deductive organization of
the stimuli can be considered the fundamental elements remediated by the
verbalization method.

Such verbal expression can force the person to use a cognitive strategy that
allows interpretation of the incoming stimulus on the basis of context and previous experience. The act of verbal expression can serve to isolate and "bypass"
the interference of deficits on cognitive functioning. Alternative or complementary hypotheses that may explain the effectiveness of verbalization include
reinforcement of working memory or attentional or motivational components.

An interesting further explanation could be that linguistically coded
thoughts support metacognition and the narrative of self. Metacognitive processes (i.e., the "knowing about knowing"), which focus on building knowledge and ability to use problem-solving strategies, are an interesting and
promising area for cognitive remediation research and practice. The metacognitive processes of self-monitoring and self-regulation are the fundamental determinants of successful functioning in the real world (Stratta et al. 2009).

Verbalization could lead to the use of metacognitive processes for behavioral monitoring and control: monitoring to subjectively evaluate the correct-

ness of the possible responses and control of one's own cognitive performance on the basis of the monitoring result (Stratta et al. 1994, 1997). Thus, verbalization could allow adequate feedback and connection between thoughts and actions.

The effectiveness of the verbalization method in a substantial proportion of people with schizophrenia has been confirmed by independent studies. The method also can allow clinicians to distinguish between patients who are likely to profit from a proposed strategy (i.e., to develop and use a conceptual approach, allowing performance remediation) and those who are unlikely to profit and whose condition might even be worsened by the strategy. Such patients show an earlier age at onset and more negative symptoms (Stratta et al. 1997).

Task Simplification

Simplification consists of reducing the task complexity to improve learning. Task simplification is usually used in combination with the scaffolding method.

Scaffolding and Errorless Learning

The scaffolding method involves enrichment of the impaired functional domain through provision of targeted information about the specific deficit the person shows during the task performance. This method allows the person to make use of skills that are still intact, with temporary support offered when and where necessary. The instructor's role is to assist the subject in grasping the fundamental characteristics of the task and, through a Socratic "maieutic" process, obtaining the correct solution to the problem.

Like scaffolding, errorless learning is borrowed from ethological studies and resembles methods used in the rehabilitation of patients with especially severe memory deficits following TBI. Errorless learning is based on the assumption that the errors implicitly remembered would interfere with the registration of correct items to be remembered; implicit memory, less damaged in schizophrenia than explicit memory, is likely more involved. However, the effectiveness of this method could be the result of a better use of residual explicit memory rather than an intact implicit memory. A main difference from the scaffolding method is a greater involvement of the subject, with important benefits to self-esteem.

Cognitive Remediation Protocols

Several cognitive remediation protocols have been used and evaluated in randomized controlled trials (see also Chapter 5, "Cognition and Schizophrenia," by Strik and colleagues, in this volume):

- *Integrated Psychological Therapy,* first to be developed, combines cognitive remediation and social skills training. It includes five subprograms of increasing complexity; the first three target neurocognitive and social cognitive functioning (cognitive differentiation, social perception, verbal communication), whereas the last two target social competence (social skills and interpersonal problem solving) (Roder et al. 2006, 2010).
- *Cognitive remediation therapy* consists of three modules designed to improve cognitive flexibility, working memory, and planning, with the aim of helping the person to develop his or her own strategies for solving problems, with a therapist providing guidelines for responding as needed (Wykes and Reeder 2005).
- *Neuropsychological Educational Approach to Remediation (NEAR)* is founded on strategy-based methods of learning rather than drill and practice exercises and is designed to stimulate intrinsic motivation and task engagement (Medalia et al. 2002).
- *Neurocognitive enhancement therapy* uses software programs designed to train attention, memory, and executive functions for cognitive remediation and vocational rehabilitation (Bell et al. 2007).
- *Cognitive adaptation training* is not really a cognitive remediation program but rather a compensatory method in which environmental supports and adaptations (signs, checklists, and medication containers with alarms) are used in association with target behaviors (taking medication; taking care of living quarters) (Velligan et al. 2008).

Heterogeneity of Cognitive Deficits and Prediction of Best Outcome

A fundamental principle of psychiatric rehabilitation is that selection of interventions must be guided by the person's individual strengths and weaknesses. A first essential point is therefore the assessment of rehabilitation appropriateness at a certain stage of the subject's life.

The success of a rehabilitation procedure derives from identification of subject characteristics—that is, the cognitive factors limiting the person's functionality, the cognitive strengths to be focused on in the intervention, and the weaknesses to be bypassed.

Although we are still far from achieving a meaningful integration of neuro-cognitive science observations into psychiatric diagnosis, the results of neuro-cognitive assessments may provide useful guidance in the rehabilitation process. For instance, through the verbalization method (see "Verbalization" subsection earlier in this section), it is possible to identify different subgroups of patients who are likely to benefit from different rehabilitation protocols. Distinguishing samples by verbalization also could identify an association with different drug treatments (Rossi et al. 2006). In regard to sample selection, the ability to im-prove one's performance on a task such as the WCST could be used as a pre-dictor of treatment outcome as well as an indication for a specific strategy and method of cognitive rehabilitation (Stratta et al. 1997). Those subjects who demonstrated improved WCST performance in response to cognitive interven-tion are likely able to use alternative strategies that allow them to "bypass" their deficits, as opposed to those who did not achieve remediation. These two groups may not be able to use the same rehabilitation protocols, but instead would benefit from different training procedures. Thus, knowledge of patient characteristics is fundamental to prediction of outcome.

Moreover, cognitive remediation interventions have been shown to achieve better results in association with other rehabilitative treatments. Results of a study by Cavallaro et al. (2009) confirmed that the addition of cognitive reme-diation to standard rehabilitation treatment of schizophrenia produced en-hanced neuropsychological benefits and increased the effects of the long-term rehabilitation program in terms of functional outcomes.

Processes and "active ingredients" able to produce improvements in pa-tients' global functioning also must be considered: motivation, regular partici-pation in the program, training session intensity, patients' work style, therapeu-tic alliance characteristics, therapists' characteristics, coaching strategies, phase of illness, self-esteem, and negative and affective symptomatology. The need to study what elements constitute the "ingredients" of a remedial therapy is clear.

It is essential to identify appropriate outcome measures that reflect a tan-gible change in cognitive functioning in daily life, particularly social life. The relevance of outcomes other than cognitive ones also should be considered; for

Table 10–3.   Factors to be considered in subject selection for best outcome prediction

Characteristics of cognitive impairment: verbalization, metacognitive evaluation

Association with other treatments: pharmacological treatment, psychosocial rehabilitation

Psychological factors: self-esteem, neuroticism

Phase of illness: high-risk population, recent-onset patients

instance, improvement of self-esteem, which has been observed after cognitive remediation treatment, could be considered an important outcome likely proximal to onset and symptomatology rather than an epiphenomenon. Psychological factors (e.g., negative beliefs about the self) may confer vulnerability to psychosis in people at ultra-high risk (Morrison et al. 2006); low self-esteem and high neuroticism are risk factors for psychosis (Krabbendam et al. 2002). Combinations of a pessimistic thinking style (e.g., low self-esteem, pessimistic explanatory style, negative emotion) and cognitive impairments are involved in paranoid delusions (Bentall et al. 2009).

These considerations could help to identify which cognitive remediation interventions are likely to be most effective for which patients (Table 10–3).

Conclusion

The importance of social dysfunction in the course of schizophrenia suggests that any interventions, psychosocial or pharmacological, must influence social functioning to have a positive effect on long-term outcome. Despite the availability of new pharmacological treatments, psychosocial interventions are needed to ensure the best psychosocial functioning achievable (Mueser and McGurk 2004). Specifically, the effects of cognitive remediation are relevant and promising in several contexts of care and open new perspectives for beneficial interaction with vocational rehabilitation. However, questions remain regarding specific therapeutic ingredients, synergistic effects, indications, and generalization of cognitive improvement. Future research should reveal whether the psychosocial and cognitive rehabilitation programs that are drawing the attention of many researchers and clinicians have a greater effect than other kinds of intervention.

References

Álvarez-Jiménez M, Hetrick SE, Gonzalez-Blanch C, et al: Non-pharmacological management of antipsychotic-induced weight gain: systematic review and 2009 PORT Psychosocial Treatment Recommendations meta-analysis of randomized controlled trials. Br J Psychiatry 193:101–107, 2008

American Psychiatric Association: Diagnostic and Statistical Manual of Mental Disorders, 4th Edition, Text Revision. Washington, DC, American Psychiatric Association, 2000

Anthony WA: Integrating psychiatric rehabilitation into managed care. Psychiatr Rehabil J 20:39–44, 1996

Anthony WA, Liberman RP: The practice of psychiatric rehabilitation: historical, conceptual, and research base. Schizophr Bull 2:542–559, 1986

Baker A, Bucci S, Lewin TJ, et al: Cognitive-behavioural therapy for substance use disorders in people with psychotic disorders: randomised controlled trial. Br J Psychiatry 188:439–448, 2006

Bazzoni A, Morosini P, Polidori G, et al: [Group cognitive behavior therapy in the routine care at a Psychiatric Ward of Diagnosis and Treatment] [in Italian]. Epidemiol Psichiatr Soc 10:27–36, 2001

Bell M, Fiszdon J, Greig T, et al: Neurocognitive enhancement therapy with work therapy in schizophrenia: 6-month follow-up of neuropsychological performance. J Rehabil Res Dev 44:761–770, 2007

Bellack AS: Skills training for people with severe mental illness. Psychiatr Rehabil J 27:375–391, 2004

Bentall RP, Rowse G, Shryane N, et al: The cognitive and affective structure of paranoid delusions: a transdiagnostic investigation of patients with schizophrenia spectrum disorders and depression. Arch Gen Psychiatry 66:236–247, 2009

Brekke J, Kay DD, Lee KS, et al: Biosocial pathways to functional outcome in schizophrenia. Schizophr Res 80:213–225, 2005

Burns T, Catty J, Becker T, et al: The effectiveness of supported employment for people with severe mental illness: a randomised controlled trial. Lancet 370:1146–1152, 2007

Cavallaro R, Anselmetti S, Poletti S, et al: Computer-aided neurocognitive remediation as an enhancing strategy for schizophrenia rehabilitation. Psychiatry Res 169:191–196, 2009

Cerroni G, Tempesta D, Riccardi I, et al: [Facial emotion recognition in schizophrenia and depression] [in Italian]. Epidemiol Psichiatr Soc 16:179–182, 2007

Choi J, Kurtz MM: A comparison of remediation techniques on the Wisconsin Card Sorting Test in schizophrenia. Schizophr Res 107:76–82, 2009

Cleary M, Hunt GE, Matheson SL, et al: Psychosocial interventions for people with both severe mental illness and substance misuse. Cochrane Database of Systematic Reviews 2008, Issue 1. Art. No.: CD001088. DOI: 10.1002/14651858. CD001088.pub2.

Cook JA, Leff HS, Blyler CR, et al: Results of a multisite randomized trial of supported employment interventions for individuals with severe mental illness. Arch Gen Psychiatry 62:505–512, 2005

Diller L: Neuropsychological rehabilitation, in Neuropsychological Rehabilitation. Edited by Meier M, Benton A, Diller L. New York, Guilford, 1987, pp 3–18

Dixon LB, Dickerson F, Bellack AS, et al: The 2009 schizophrenia PORT psychosocial treatment recommendations and summary statements. Schizophr Bull 36:48–70, 2010

Durham RC, Guthrie M, Morton RV, et al: Tayside-Fife clinical trial of cognitive-behavioural therapy for medication-resistant psychotic symptoms: results to 3-month follow- up. Br J Psychiatry 182:303–311, 2003

Garety PA, Fowler D, Kuipers E: Cognitive-behavioral therapy for medication-resistant symptoms. Schizophr Bull 26:73–86, 2000

Glynn SM, Marder SR, Liberman RP, et al: Supplementing clinic-based skills training with manual-based community support sessions: effects on social adjustment of patients with schizophrenia. Am J Psychiatry 159:829–837, 2002

Granholm E, McQuaid JR, McClure FS, et al: A randomized, controlled trial of cognitive behavioral social skills training for middle-aged and older outpatients with chronic schizophrenia. Am J Psychiatry 162:520–529, 2005

Gumley A, O'Grady M, McNay L, et al: Early intervention for relapse in schizophrenia: results of a 12-month randomized controlled trial of cognitive behavioural therapy. Psychol Med 33:419–431, 2003

Horan WP, Kern RS, Green MF, et al: Social cognitive training for individuals with schizophrenia: emerging evidence. Am J Psychiatr Rehabil 11:205–252, 2008

Jaeger J, Berns S: Neuropsychological management, treatment, and rehabilitation of psychiatric patients, in Assessment of Neuropsychological Functions in Psychiatric Disorders. Edited by Calev A. Washington, DC, American Psychiatric Press, 1999, pp 447–480

Jones C, Cormac I, Silveira da Mota Neto JI, et al: Cognitive behaviour therapy for schizophrenia. Cochrane Database of Systematic Reviews 2004, Issue 4. Art. No.: CD000524. DOI: 10.1002/14651858.CD000524.pub2.

Kayser N, Sarfati Y, Besche C, et al: Elaboration of a rehabilitation method based on a pathogenetic hypothesis of "theory of mind" impairment in schizophrenia. Neuropsychol Rehabil 16:83–95, 2006

Keefe RS, Eesley CE, Poe MP: Defining a cognitive function decrement in schizophrenia. Biol Psychiatry 57:688–691, 2005

Kern RS, Glynn SM, Horan WP, et al: Psychosocial treatments to promote functional recovery in schizophrenia. Schizophr Bull 35:347–361, 2009

Kopelowicz A, Liberman RP, Zarate R: Recent advances in social skills training for schizophrenia. Schizophr Bull 32:12–23, 2006

Krabbendam L, Janssen I, Bak M, et al: Neuroticism and low self-esteem as risk factors for psychosis. Soc Psychiatry Psychiatr Epidemiol 37:1–6, 2002

Krabbendam L, Aleman A: Cognitive rehabilitation in schizophrenia: a quantitative analysis of controlled studies. Psychopharmacology (Berl) 169:376–382, 2003

Kurtz MM, Mueser KT: A meta-analysis of controlled research on social skills training for schizophrenia. J Consult Clin Psychol 76:491–504, 2008

Kurtz MM, Moberg PJ, Gur RC, et al: Approaches to cognitive remediation of neuro-psychological deficits in schizophrenia: a review and meta-analysis. Neuropsychol Rev 11:197–210, 2001

Lehman AF, Goldberg R, Dixon LB, et al: Improving employment outcomes for persons with severe mental illnesses. Arch Gen Psychiatry 59:165–172, 2002

Leucht S, Corves C, Arbter D, et al: Second-generation versus first-generation antipsychotic drugs for schizophrenia: a meta-analysis. Lancet 373:31–41, 2009

Liberman RP, Kopelowicz A, Silverstein SM: Psychiatric rehabilitation, in Kaplan and Sadock's Comprehensive Textbook of Psychiatry, 8th Edition. Edited by Sadock BJ, Sadock VA. Baltimore, MD, Lippincott Williams & Wilkins, 2005, pp 3884–3930

Lysaker PH, Buck KD: Metacognition in schizophrenia spectrum disorders: methods of assessing metacognition within narrative and links with neurocognition. Italian Journal of Psychopathology 15:1–11, 2008

Lysaker PH, Dimaggio G, Carcione A, et al: Metacognition and schizophrenia: the capacity for self-reflectivity as a predictor for prospective assessments of work performance over six months. Schizophr Res 122:124–130, 2010

Mangrum LF, Spence RT, Lopez M: Integrated versus parallel treatment of co-occurring psychiatric and substance use disorders. J Subst Abuse Treat 30:79–84, 2006

Marronaro M, Riccardi I, Pacifico R, et al: Cognitive remediation: beyond psychosis? Italian Journal of Psychopathology 15:13–24, 2009

Marshall M, Lockwood A: Assertive community treatment for people with severe mental disorders. Cochrane Database of Systematic Reviews 1998, Issue 2. Art. No.: CD001089. DOI: 10.1002/14651858.CD001089.

McFarlane WR, Dushay RA, Deakins SM, et al: Employment outcomes in family aided assertive community treatment. Am J Orthopsychiatry 70:203–214, 2000

McGurk SR, Twamley EW, Sitzer DI, et al: A meta-analysis of cognitive remediation in schizophrenia. Am J Psychiatry 164:1791–1802, 2007

Medalia A, Revheim N, Casey M: Remediation of problem-solving skills in schizophrenia: evidence of persistent effect. Schizophr Res 57:165–171, 2002

Mirabilio D, Di Tommaso S, Riccardi I, et al: Predictors of social cognition in patients with schizophrenia. Neuropsychiatr Dis Treat 2:571–576, 2006

Morrison AP, French P, Lewis SV, et al: Psychological factors in people at ultra-high risk of psychosis: comparisons with non-patients and associations with symptoms. Psychol Med 36:1395–1404, 2006

Mueser KT, McGurk SR: Schizophrenia. Lancet 363:2063–2072, 2004

Penn DL, Addington J, Pinkham A: Social cognitive impairments, in The American Psychiatric Publishing Textbook of Schizophrenia. Edited by Lieberman JA, Stroup TS, Perkins DO. Washington, DC, American Psychiatric Publishing, 2006, pp 261–274

Pfammatter M, Junghan UM, Brenner HD: Efficacy of psychological therapy in schizophrenia: conclusions from meta-analyses. Schizophr Bull 32 (suppl 1):S64–S80, 2006

Pilling S, Bebbington P, Kuipers E, et al: Psychological treatments in schizophrenia, I: meta-analysis of family intervention and cognitive behaviour therapy. Psychol Med 32:763–782, 2002

Pitschel-Walz G, Leucht S, Bauml J, et al: The effect of family interventions on relapse and rehospitalization in schizophrenia—a meta-analysis. Schizophr Bull 27:73–92, 2001

Riccardi I, Stratta P, Mirabilio D, et al: La comprensione dell'ironia in persone affette da disturbo schizofrenico. Rivista Italiana di Psichiatria 42:1, 2007

Roder V, Mueller DR, Mueser KT, et al: Integrated psychological treatment (IPT) for schizophrenia: it is effective? Schizophr Bull 32:81–93, 2006

Roder V, Müller D, Brenner HD, et al: Integrated Psychological Therapy (IPT) for the Treatment of Neurocognition, Social Cognition and Social Competency in Schizophrenia Patients. Göttingen, Germany, Hogrefe & Huber, 2010

Rossi A, Daneluzzo E, Tomassini A, et al: The effect of verbalization strategy on Wisconsin Card Sorting Test performance in schizophrenic patients receiving classical or atypical antipsychotics. BMC Psychiatry 6:3, 2006

Russell TA, Chu E, Phillips ML: A pilot study to investigate the effectiveness of emotion recognition remediation in schizophrenia using the micro-expression training tool. Br J Clin Psychol 45:579–583, 2006

Sensky T, Turkington D, Kingdon D, et al: A randomized controlled trial of cognitive-behavioral therapy for persistent symptoms in schizophrenia resistant to medication. Arch Gen Psychiatry 57:165–172, 2000

Sohlberg MM, Mateer CA: Introduction to Cognitive Rehabilitation: Theory and Practice. New York, Guilford, 1989

Stip E, Rialle V: Environmental cognitive remediation in schizophrenia: ethical implications of "smart home" technology. Can J Psychiatry 50:281–291, 2005

Stratta P, Rossi A: [Executive function remediation in schizophrenia: possible strategies and methods] [in Italian]. Epidemiol Psichiatr Soc 13:55–65, 2004

Stratta P, Mancini F, Mattei P, et al: Information processing strategy to remediate Wisconsin Card Sorting Test performance in schizophrenia: a pilot study. Am J Psychiatry 151:915–918, 1994

Stratta P, Mancini F, Mattei P, et al: Remediation of Wisconsin Card Sorting Test performance in schizophrenia: a controlled study. Psychopathology 30:59–66, 1997

Stratta P, Riccardi I, Mirabilio D, et al: Exploration of irony appreciation in schizophrenia: a replication study on an Italian sample. Eur Arch Psychiatry Clin Neurosci 257:337–339, 2007

Stratta P, Daneluzzo E, Riccardi I, et al: Metacognitive ability and social functioning are related in persons with schizophrenic disorder. Schizophr Res 108:301–302, 2009

Szoke A, Trandafir A, Dupont ME, et al: Longitudinal studies of cognition in schizophrenia: meta-analysis. Br J Psychiatry 192:248–257, 2008

Tarrier N, Wykes T: Is there evidence that cognitive behaviour therapy is an effective treatment for schizophrenia? A cautious or cautionary tale? Behav Res Ther 42:1377–1401, 2004

Trower P, Birchwood M, Meaden A, et al: Cognitive therapy for command hallucinations: randomised controlled trial. Br J Psychiatry 184:312–320, 2004

Turkington D, Sensky T, Scott J, et al: A randomized controlled trial of cognitive-behavior therapy for persistent symptoms in schizophrenia: a five-year follow-up. Schizophr Res 98:1–7, 2008

Twamley EW, Jeste DV, Bellack AS: A review of cognitive training in schizophrenia. Schizophr Bull 29:359–382, 2003

Vallée C: Journée de Formation sur l'Approche de la Réadaptation Psychosociale. Organisés par le Service d'Ergothérapie du CHUM. Montreal, QC, Canada, Organisés par le Service d'Ergothérapie du CHUM, 2001

Velligan DI, Diamond PM, Mintz J, et al: The use of individually tailored environmental supports to improve medication adherence and outcomes in schizophrenia. Schizophr Bull 34:483–493, 2008

Weber M, Wyne K: A cognitive/behavioral group intervention for weight loss in patients treated with atypical antipsychotics. Schizophr Res 83:95–101, 2006

Wykes T, Reeder C: Cognitive Remediation Therapy for Schizophrenia: Theory and Practice. New York, Routledge, 2005

Wykes T, Hayward P, Thomas N, et al: What are the effects of group cognitive behaviour therapy for voices? A randomised control trial. Schizophr Res 77:201–210, 2005

Wykes T, Steel C, Everitt B, et al: Cognitive behaviour therapy for schizophrenia: effect sizes, clinical models, and methodological rigor. Schizophr Bull 34:523–537, 2008

Wykes T, Huddy V, Cellard C, et al: A meta-analysis of cognitive remediation for schizophrenia: methodology and effect sizes. Am J Psychiatry 168:472–485, 2011

Xiang YT, Weng YZ, Li WY, et al: Efficacy of the Community Re-Entry Module for patients with schizophrenia in Beijing, China: outcome at 2-year follow-up. Br J Psychiatry 190:49–56, 2007

11

Family Issues and Treatment in Schizophrenia

Amy L. Drapalski, Ph.D.

Lisa B. Dixon, M.D., M.P.H.

Although many families provide considerable emotional, financial, and practical support to relatives with schizophrenia, few have access to resources and services that could help them more effectively support their relative and better manage the burden, stress, and distress often associated with their caregiver role. Several effective evidence-based interventions have been developed to provide the families of individuals with schizophrenia with the information, education, and support necessary to help them effectively support their ill relative and minimize the effect of the illness on family functioning. However, few families participate in formal family programs or services or are regularly involved in their relative's ongoing clinical care. In this chapter, we discuss the potential effect of schizophrenia on the family and specific factors that may influence family needs, describe several evidence-based family interventions and possible ways to involve families in ongoing care, and propose potential strategies for working with patients and family members that minimize common barriers and promote greater family involvement.

Effect of Mental illness on the Family

Families often play a significant role in the lives of the individuals with schizophrenia. Family members typically provide ongoing emotional support, help ill relatives cope with symptoms, and assist with daily functioning. Moreover, family members often initiate and facilitate treatment when symptoms emerge or worsen and provide practical assistance, including transportation, housing, and financial support.

Despite many rewarding aspects of serving as a caregiver or support person, the time and effort often required to support an individual with schizophrenia can be overwhelming and, at times, emotionally taxing (Dixon et al. 2001b). This may be particularly true when an ill relative is not psychiatrically stable, when hospitalization is necessary, or when a family member has served as the primary caregiver for a substantial period of time. The additional stress that may result can lead to objective and subjective family burden. *Objective burden* refers to disruptions in the family unit, directly attributable to having a family member with a mental illness. Often observable, objective burden typically includes changes in family relationships and roles, daily routines, and financial status created by the additional responsibilities associated with the caregiver role (Hackman and Dixon 2008).

One potential consequence of objective burden for families is a decline in the number and quality of social relationships and fewer opportunities for participation in social activities, which can weaken or limit the family's access to or use of social supports. Reduced participation in social activities and subsequent reductions in social support may be a consequence of time limitations resulting from the growing demands of the caregiver role. Alternatively, this reduction may be directly attributable to stigma. Family members of individuals with schizophrenia and other mental illnesses may be subject to "courtesy stigma" or secondhand stigma, stigma and discrimination experienced as a direct result of their relationship to the person with a mental illness (Larson and Corrigan 2008). Fear of being treated differently, being blamed for, or in some cases being rejected because of a family member's illness can deter families from disclosing a relative's illness and its effects to others, lead them to actively avoid social situations and interactions, or cause them to distance themselves from members of their social support network.

Subjective burden, the psychological and emotional effect of schizophrenia on family members, is also common. Subjective burden often manifests as increased psychological distress (e.g., anxiety and depression) and is particularly evident among family members who are primary caregivers and relatives of those with first onset of psychosis (Lefley 1989). It is not surprising that family members experience anxiety associated with concerns regarding the safety, health, and well-being of their relative; their ability to help their relative access appropriate services; and planning for their relative's future care. At times, family members also may experience anxiety because their relative's behavior causes concern about their own safety or the safety of other family members. In addition, family members often experience a sense of grief, loss, and, at times, anger and frustration in response to the additional responsibilities placed on them as a result of their caregiver role and challenges they face in supporting their relative and ensuring that their relative is able to access the services needed. Family members often struggle to come to terms with their own grief and sense of loss over changing expectations concerning a relative's functioning, capacities, and future goals, in addition to trying to find ways to help their ill relative cope with his or her own feelings of grief and loss (Drapalski et al. 2009).

Family Issues and Needs

Given the substantial effect having a family member with schizophrenia can have on the family, understanding what information and assistance the family may need to support their relative and maintain their own health and well-being is extremely important. Previous studies suggested the need for education and information in several areas, including mental illness and mental health treatments, strategies for assisting an ill relative cope with his or her illness, tools to help the family better cope with problem behaviors, and better problem-solving skills (Hatfield 1978; Johnson 1984; Lefley 1989; Winefield and Harvey 1994). The need for assistance in helping the family better understand the structure of the mental health system, the roles and functions of various mental health providers, and how to navigate the mental health system to ensure that their needs and the needs of their ill relative are met (Drapalski et al. 2008) also has been noted, as well as the need for information on community resources (e.g., housing, employment), social and recreational programs, and planning for the future (Drapalski et al. 2008; Smith 2003). Although studies of family needs highlight the need for education and information in a variety of areas, these studies are based largely on reports from parents of adult children with schizophrenia. Consequently, these findings may not accurately reflect the needs of all family members (e.g., spouses, children) and suggest that other factors, such as relationship to the ill relative, stage of illness and recovery, and culture, should be considered.

Considerations When Determining the Needs of the Family

Family Relationships

Although parents traditionally have been viewed as serving as the primary caregivers for individuals with schizophrenia, other family members often play an important and sometimes primary role in supporting an individual with schizophrenia. Many individuals with schizophrenia are married or are in long-term relationships, and some have children (Hackman and Dixon 2008). Others have siblings or other family members, such as cousins, aunts, or uncles, who provide substantial support. Although most family members will require education, assistance, and support, the needs of family members can differ considerably depending on the role they play and the type of support they provide.

Parents

As noted previously, parents often serve as the primary caregivers for individuals with schizophrenia. Consequently, they may need information on and assistance with accessing resources to help foster independence and self-sufficiency in their child. Parents experience worry and concern regarding who will care for their child when they are gone and, as such, typically require assistance with planning for their child's future care, particularly as the parents get older (Smith 2003).

Spouses and Significant Others

Although rates of marriage among individuals with schizophrenia are somewhat lower than rates among the general population and among individuals with other mental illnesses, studies show that many individuals with schizophrenia (approximately 50% or more) have been married at some point during their life (Lehman and Steinwachs 1998; MacCabe et al. 2009; Thara and Srinivasan 1997). Spouses or significant others of individuals with schizophrenia may experience an even greater burden than parents; however, they are less likely to seek services and, as a result, are less likely to have their needs addressed (Jungbauer et al. 2004). Onset of schizophrenia or exacerbation of symptoms can have a substantial effect on a romantic relationship, particularly when the illness develops during the course of the marriage or at the beginning of a relationship or when a partner becomes threatening or violent as a consequence of the illness. In contrast to familial relationships, romantic relationships are often based on certain assumptions and expectations concerning individual roles and responsibilities, mutual understanding and support, and future goals and plans, all of which may be challenged when a spouse or significant other develops a mental illness (Jungbauer et al. 2004).

Illness may prevent an individual with schizophrenia from working for periods of time, placing the burden of financially supporting the family on the spouse. Roles may shift from that of a partner to one of a caregiver, with responsibilities previously shared within the relationship suddenly falling on the well partner. Unique to the spousal relationship is the potential for issues concerning intimacy and mutual support to arise (Glynn et al. 2006). Individuals with schizophrenia may experience changes in their sexuality and sexual interest as a result of side effects of medication or disinterest as a consequence of negative symptoms (Jungbauer et al. 2004). Alternatively, sexual disinterest on the part of spouses or significant others also may occur as the spouse takes on a caregiver role rather than serving as an equal partner within the relationship. Finally, opportunities for mutual support previously provided within the context of the relationship may be limited (Jungbauer et al. 2004). Thus, because of these unique needs, spouses and significant others may need more information and support to cope with emotional, social, and financial losses associated with their partner's illness, with a particular emphasis on the effect of the illness on the relationship, intimacy concerns, and loss of support.

Siblings

Siblings may have concerns about becoming ill themselves or passing on "bad genes" to their family, may harbor negative feelings toward their ill sibling because of past experiences, or may experience guilt associated with not having developed the illness (i.e., survivor guilt) (Glynn et al. 2006; Stalberg et al. 2004). Consequently, some siblings may use ineffective coping strategies such as avoidance, isolation, and prolonged grieving to deal with a sibling's illness (Stalberg et al. 2004). As such, siblings may benefit from education on mental illness and its etiology and the development of more effective strategies for coping with their sibling's illness and its effect on the sibling relationship. Moreover, as parents become older and less able to handle the responsibilities associated with caring for an ill child, siblings often assume the role of the caregiver. As such, siblings who had previously played a less central role in supporting a brother or sister may need information to help them gain a better understanding of their sibling's illness, current treatment and recovery goals, and how to access additional services that may be needed moving forward, including planning for future care, community resources, and vocational, housing, and other rehabilitation services (Friedrich et al. 2008).

Children

Studies have shown that more than one-third of individuals with schizophrenia have children (Hackman and Dixon 2008). Although family members often attempt to shelter children from disruptions that may be caused by the parent's illness, children often experience the same feelings of instability, confusion, embarrassment, and, sometimes, fear associated with the changes they notice in their parent's behavior and disruptions in the family associated with an emerging illness as do other family members. However, children of individuals with schizophrenia often have limited understanding or knowledge of schizophrenia and its effects. Thus, adult children of individuals with schizophrenia may have an even greater need for illness education, particularly with regard to the symptoms associated with schizophrenia and how those symptoms may influence an individual's behavior. Moreover, children may need assistance integrating this new knowledge into their understanding of prior childhood experiences and coming to terms with how those experiences have affected their relationship with their parent.

Stage of Illness and Recovery Status

The stage of illness and current recovery status of an ill family member also may influence family needs. Family members of individuals with emerging psychosis often have limited knowledge and understanding of psychosis and its treatment and, as such, are often unaware of when and how to access mental health services. Thus, these families may require information and education on mental illness, its etiology, and its course; treatments and services available to the ill relative and the family; and how families can help their relative access mental health services (Addington and Burnett 2004). Given this limited knowledge, more active outreach on the part of the clinician may be required to engage families of individuals in the early stages of illness. Diagnostic uncertainty and a lack of clarity with regard to illness course are also common among individuals in the early stage of illness. As such, the information provided to families may need to be less illness-specific and should include information on the diagnostic process and the potential variability in the course of the illness among individuals with schizophrenia (Addington and Burnett 2004).

Families of individuals experiencing a reemergence or exacerbation of symptoms may benefit from information on coping strategies and relapse prevention as well as greater support from mental health providers to ensure that the family member is receiving the services needed to prevent worsening of symptoms or hospitalization (Glynn et al. 2006). In contrast, families of individuals who have made significant progress in their recovery may require more targeted information aimed at helping the individual achieve personal recovery goals. This may include information on vocational and educational programs and services, developing and maintaining social relationships, problem-solving around a particular issue or concern, increasing participation in social and leisure activities and hobbies, opportunities for housing and independent living, or simply working with individuals and family members to help identify recovery goals and next steps (Drapalski et al. 2009).

Culture

Cultural influences also must be taken into account when working with the families of individuals with schizophrenia. Most family interventions are based largely on Western values and norms, and studies of their effectiveness were conducted primarily with Caucasian participants. As a result, many of these interventions are based on the notion that the mental health system is the primary means through which individuals with mental illness receive care, and the primary goal of treatment is to increase independence and self-sufficiency (Snowden 2007; Xiong et al. 1994). However, these views are often in sharp contrast to the values and norms of many other cultures.

Conceptualizations of mental illness, treatment goals and expected treatment outcomes, comfort with different treatment strategies, and the perceived role of the family in an individual's mental health treatment differ substantially from culture to culture. For example, the family tends to play a more important role in Latino, Asian American, and African American communities when compared with white communities. The emphasis placed on family in these communities may reflect a greater sense of collectivism (Snowden 2007). This focus on collectivism may result in families placing greater value on family relationships and support, which instills a sense of obligation or responsibility to care for family members, despite the additional burden that that responsibility may create (Guada et al. 2009; Snowden 2007). As a result, families that place greater emphasis on collectivism may enter treatment with the expectation that family members will be involved in all aspects of care. Moreover, Latino, Asian American, and African American individuals with schizophrenia are more apt to live with family than are Caucasian schizophrenic patients and thus often receive greater instrumental or practical assistance from family (Snowden 2007). Therefore, culture can substantially affect the acceptability and effectiveness of family services, suggesting the need to adapt these services so they are more in line with the families' cultural expectations and norms.

Family Services and Programs

Programs have been developed in an attempt to address the needs of the family of individuals with schizophrenia. Despite differing somewhat in their approach to providing services, each program offers potential benefits and opportunities to directly target and address the individual needs of the family. In addition to formal family programs, more informal family involvement in the treatment of individuals with schizophrenia has proven to be beneficial. Thus, when working with individuals with schizophrenia and their families, treatment providers should be aware of the services available to the family members and the ways in which family can be involved in the care of the individuals with whom they work.

Family Psychoeducation Programs

Family psychoeducation programs were originally developed with the goal of reducing expressed emotion by improving family communication and problem-solving skills. Facilitated by a mental health professional, most family psychoeducation programs include both the patient and the family member and offer education, communication and problem-solving skill building, and mutual support (Cuijpers 1999), although the manner in which these are provided varies depending on the format and structure of the particular program (e.g., individual vs. group format; location where the program is held; length of the intervention; whether the ill relative is involved). Two of the most commonly used family psychoeducation programs—behavioral family therapy (Mueser and Glynn 1999) and multifamily group therapy (McFarlane 2002b)—clearly reflect these differences.

In behavioral family therapy, sessions are conducted with an individual family, with sessions held on a weekly or biweekly basis for 9–12 months. After conducting an assessment of individual and family strengths, weaknesses, needs, and treatment goals, behavioral family therapy progresses in a fairly standard sequence. Initially, sessions focus on the provision of education on schizophrenia, its treatment, and other topics of relevance to the family and then transition to communication skills training, followed by problem-solving skills training, and, finally, assistance in helping the family manage problems or goals unique to the individual and/or family (Mueser and Glynn 1999). Alternatively, multifamily group therapy involves several families meeting as a group for 9 months to 2–3 years. Similar to behavioral family therapy, multifamily groups are led by a mental health professional, with group sessions focused on providing education, support, and problem-solving skill building. Multifamily group therapy begins with several sessions focused on helping the facilitator join and build an alliance with the individual and the family. Joining sessions are followed by a half-day or day-long workshop aimed at providing the individual and his or her family members with educa-tion about schizophrenia, its etiology, and its treatment. On completion of the educational workshop, families participate in group sessions, held on a bi-monthly basis, during which families receive additional education and infor-mation, mutual support, and group-based problem-solving skills building (McFarlane 2002a).

Regardless of the manner in which family psychoeducation programs are offered, the benefits of family participation in family psychoeducation pro-grams for individuals with schizophrenia are evident. Most notable is that family participation in family psychoeducation programs that last 6 months or longer has consistently been shown to be associated with significantly lower rates of relapse and rehospitalization in individuals with schizophrenia with a recent illness exacerbation (Baucom et al. 1998; Pitschel-Walz et al. 2001). In fact, meta-analyses of family psychoeducation programs suggest that partici-pation in interventions for 6 months or more can reduce relapse rates by as much as 50% (Baucom et al. 1998). Other benefits of family participation in family psychoeducation programs include improved treatment adherence (Falloon et al. 1985), social functioning (Montero et al. 2001), employment rates (McFarlane et al. 2000), and negative symptoms (Dyck et al. 2000) in the relative with schizophrenia. For family members, participation in family psychoeducation programs was associated with lower levels of subjective bur-den (Falloon and Pederson 1985); improved life satisfaction, knowledge, hope, and empowerment (Resnick et al. 2004); and better family functioning (Cuijpers 1999; Murray-Swank and Dixon 2005) compared with those who did not participate in family psychoeducation programs (see Table 11–1).

Although substantial evidence indicates the effectiveness of family psycho-education programs for individuals with recent symptom exacerbation, the evi-dence for individuals who are currently psychiatrically stable has been mixed (Dixon et al. 2010), with some studies finding that individuals whose families participated in family psychoeducation programs had fewer hospitalizations and lower relapse rates (Bradley et al. 2006; Dyck et al. 2002; Ran et al. 2003) but others finding no differences (Dyck et al. 2000; Magliano et al. 2006). Al-though the evidence for the effectiveness of family psychoeducation programs for more psychiatrically stable individuals is less clear, other patient and family benefits have been noted and warrant family participation in family psychoedu-cation programs. These benefits include fewer psychiatric symptoms (Dyck et

Table 11–1.   Potential benefits of family psychoeducation for individuals with schizophrenia and their families

Benefits to the patient	Benefits to the family member
• Lower rehospitalization and relapse rates (Baucom et al. 1998; Pitschel-Walz et al. 2001)	• Lower level of subjective burden (Falloon and Pederson 1985)
• Improved treatment adherence (Falloon et al. 1985; Ran et al. 2003; Zhang et al. 1993)	• Improved life satisfaction, hope, and empowerment (Resnick et al. 2004)
• Better social (Magliano et al. 2006; Montero et al. 2001) and vocational functioning (Magliano et al. 2006)	• Greater knowledge of schizophrenia (Ran et al. 2003; Resnick et al. 2004)
• Increased rates of employment (McFarlane et al. 2000)	• Better family functioning and improved family relationships (Cuijpers 1999; Murray-Swank and Dixon 2005; Ran et al. 2003)
• Fewer psychiatric symptoms (Dyck et al. 2000)	

al. 2000), improved social and vocational functioning (Magliano et al. 2006), and better treatment adherence (Ran et al. 2003; Zhang et al. 1993) in individuals with schizophrenia and greater knowledge of schizophrenia (Ran et al. 2003), improved family relationships (Ran et al. 2003), and more positive perceptions of professional and social support among family members (Magliano et al. 2006). Given the apparent benefits of these programs, the Schizophrenia Patient Outcomes Research Team (PORT) has recommended that individuals with schizophrenia and their families be offered family interventions that are at least 6–9 months in length (Dixon et al. 2010).

Brief Family Educational Groups

Because of the training and long-term commitment on the part of the provider, patient, and family, offering long-term family psychoeducational programs like behavioral family therapy and multifamily group therapy may not be feasible or practical for some mental health providers or mental health systems. Moreover, some families may not have the interest or capacity to be involved in longer family psychoeducation programs, and others may not require such intensive family services. Thus, brief educational programs (those lasting less than 6 months) can be offered to families when longer interventions are not feasible, readily available, or of interest to families (Drapalski et al. 2009). Similar to longer family psychoeducation programs, brief educational programs are typically led by a mental health professional and include sessions that focus on providing families with education, improving communication and problem-solving skills, and increasing opportunities for mutual support. However, brief educational programs are often time-limited (e.g., 6 weeks, 10 weeks) and can occur with or without the patient present.

Shorter programs appear to have limited effect on relapse and rehospitalization rates when compared with longer programs, but several important benefits to participation in brief educational programs have been documented. Participation in brief educational programs has been shown to lead to increased knowledge of schizophrenia, more positive perceptions of mental health providers and the mental health system (Posner et al. 1992), and reduced family burden and distress (Cuijpers 1999). Benefits to the individual with schizophrenia have included reduced symptoms (Merinder et al. 1999), better self-care, more social and vocational interest (Magliano et al. 2006; Xiong et al. 1994), and better treatment adherence (Pitschel-Walz et al. 2006; Xiong et al. 1994). Thus, brief educational interventions may serve as an alternative strategy for increasing knowledge, reducing family burden and distress, and improving patient outcomes when longer interventions may not be feasible or warranted (Drapalski et al. 2009). Consequently, updated PORT recommendations suggest that family interventions lasting less than 6 months but at least four sessions be offered to these families (Dixon et al. 2010)

Brief Consultation

Brief consultation represents another alternative to working with families. Brief consultation typically involves a mental health professional (either the patient's mental health provider or a different provider) meeting with the family with the goal of identifying a specific family problem and developing a plan for addressing that problem (Family Institute for Education, Practice and Research, and New York State Office of Mental Health, unpublished manuscript, Department of Psychiatry, University of Rochester, Rochester, NY, 2007). Consultation can last anywhere from one to five sessions and occur with or without the patient present. Although the content is largely dependent on the needs of the family, family consultation often includes some education and problem solving. Initial sessions tend to focus on assessing family needs and working with the family to identify a specific problem to be addressed within the context of the consultation. Within this session, the consultant provides information on possible ways in which the problem could be addressed and helps the family to identify one particular strategy they would like to use to address that goal (Family Institute for Education, Practice and Research, and New York State Office of Mental Health, unpublished manuscript, 2007). When needed, subsequent sessions focus on implementing ways to resolve the specific problem or issue identified by the family (e.g., education, coping skills development, referrals to community resources). Once the problem has been resolved, the consultation is terminated, with the understanding that if another problem or need should arise in the future, a new consultation can be initiated.

For example, during an initial consultation session in which a patient and family member are present, it may become apparent that one of the most pressing problems is increasing arguments and conflicts between the patient and the family members regarding treatment decisions. After discussing potential options for addressing this problem, the patient and family member decide to address this problem by finding more effective ways to communicate with each other. A decision is then made that the patient, family member, and consultant will meet for several sessions, with each session focused on helping the family to develop more effective communication and conflict resolution skills. This might involve several sessions in which the consultant teaches them specific skills to communicate more effectively with one another regarding treatment decisions, including listening to another point of view, agreeing to disagree, and compromise and negotiation. Alternatively, consultation may be conducted with the family only and may be relatively short. For example, it may become clear during the initial session that the family member needs additional information about his or her relative's illness, ways to cope with the effects the illness has on the family, and how to care for his or her own health and well-being and could benefit from the support of others in a similar situation. After presenting several possible options for addressing those concerns, the family member decides that attending a peer-led educational and support group would best meet his or her current needs. The consultant would then provide the family member with contact information for the program and develop a plan for helping the family member contact the program and initiate participation.

To date, only a few studies have examined the effectiveness of family consultation. However, these studies found that family consultation increased family members' self-efficacy or perception of their ability to successfully cope with the effects of their relative's mental illness (Solomon et al. 1996, 1997), suggesting that family consultation may help family members learn strategies or skills for coping with particular problems or issues associated with a relative's illness. Greater knowledge of these skills may serve to increase a family member's confidence in his or her ability to cope with the effects of the illness, which may improve the quality of the family relationship. Although additional research is needed to more clearly determine the effect of family consultation on both patient and family outcomes, family consultation may be useful when a specific, circumscribed problem or issue can be addressed in a relatively short time or when the patient is not interested in participating with the family.

Community-Based, Peer-Led Programs

One of the most well-known peer-led educational programs for families is the National Alliance on Mental Illness's (NAMI) Family-to-Family Education Program. Based on theories of stress, coping, and adaptation (Dixon et al. 2001b), the goal of the Family-to-Family Education Program is to improve the well-being of the family by providing classes that focus on information on mental illness and mental health treatments; improving communication and problem-solving skills; understanding the personal effect of the illness on the family; and information on and assistance with potential ways to advocate for an ill relative (Murray-Swank and Dixon 2005). In addition to the information and education provided in the classes, the course allows the opportunity for mutual understanding and support. The Family-to-Family Education Program is delivered by trained volunteers who have a family member with a mental illness. Classes are held on a weekly basis for 12 weeks and last approximately 2–3 hours. Classes are free and available to any individual with a family member with serious mental illness.

Similarly, Journey of Hope is a free 8-week course, led by trained family members and available to caregivers of individuals with a mental illness. The course is held once a week for 1.5–2 hours and focuses on providing education, skills building, and mutual support. Classes focus on the etiology and treatment of mental illnesses, communication and problem-solving skill development, better understanding of the mental health services system and how to access services, normalizing family members' reactions to the illness, and strategies for coping with the effects of the illness (Pickett-Schenk et al. 2006b).

Participation in the Family-to-Family Education Program was shown to be associated with several positive outcomes, including reduced subjective burden and worry, greater empowerment, more knowledge of serious mental illness and the mental health system, and better self-care among family members (Dixon et al. 2001a, 2001b; Dixon et al. 2004). Similarly, family members who participated in Journey of Hope had greater knowledge of mental illness, greater satisfaction with the care they provided to their ill relative, less need for information about family problem solving and communication and ways to help improve their relative's social interaction and activity, and fewer depressive symptoms (Pickett-Schenk et al. 2006a, 2006b, 2008). Community-based, peer-led programs may be particularly useful when the ill relative is not consistently involved in treatment or not interested in participating in a family program but the family is clearly in need of services, when the family prefers to receive services in the community rather than in a mental health clinic, or when the family would benefit from both education and mutual support.

Family Involvement in Ongoing Clinical Care

Involving family in a patient's ongoing mental health care also can be of benefit, with even minimal family-provider contact producing positive effects. Family involvement can involve intermittent telephone contacts to families, a family member's attendance for part of an individual session or during treatment planning, or separate meetings with the patients and family members to address specific needs. Efforts to involve family members often require little time on the part of providers but can be extremely useful for patients, families, and providers alike (Dixon et al. 2000). More informal family-provider contact offers opportunities for helping family members learn more about schizophrenia and its treatment, identify strategies and develop skills to assist them in helping their relative cope with symptoms and improve the family relationship, and obtain much-needed support.

Family involvement can also be useful in helping the clinician provide the most effective and appropriate treatment. Family members often spend considerably more time with patients than with their clinicians. Therefore, family members often have knowledge of the individual's functioning outside of the treatment setting; the history and course of the relative's illness, including factors associated with the worsening of symptoms; and personal strengths, interests and talents, and coping skills that could aid in treatment planning. Moreover, by actively collaborating and working with family members and patients, treatment providers can ensure that the treatment correctly reflects the individual's needs and goals and can identify ways in which the family may support progress toward treatment goals (Drapalski et al. 2009). Finally, more informal contact also may give clinicians the opportunity to provide families with information on the benefits of family involvement and the availability of more formal family programs and supports that may be useful to the family.

Involving Families in Care

Discussing and Initiating Family Involvement With Patients

Many individuals with schizophrenia are unaware of the programs available to patients and family members, their ability to have family involved in their care, and the potential benefits of their involvement; however, studies have shown that when asked, as many as two-thirds of individuals with schizophrenia express interest in having one or more family members involved in their treatment (Murray-Swank et al. 2007). Given this lack of knowledge, most individuals with schizophrenia are unlikely to initiate a conversation about family involvement with their clinician, thus placing the responsibility for initiating this conversation on the clinician. Engaging patients in a discussion of family involvement affords the clinician the opportunity to gain a better understanding of the individual's support system, assess the patient's interest in having family involved, and determine which services would benefit the patient most. In addition, initiating a discussion of family involvement allows the clinician to provide the patient with information on the benefits of family involvement and available services, which can help the patient to make a more informed decision about if and how they would like their family involved

(Drapalski et al. 2009). For example, a clinician can initiate a conversation about family involvement by gathering information about the patient's family and support network and the patient's perception of the family's understanding and knowledge of the patient's illness and treatment. The following are examples of questions that can be used to initiate and facilitate this discussion (S. M. Glynn, A. N. Cohen, A. Murray-Swank, et al., "Family Member Provider Outreach [FMPO] Manual," unpublished manual, Baltimore, MD, VA Maryland Health Care System, 2010):

- Tell me about your family. Are there any other individuals you consider to be "like" family to you?
- What are your family's thoughts or understanding of your difficulties? What do they think led up to you needing treatment?
- How does your family feel about you getting mental health treatment?
- What is their understanding of the goals you have for your recovery and treatment?

Once a clinician has gained a better understanding of the patient's family and the family's perception of the patient's illness, the clinician can then work with the patient to explore the potential benefits of involving family. The following questions can be used to explore the potential benefits of having family more involved (S. M. Glynn, A. N. Cohen, A. Murray-Swank, et al., "Family Member Provider Outreach [FMPO] Manual," unpublished manual, Baltimore, MD, VA Maryland Health Care System, 2010):

- What might be some benefits to having your family more involved in your care? To having them understand your difficulties a little better?
- How could your family help you work toward the goals you have for your recovery and treatment?
- What do you think your family might need to assist you in achieving your goals?
- How has your family supported you in the past? How do you think they could support you with your new goals?
- Have you wanted your family to have a chance to talk with your treatment team, psychiatrist, and other mental health providers? How would contact with the treatment team be helpful for your family? For you?

Patient Barriers to Family Involvement

Most individuals with schizophrenia will be agreeable to family involvement, but some individuals may express hesitation or reluctance to involving family in their care. Reasons for this reluctance often reflect several commonly cited barriers to family involvement, including limited knowledge about the availability of family programs, the possibility of family involvement, and the potential benefits of including family in care; concerns about privacy; concerns about overinvolvement of family and subsequent loss of independence; fear of stigma; and concerns that greater involvement will create additional family burden or family conflict (Dixon et al. 2001a; Murray-Swank and Dixon 2005). However, many of these concerns or barriers can be allayed by discussing the individual's concerns about family involvement and educating patients about family involvement and family services.

When patients are concerned that health information will be disclosed without their knowledge or consent, providers can work with the patient to clearly outline what information can and cannot be shared with family (Murray-Swank and Dixon 2005). Some individuals are concerned that family will become overinvolved in their care, which may lead to diminished autonomy and independence, particularly with regard to treatment decisions. Discussing and clearly outlining the role that the patient would like the family to play in treatment may alleviate some of these concerns. Fear of being stigmatized or treated differently if a family member knew more about their illness, symptoms, and treatment also may deter individuals from involving family (McFarlane et al. 2003). Although increasing the family's knowledge about their relative's illness may have potential disadvantages, clinicians can help the patient to explore the potential benefits to having family know more about his or her illness and treatment. These benefits can include greater knowledge of warning signs or symptoms that may help the family member to identify when the patient may need additional support from providers to maintain health and prevent hospitalization, gain better understanding of ways to assist the ill relative in coping with symptoms, or provide assistance in remembering to take medications or attend appointments.

Many individuals with schizophrenia often feel as though they are already a substantial burden on family members. Asking family to be more involved in their care or to participate in family services would increase that burden, which many individuals with schizophrenia are reluctant to do (Murray-Swank et al. 2007). Patients often cite concerns about the time commitment participation would involve, adding to their relative's already hefty responsibilities, and particularly in the case of siblings and children, reluctance to burden the family member with the patient's problems because of the family member's responsibility to his or her own family. Finally, unresolved symptoms may serve as a barrier to family involvement. Individuals experiencing symptoms of paranoia may be suspicious of family members or have specific delusions related to family members, which may affect their willingness to have their family involved. Thus, it is important for providers to explore and address these concerns with patients and help them to overcome concerns about having family members or other supportive individuals involved.

Discussing and Initiating Family Involvement With Families

Although many individuals with schizophrenia are interested in having family members involved in their care, most family members do not receive family services, and few report having any contact with their relative's treatment providers (Dixon et al. 2000; Resnick et al. 2005). Many family members are unaware of the services available to family members of individuals with mental illness and the ability to be more involved in the relative's care. Even when families are interested in involvement, lack of knowledge about the mental health system and their relative's treatment providers often precludes involvement. Thus, engaging families in care may require more active outreach and effort on the part of providers. Moreover, once initial contact has been made, providers should attempt to assess the family members' knowledge and understanding of their relative's illness and what programs or services the family may need to continue to support both their relative and their own health and wellness. The following are examples of questions that can be used to that end (S.M. Glynn, A.N. Cohen, A. Murray-Swank, et al., "Family Member Provider Outreach [FMPO] Manual," unpublished manual, Baltimore, MD, VA Maryland Health Care System, 2010).

- What are your thoughts about your relative's current problems and goals? How do you feel you might be able to help him or her with those problems and goals?
- Are there any concerns you have about his or her treatment?

- What do you think you might need to help your family member with these problems and goals?
- Are there other things you would like to be different or better for your family member? What do you think you might need to make that happen?

Family Barriers to Involvement

Even with knowledge of mental illness, mental health treatments, and available family services, family members of individuals with schizophrenia may be reluctant or ambivalent about involvement in their relative's care. Common family-related barriers to involvement include concerns about confidentiality and privacy; previous negative experiences with the mental health system; and practical or instrumental factors (Dixon et al. 2001a; Murray-Swank and Dixon 2005). If patients have not discussed their interest in family involvement with their family members, family members may not broach the subject out of respect for the individuals' privacy. Family members may feel more comfortable being involved when their relative has expressed interest in having them be a part of the care and discussed the possibility of clinician-family contact.

Stigma associated with mental illness and prior negative experiences with mental health providers and the mental health system also may deter family involvement. As mentioned previously, families may conceal a relative's illness from others out of fear that they will be blamed or in some way be held responsible for their relative's current mental health problems (McFarlane et al. 2003). Moreover, many family members report prior negative experiences with the mental health system and mental health providers. In many cases, the first and sometimes only family contact with a mental health provider occurs within the context of a hospitalization. Hospitalizing a relative can be a frightening and distressing experience, particularly early in the illness when family members have even less understanding of their relative's illness or when involuntary hospitalization is required. Family members may feel thwarted in their efforts to speak with mental health providers, obtain information about their relative's well-being, and be involved in decisions concerning their relative's future care and treatment. These experiences may lead to distrust of the mental health system and, subsequently, greater reluctance to be involved in future care. By reaching out to families, providers may be able to correct some of the misperceptions that may contribute to perceived stigma and minimize the effect of prior negative experiences with mental health providers, which may increase the family's willingness to be involved (McFarlane et al. 2003; Murray-Swank and Dixon 2005).

Finally, more practical barriers, such as lack of time, energy, and transportation, may prevent family members from being involved in a relative's care (Cohen et al. 2008; Murray-Swank and Dixon 2005). Work and family schedules may conflict with traditional clinic hours, requiring clinicians and mental health systems to think more flexibly about when, where, and how they offer family services. Instituting evening and/or weekend hours, offering telephone and/or in-home sessions, mailing educational materials or other information to family members, and supplementing in-person meetings with telephone contacts are all potential strategies for overcoming practical barriers to involvement that family members often experience (Cohen et al. 2008). Discussing all the possible options and tailoring family involvement to better meet the needs and preferences of the family can help clinicians to overcome barriers to family involvement and increase the likelihood that the family will stay involved.

Conclusion

Families of individuals with schizophrenia often require considerable information, education, and support in order for them to continue to support their ill relative in recovery from mental illness. Several programs have been developed in an effort to meet the diverse needs of these families. Although participation in these programs has been shown to be associated with benefits, few families participate in these programs, and many have little to no involvement in their relative's ongoing clinical care. Many individuals with schizophrenia are interested in having their family more involved in their care; however, lack of knowledge about available family programs, the possibility of having their family involved in their ongoing treatment, and the potential benefits of family involvement often precludes family involvement. By engaging individuals with schizophrenia and their families in a discussion regarding family involvement, providers can help patients and families to identify their needs and goals, determine which services would best address those needs, and discover and, subsequently, overcome any patient or family barriers to involvement. Thus, this discussion may increase the likelihood of family involvement, which may lead to better outcomes for both the patient and the family.

Suggested Readings

Books/Manuals

Froggatt D, Fadden G, Johnson DL, et al: Families as Partners in Care: A Guidebook for Implementing Family Work. Toronto, ON, Canada, World Fellowship for Schizophrenia and Allied Disorders, 2007

Jones S, Hayward P: Coping With Schizophrenia: A Guide for Patients, Families, and Carers. Oxford, UK, Oneworld Publications, 2004

McFarlane WR: Multifamily Groups in the Treatment of Severe Psychiatric Disorders. New York, Guilford, 2002

Mueser KT, Gingerich S: The Complete Family Guide to Schizophrenia: Helping Your Loved One Get the Most Out of Life. New York, Guilford, 2006

Mueser KT, Glynn SM: Behavioral Family Therapy for Psychiatric Disorders, 2nd Edition. Oakland, CA, New Harbinger Publications, 1999

Articles

Cohen A, Glynn SM, Murray-Swank AB, et al: The family forum: directions for the implementation of family psychoeducation for severe mental illness. Psychiatr Serv 59:40–48, 2008

Drapalski AL, Leith J, Dixon L: Involving families in the care of persons with schizophrenia and other serious mental illnesses: history, evidence, and recommendations. Clin Schizophr Related Psychoses 3:39–49, 2009

Murray-Swank A, Dixon LB, Stewart B: Practical interviewing strategies for building an alliance with the families of patients who have severe mental illness. Psychiatr Clin North Am 30:167–180, 2007

Relevant Web Sites/Resources

National Alliance on Mental Illness: www.nami.org

National Alliance on Mental Illness of New York State (NAMI-NYS): Family Survival Handbook: Reaching Mental Health Recovery Together (A Joint Collaboration between Family Institute for Education, Practice & Research, NAMI-NYS, and New York State Office of Mental Health). June 17, 2009. Available at: http://www.naminys.org/family-toolkit. Accessed September 2011.

The New York Family Institute for Education, Practice and Research: www.nysfamily-institute.org

Substance Abuse and Mental Health Administration: Family Psychoeducation Evidence-Based Practices (EBP) KIT. March 2010. Available at: http://store.samhsa.

gov/product/Family-Psychoeducation-Evidence-Based-Practices-EBP-KIT/
SMA09-4423. Accessed August 23, 2011

References

Addington J, Burnett P: Working with families in the early stages of psychosis, in Psychological Interventions in Early Psychosis: A Treatment Manual. Edited by Gleeson JFM, McGorry PD. West Sussex, UK, Wiley, 2004, pp 99–116

Baucom DH, Shoham V, Mueser KT, et al: Empirically supported couple and family interventions for marital distress and adult mental health problems. J Consult Clin Psychol 66:53–58, 1998

Bradley GM, Couchman GM, Perlesz A, et al: Multiple-family group treatment for English and Vietnamese-speaking families living with schizophrenia. Psychiatr Serv 57:521–530, 2006

Cohen A, Glynn SM, Murray-Swank AB, et al: The family forum: directions for the implementation of family psychoeducation for severe mental illness. Psychiatr Serv 59:40–48, 2008

Cuijpers P: The effects of family intervention on relatives' burden: a meta-analysis. J Ment Health 8:275–285, 1999

Dixon L, Lucksted A, Stewart B, et al: Therapists' contacts with family members of persons with severe mental illness in a community treatment program. Psychiatr Serv 51:1449–1451, 2000

Dixon L, McFarlane WR, Lefley H, et al: Evidence-based practices for services to families of people with psychiatric disabilities. Psychiatr Serv 52:903–910, 2001a

Dixon L, Stewart B, Burland J, et al: Pilot study of the effectiveness of the Family-to-Family Education Program. Psychiatr Serv 52:965–967, 2001b

Dixon L, Lucksted A, Stewart B, et al: Outcomes of the peer-taught 12-week Family-to-Family Education Program for severe mental illness. Acta Psychiatr Scand 109:207–215, 2004

Dixon LB, Dickerson F, Bellack AS, et al: The 2009 Schizophrenia PORT psychosocial treatment recommendations and summary statements. Schizophr Bull 36:48–70, 2010

Drapalski AL, Marshall T, Seybolt D, et al: The unmet needs of families of adults with mental illness and preferences regarding family services. Psychiatr Serv 59:655–662, 2008

Drapalski AL, Leith J, Dixon L: Involving families in the care of persons with schizophrenia and other serious mental illnesses: history, evidence, and recommendations. Clin Schizophr Related Psychoses 3:39–49, 2009

Dyck D, Short R, Hendryx M, et al: Management of negative symptoms among patients with schizophrenia attending multiple-family groups. Psychiatr Serv 51:513–519, 2000

Dyck DG, Hendryz MS, Short RA, et al: Service use among patients with schizophrenia in psychoeducational multiple-family group treatment. Psychiatr Serv 53:749–754, 2002

Falloon IR, Pederson J: Family management in the prevention of morbidity of schizophrenia: the adjustment of the family unit. Br J Psychiatry 147:156–163, 1985

Falloon IR, Boyd JL, McGill CW, et al: Family management in the prevention of morbidity of schizophrenia: clinical outcome of a two-year longitudinal study. Arch Gen Psychiatry 42:887–896, 1985

Friedrich RM, Lively S, Rubenstein LM: Sibling's coping strategies and mental health services: a national study of siblings of persons with schizophrenia. Psychiatr Serv 59:261–267, 2008

Glynn SM, Cohen AN, Dixon LB, et al: The potential impact of the recovery movement on family interventions for schizophrenia: opportunities and obstacles. Schizophr Bull 32:451–463, 2006

Guada J, Brekke JS, Floyd R, et al: The relationship among perceived criticism, family contact, and consumer clinical and psychosocial functioning for African-American consumers with schizophrenia. Community Ment Health J 45:106–116, 2009

Hackman A, Dixon L: Issues in family services for persons with schizophrenia. Psychiatric Times, 2008. Available at: www.psychiatrictimes.com/showArticle.jhtml?articleID=206900852. Accessed April 11, 2011.

Hatfield AB: Psychological costs of schizophrenia to the family. Soc Work 23:355–359, 1978

Johnson D: The needs of the chronically mentally ill: as seen by the consumer, in The Chronically Mentally Ill: Research and Services. Edited by Mirabi M, Feldman L. New York, Spectrum Publications, 1984, pp 45–48

Jungbauer J, Wittmund B, Dietrich S, et al: The disregarded caregivers: subjective burden in spouses of schizophrenia patients. Schizophr Bull 30:665–675, 2004

Larson J, Corrigan P: The stigma of families with mental illness. Acad Psychiatry 32:87–91, 2008

Lefley HP: Family burden and family stigma in major mental illness. Am Psychol 44:556–560, 1989

Lehman AF, Steinwachs DM: Patterns of usual care for schizophrenia: initial results from the Schizophrenia Patients Outcomes Research Team survey. Schizophr Bull 24:11–20, 1998

MacCabe JH, Koupil I, Leon DA: Lifetime reproductive output over two generations in patients with psychosis and their unaffected siblings: the Uppsala 1915–1929 birth cohort multigenerational study. Psychol Med 39:1667–1676, 2009

Magliano L, Fiorillo A, Malangone C, et al: Patient functioning and family burden in a controlled, real-world trial of family psychoeducation for schizophrenia. Psychiatr Serv 57:1784–1791, 2006

McFarlane WR: Empirical studies of outcome in multifamily groups, in Multifamily Groups in the Treatment of Severe Psychiatric Disorders. Edited by McFarlane WR. New York, Guilford, 2002a, pp 49–70

McFarlane WR: Multifamily Groups in the Treatment of Severe Psychiatric Disorders. New York, Guilford, 2002b

McFarlane WR, Dushay RA, Deakins SM, et al: Employment outcomes in family-aided assertive community treatment. Am J Orthopsychiatry 70:203–214, 2000

McFarlane WR, Dixon L, Lukens E, et al: Family psychoeducation and schizophrenia: a review of the literature. J Marital Fam Ther 29:223–245, 2003

Merinder LB, Viuff AG, Laugensen HD, et al: Patient and relative education in community psychiatry: a randomized controlled trial regarding its effectiveness. Soc Psychiatry Psychiatr Epidemiol 34:287–294, 1999

Montero I, Asencio A, Hernandez I, et al: Two strategies for family intervention in schizophrenia: a randomized trial in a Mediterranean environment. Schizophr Bull 27:661–670, 2001

Mueser KT, Glynn SM: Behavioral Family Therapy for Psychiatric Disorders, 2nd Edition. Oakland, CA, New Harbinger Publications, 1999

Murray-Swank A, Dixon L: Evidence based practices for working with families of individuals with serious mental illness, in Evidence-Based Mental Health Practice: A Textbook. Edited by Drake R, Merrens M, Lynde D. New York, WW Norton, 2005, pp 424–452

Murray-Swank A, Glynn S, Cohen AN, et al: Family contact, experience of family relationships, and views about family involvement in treatment among VA consumers with serious mental illness. J Rehabil Res Dev 44:801–812, 2007

Pickett-Schenk SA, Bennett C, Cook JA, et al: Changes in caregiving satisfaction and information needs among relatives of adults with mental illness: results of a randomized evaluation of a family-led education intervention. Am J Orthopsychiatry 76:545–553, 2006a

Pickett-Schenk SA, Cook JA, Steigman P, et al: Psychological well-being and relationship outcomes in a randomized study of family-led education. Arch Gen Psychiatry 63:1043–1050, 2006b

Pickett-Schenk SA, Lippincott RC, Bennett C, et al: Improving knowledge about mental illness through family led education: the journey of hope. Psychiatr Serv 59:49–56, 2008

Pitschel-Walz G, Leucht S, Bauml J, et al: The effect of family interventions on relapse and rehospitalization in schizophrenia—a meta-analysis. Schizophr Bull 21:73–92, 2001

Pitschel-Walz G, Bauml J, Bender W, et al: Psychoeducation and compliance in the treatment of schizophrenia: results of the Munich Psychosis Information Project Study. J Clin Psychiatry 67:443–452, 2006

Posner CM, Wilson KG, Kral MJ, et al: Family psychoeducational support groups in schizophrenia. Am J Orthopsychiatry 62:206–218, 1992

Ran MS, Xiang MZ, Chan CL, et al: Effectiveness of psychoeducational intervention for rural Chinese families experiencing schizophrenia—a randomized controlled trial. Soc Psychiatry Psychiatr Epidemiol 38:69–75, 2003

Resnick SG, Rosenheck RA, Lehman AF: An exploratory analysis of correlates of recovery. Psychiatr Serv 55:540–547, 2004

Resnick SG, Rosenheck RA, Dixon L, et al: Correlates of family contact with the mental health system: allocation of a scarce resource. Ment Health Serv Res 7:113–121, 2005

Smith GC: Patterns and predictors of service use and unmet needs among aging families of adults with severe mental illness. Psychiatr Serv 4:871–877, 2003

Snowden LR: Explaining mental health treatment disparities: ethnic and cultural differences in family involvement. Cult Med Psychiatry 31:389–402, 2007

Solomon P, Draine J, Mannion E, et al: Impact of brief family psychoeducation on self-efficacy. Schizophr Bull 22:41–50, 1996

Solomon P, Draine J, Mannion E, et al: Effectiveness of two models of brief family education: retention of gains by family members of adults with serious mental illness. Am J Orthopsychiatry 67:177–186, 1997

Stalberg G, Ekerwald H, Hultman CM: At issue: siblings of patients with schizophrenia: sibling bond, coping patterns, and fear of possible schizophrenia heredity. Schizophr Bull 30:445–458, 2004

Thara R, Srinivasan TN: Outcome of marriage in schizophrenia. Soc Psychiatry Psychiatr Epidemiol 32:416–420, 1997

Winefield H, Harvey E: Needs of family caregivers in chronic schizophrenia. Schizophr Bull 20:557–566, 1994

Xiong W, Phillips MR, Hu X, et al: Family based intervention for schizophrenic patients in China: a randomized controlled trial. Br J Psychiatry 165:239–247, 1994

Zhang M, Yan C, Ye J: Effectiveness of psychoeducation of relatives of schizophrenia patients: a prospective cohort study in five cities in China. Int J Ment Health 22:47–59, 1993

12

Remission in Schizophrenia

Laine M. Young-Walker, M.D.

Alan J. Mendelowitz, M.D.

John Lauriello, M.D.

The treatment of schizophrenia has evolved significantly since the diagnosis was first established 100 years ago. This evolution was fueled by advances in psychopharmacology, a better identification and understanding of psychosocial deficits, and the development of remediation techniques. However, the early conceptualization of schizophrenia by Emil Kraepelin at the turn of the twentieth century as "dementia praecox," or a progressive deteriorating illness, persists. Schizophrenia is still often perceived as an illness in which one is never able to reachieve the previous level of psychosocial functioning.

Until recently, there has not been significant interest in defining remission in schizophrenia. This disinterest lay in the clinical perception that positive, negative, and cognitive deficits continued to progress over time, and therefore, the idea of a patient stabilizing and remitting was considered impossible. Furthermore, even with data that suggested that some positive symptoms improved over time, the belief was that negative and cognitive symptoms remained, and the patients *never* regained their premorbid status. The result of these clinical impressions was that the goal for proposed treatment became getting patients "better," with a decrease in acute symptoms, as opposed to the goal of attempting to achieve a period of significant sustained improvement or "remission." One could argue that the dogged pursuit of control of positive symptoms was so extreme in the late twentieth century that patients were expected to tolerate debilitating side effects to maximally reduce hallucinations and paranoia. This is illustrated in the following case:

> Bill, a 21-year-old white man, was admitted to the inpatient psychiatric ward after being found screaming in the dormitory courtyard at his university. He believed that he was possessed by the devil and that the end of the world was near. In the psychiatric hospital, he was given antipsychotic medication, and his dose was escalated until he no longer heard voices or believed that he was possessed. However, the given dose left Bill slowed down and rigid, and he was administered anticholinergic medication that partially ameliorated these side effects. He did not feel that he could "think well enough" to complete his classes and left school to return home with his parents.

With the advent of newer effective antipsychotic medications that produce fewer neurological side effects and greater attention to clinical improvement in multiple symptom domains, the concept of remission in schizophrenia began to emerge.

Response, Remission, and Recovery

The concept of remission in medical and psychiatric illness is an important one. Although the term *remission* is used in other illnesses, it is a relatively new construct in the treatment of schizophrenia. *Remission* needs to be defined and differentiated from the concepts of *improvement* and *response.* One example would be the concept of improvement, response, and remission in an illness such as cancer. In cancer, any change for the better in the patient's tumor load or clinical condition would be considered an *improvement.* When patients show a significant amount of a priori–defined improvement, they are said to have had a *response* to treatment, and if and when they meet an a priori–defined criterion for having no more detectable cancer cells in their body, they have achieved *remission*. This does not imply that the patients are "cured" or that relapse is not still a risk. In fact, patients may be asked to continue some form of chemotherapy to maintain their remitted state. To understand this in psychiatry, let us use an example from the treatment of depression.

Response

When one discusses the concept of *response* in a clinical trial, it is similar but not wholly equated to the clinical construct of *improvement*. In the treatment of depression, *improvement* or "better" is the change in a positive direction of clinical meaningful symptoms; in other words, at the patient level, "feeling better." In a clinical trial, this clinical improvement must be given an a priori definition of what constitutes meaningful clinical improvement. Continuing with this example, a patient may feel better when sleep appetite and mood have improved and he or she feels that he or she can return to work. A research definition of improvement defined as *response* would be a 50% reduction in the score on a depression rating scale, such as the Hamilton Rating Scale for Depression.

However, differences exist between being "better," having a "response," and being "well," which we define as "remission." Patients may feel "better" enough to go back to work, but "well" is when they feel like their "old selves" before the depressive episode. The research term for well is *remission*. This again needs to be defined with operational criteria so it can be used and replicated across studies, populations, and treatments. When one discusses the concept of "remission" in depression, it is often defined as a final Hamilton Rating Scale for Depression score of less than 8.

When evaluating these concepts in the treatment of schizophrenia, we must define similar terms. Schizophrenia is a complex illness with several areas of deficits (see Lauriello et al., "Introduction to Schizophrenia," Chapter 1 in this volume). In DSM-IV-TR (American Psychiatric Association 2000), Criterion A for schizophrenia is two (or more) of the following five symptoms: delusions, hallucinations, thought disorder, negative symptoms, and catatonic behavior. Patients with schizophrenia may have a combination of positive symptoms (delusions, hallucinations, thought disorder), negative symptoms (amotivation, anhedonia, social isolation, flattening of affect), cognitive symptoms (such as difficulty in executive functions), and disorganized behaviors, all of which result in difficulty in social and occupational functioning.

In industry pharmacological clinical trials of patients with schizophrenia, *response* is often defined as a 20% reduction (i.e., improvement) on either the Brief Psychiatric Rating Scale (BPRS; Overall and Gorham 1962) or the Positive and Negative Syndrome Scale (PANSS) score (Kay et al. 1988). These scores, although useful for the approval of new medications by governmental regulatory agencies, inadequately capture all of the symptom domains. The BPRS is strongly weighted to positive symptoms, whereas the PANSS covers both positive and negative symptoms but fails to fully include cognitive symptoms and social functioning.

> Anne had tried a variety of antipsychotic medications with minimal improvement of her symptoms, which mainly consisted of disorganized and bizarre behaviors. She would often talk in "gibberish" and make odd circular movements with her hands. Within seconds, she would go from sitting in a chair to racing down the hallway. Anne finally was given clozapine, which resulted in a definite improvement in the organization of her thoughts, fewer odd mannerisms, and less impulsive behavior. Despite this positive response, Anne still needed live-in staff at her apartment and required redirection when necessary.

Remission

In attempting to define *remission* in schizophrenia, it is vital that as many domains as possible be included in our definition. This requires two definitions for remission—one that can be used when retrospectively evaluating older studies and a new one that can be created to prospectively evaluate patients.

Several attempts have been made over the last 15 years to begin to study criteria for potential remission in schizophrenia. These attempts require both a set of criteria that quantify improvement that is clinically meaningful and a time criterion to confirm that this improvement is sustained. In addition, clinical studies report that patients in their first episode, or first 2 years of the illness, may have better responses to treatment than do patients who have been chronically ill. As a result, early attempts to define remission often have viewed these two populations independently.

In 1993, J. Lieberman et al. looked at early-episode, acutely ill patients with schizophrenia and created a set of remission criteria that included a score of 3 or less on psychotic and disorganization items. In addition, patients needed a score of less than 3 on the Clinical Global Impressions Scale, a 7-point scale that assesses overall illness. Lieberman and colleagues also added a time criterion that this improvement had to be maintained for 8 weeks (J. Lieberman et al. 1993). In a similar population of acutely ill patients, Eaton et al. (1998) used the "absence" of positive symptoms and extreme psychomotor disorder and extended the time criterion to 3 months. In evaluating studies in which chronic patients received treatment, R. P. Lieberman et al. (2002) used criteria similar to the first-episode criteria of J. Lieberman et al. (1993); however, they were more lenient with the symptom severity by allowing patients to have BPRS items up to a severity of 4 (moderate), and they extended the time criterion from 8 weeks to 24 months. Curtis et al. (2001), in an effort to further operationalize these criteria, defined the various areas of symptom remission and functioning and proposed a remission definition that included multiple factors:

- A BPRS total score of less than 30
- Scores of less than 3 (moderate) on multiple negative symptom items from the Scale for the Assessment of Negative Symptoms (SANS)
- A Global Assessment of Functioning (GAF) score of at least 60
- No psychotic symptoms for 1 month
- No hospitalizations for 3 months
- No more than one "residual symptom"
- Presence of employment and association with friends

These criteria from Curtis et al. (2001) are perhaps the most comprehensive definition but are difficult to use retrospectively and require extensive evaluation, as well as additional clinical informants.

Because the differing remission criteria could result in diagnostic confusion, a work group was created to attempt to create an operational definition that could be used both retrospectively when evaluating older studies and prospectively. This group, the Remission in Schizophrenia Working Group, published these refined criteria in 2005 in the *American Journal of Psychiatry* (Andreasen et al. 2005). Core elements of the group's approach were to set thresholds that must be obtained as opposed to a certain percentage of change. As the authors stated: "The working group chose to define remission as a state in which patients have experienced an improvement…that any remaining symptoms are of such low intensity that they no longer interfere significantly with behavior" (p. 447). These criteria require that patients maintain scores of mild or less in three dimensions of psychopathology:

1. Psychoticism includes the DSM-IV-TR Criterion A of delusions and hallucinations.
2. Disorganization includes the DSM-IV-TR Criterion A of disorganized speech and disorganized behavior.
3. Negative symptoms consists of all the ▬ tive symptom items (e.g., avolition, flattening of affect, asociality, anhedonia).

An additional requirement is that the improvement must be maintained for a period of 6 months. Unlike the Curtis et al. (2001) criteria, the Remission in Schizophrenia Working Group criteria limited the scope to the reduction of core symptoms, leaving measures of social and work functioning to be defined later as part of the recovery process.

> Gerard had received the diagnosis of schizophrenia 6 years ago. In that time, he had made steady improvement in reduction of symptoms and level of function. Gerard was interviewed by a local newspaper for an article about living with mental illness. Gerard was able to clearly describe how he occasionally heard whispers but that they did not affect his life, and he was aware that they were part of his illness. He also reported that he had developed a close group of friends, many part of the local clubhouse affiliated with the clinic he attended. He was most proud that he had obtained a part-time job as a radiology clerk at the local hospital 3 years prior. He was in charge of locating old films when requested and scanning them into a new digital imaging system. At work, he had several friends and once a week played pool with them in the evenings.

Recovery

The concepts of remission as a research instrument and clinical concept and the patient's goal of recovery must be differentiated. The idea of recovery is an emphasis on having the patient achieve what heretofore was thought to be unachievable, which is a complete recovery. Recovery denotes freedom from positive symptoms, improved negative symptoms, and successful social and vocational functioning. Recovery as a goal for every patient involves a higher level of improvement than remission. In 2002, the UCLA Criteria were developed to include improvement and recovery in four domains (R. P. Liberman et al. 2002). The level of recovery is measured by

- Symptom remission
- Appropriate role function
- Ability to perform day-to-day living tasks without supervision
- Social interactions

This level of remission must be sustained for 2 years.

It has long been believed that early diagnosis and treatment of schizophrenia should produce the best outcome and greatest chance for recovery. However, in a group of patients in their first episode of schizophrenia studied by Robinson et al. (1999), full recovery rates were found to be low—only one-eighth of those in the study met criteria for 2 or more years. Although the rate of recovery was low, this study provided predictors of recovery. These included better cognitive functioning, shorter period of psychotic symptoms prior to enrollment in the study, and more normal cerebral asymmetry.

The finding that history of psychosis serves as a predictor for recovery is an important one. This finding was initially reported by Loebel et al. (1992), and although it was not confirmed by other research groups, it is still strongly believed to be an important observation. It suggests that the longer patients with psychosis are untreated, the lower the chance for recovery. In other words, the longer one is sick before receiving initial treatment, the lower one's chance for full improvement. Conceptually, in a recovery model for psychosis, this is the most important point because it is the one area where clinicians, patients, and families can potentially have an effect. Patients with their first break of psychosis must be brought for evaluation and treatment as soon as possible. Patients who have medical problems seek treatment or their family brings them for treatment right away. However, with psychosis, because of a combination of the lack of knowledge of mental illness and the patient's lack of insight and fears of social stigma, patients are often ill for a long time before they see a mental health professional. This finding, by Robinson et al. (2004) among others, suggests that education of the public about the first episode of psychosis may have a bearing on recovery and potentially also a bearing on the percentage of patients who may be able to achieve remission.

Role of Neural Markers, Biological Correlates, and Neuroimaging in the Study of Remission

Emerging evidence indicates that neural markers of remission are present. Bodnar et al. (2010) studied neural markers of remission in first-episode schizophrenia. The definition of remission used for their study was maintaining scores of mild or less on positive and negative symptoms over 6 months (per the Remission in Schizophrenia Working Group 2005 criteria). In this study, the relation between hippocampus and amygdala volumes and early remission status was examined. The investigators compared 57 first-episode schizophrenia patients with 57 control subjects. Among the 57 first-episode schizophrenia patients, 17 had achieved remission according to the definition noted earlier. First-episode schizophrenia patients have been noted to have smaller hippocampal volume than do nonschizophrenic control subjects, but the amygdala does not appear to have smaller volumes in this population. Bodnar et al. (2010) found that the left tail of the hippocampus was smaller in nonremitted first-episode schizophrenic patients than in those who were in remission. With the emerging use of neuroimaging, these findings are promising. They give us a link to understanding the pathophysiology of schizophrenia. The use of neuroimaging may aid in early identification of patients who have a smaller hippocampal tail volume and thus who are likely to have a poorer outcome. Awareness of this outcome early in treatment may drive a search for more target-specific medications.

Altamura et al. (2005) studied some biological correlates of drug resistance in schizophrenia. Lessons learned from studying drug resistance may lead to further knowledge of biological correlates of remission. Dysfunction of dopaminergic, serotonergic, and glutamatergic brain pathways has been associated with drug resistance. An association with the inflammatory response system and hypothalamic-pituitary axis dysregulation and drug resistance is likely. Pharmacogenetics have implicated *CK* gene, dopamine type 3 receptor, and serotonin type 2A receptor polymorphisms in drug resistance. Further investigation of these biological correlates of drug resistance may provide information about remission.

Also, evidence from positron emission tomography (PET) indicates remission of "hypofrontality" with recovery from acute schizophrenia. In a study by Spence et al. (1998), subjects with schizophrenia were compared with control groups. This study had 13 subjects in acute relapse of schizophrenia and two control groups (one had 6 subjects, and the other had 5). PET was used to study dorsolateral prefrontal cortical function. The PET scans were completed while performing several movement tasks. A summary of findings from this study included hypoactivation of the left dorsolateral prefrontal cortex in the group of schizophrenia subjects in acute relapse, whereas the dorsolateral prefrontal cortex was activated in control subjects during the generation of motor acts. As the patients improved, the observed hypoactivation in the left dorsolateral prefrontal cortex was reduced. The investigators postulated that prefrontal function may improve as psychotic symptoms remit. Although this study was based on small numbers, it gives promising results for the potential use of PET scanning and evaluation of dorsolateral prefrontal cortex activation as a means of assessing remission.

Treatment Aimed at Remission

Treatment aimed at remission and recovery has been covered in several other chapters in the book, including Chapter 8, "Pharmacological Treatment of Schizophrenia," by Miyamoto and Fleischhacker, and Chapter 10, "Psychological Interventions for Schizophrenia," by Rossi and colleagues. The goals for treatment of schizophrenia include achieving a response and preventing relapse. Successfully sustaining response is critical to achieving remission and eventually attaining full recovery. Critical to sustaining response is ensuring adherence to pharmacological treatment. Depot formulations of antipsychotics may increase adherence and, therefore, may help with prevention of relapse. To meet the added functionality requirements of remission and recovery, psychosocial interventions are necessary. For coverage of these interventions, readers are directed to Chapter 10.

Conclusion

Remission is a realistic goal. The inevitability of immutable deterioration is no longer the pervasive thinking with schizophrenia. The initial description by Kraepelin that used the word "dementia" in dementia praecox suggested deterioration. In addition, the observation of many had been of a group of patients who did poorly because of multiple factors, including noncompliance and the lack of availability of treatment. However, with a new focus on symptom realms of cognitive symptoms and negative symptoms, clinicians should no longer have their treatment goals be improvement in positive symptoms but rather remission and recovery. With sustained remission, functional recovery can be attained.

Suggested Readings

Kane J: Treatment strategies to prevent relapse and encourage remission. J Clin Psychiatry 68 (suppl 14):27–30, 2007

Leucht S, Lasser R: The concepts of remission and recovery in schizophrenia. Pharmacopsychiatry 39:161–170, 2006

Leucht S, Barnes L, Kissling W, et al: Relapse prevention in schizophrenia with new-generation antipsychotics: a systematic review and explanatory meta-analysis of randomized controlled trials. Am J Psychiatry 160:1209–1222, 2003

Leucht S, Beitinger R, Kissling W: On the concept of remission in schizophrenia. Psychopharmacology (Berl) 194:453–461, 2007

Van Os J, Burns T, Cavallaro R, et al: Standardized remission criteria in schizophrenia. Acta Psychiatr Scand 113:91–95, 2006a

Van Os J, Drukker M, Campo JA, et al: Validation of remission criteria for schizophrenia. Am J Psychiatry 163:2000–2001, 2006b

References

Altamura A, Bassetti R, Elizabetta C, et al: Some biological correlates of drug resistance in schizophrenia: a multidimensional approach. World J Biol Psychiatry 6 (suppl 2): 23–30, 2005

American Psychiatric Association: Diagnostic and Statistical Manual of Mental Disorders, 4th Edition, Text Revision. Washington, DC, American Psychiatric Association, 2000

Andreasen NC, Carpenter WT Jr, Kane JM, et al: Remission in schizophrenia: proposed criteria and rationale for consensus. Am J Psychiatry 62:441–449, 2005

Bodnar M, Malla A, Czechowska Y, et al: Neural markers of remission in first-episode schizophrenia: a volumetric neuroimaging study of the hippocampus and amygdala. Schizophr Res 122:72–80, 2010

Curtis CE, Calkins ME, Grove WM, et al: Saccadic disinhibition in patients with acute and remitted schizophrenia and their first degree biological relatives. Am J Psychiatry 158:100–106, 2001

Eaton WW, Thara R, Federman E, et al: Remission and relapse in schizophrenia: the Madras Longitudinal Study. J Nerv Ment Dis 186:357–363, 1998

Kay SR, Opler LA, Lindenmeyer JP: Reliability and validity of the Positive and Negative Syndrome Scale for schizophrenics. Psychiatry Res 23:99–110, 1988

Liberman RP, Kopelowicz A, Ventura J, et al: Operational criteria and factors related to recovery from schizophrenia. Int Rev Psychiatry 14:256–272, 2002

Lieberman J, Jody D, Geisler S, et al: Time course and biologic correlates of treatment response in first-episode schizophrenia. Arch Gen Psychiatry 50:369–376, 1993

Loebel AD, Lieberman JA, Alvir JM, et al: Duration of psychosis and outcome in first-episode schizophrenia. Am J Psychiatry 149:1183–1188, 1992

Overall JE, Gorham DR: The Brief Psychiatric Rating Scale. Psychol Rep 10:799–812, 1962

Robinson D, Woerner R, Alvir JM, et al: Predictors of relapse following response from a first episode of schizophrenia or schizoaffective disorder. Arch Gen Psychiatry 53:241–247, 1999

Robinson DG, Woerner MG, McMeniman M, et al: Symptomatic and functional recovery from a first episode of schizophrenia or schizoaffective disorder. Am J Psychiatry 161:473–479, 2004

Spence S, Hirsch S, Brooks D, et al: Prefrontal cortex activity in people with schizophrenia and control subjects: evidence from positron emission tomography for remission of "hypofrontality" with recovery from acute schizophrenia. Br J Psychiatry 172:316–323, 1998

Index

*Page numbers printed in **boldface** type refer to figures or tables.*